Pharmacogenetics

Second Edition

OXFORD MONOGRAPHS ON MEDICAL GENETICS

General Editors
ARNO G. MOTULSKY   PETER S. HARPER
CHARLES SCRIVER   CHARLES J. EPSTEIN
JUDITH G. HALL

Pharmacogenetics

Second Edition

WENDELL W. WEBER, Ph.D., M.D.
Department of Pharmacology
University of Michigan Medical School
Ann Arbor

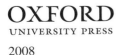

OXFORD
UNIVERSITY PRESS

2008

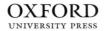

OXFORD
UNIVERSITY PRESS

Oxford University Press, Inc., publishes works that further
Oxford University's objective of excellence
in research, scholarship, and education.

Oxford   New York
Auckland   Cape Town   Dar es Salaam   Hong Kong   Karachi
Kuala Lumpur   Madrid   Melbourne   Mexico City   Nairobi
New Delhi   Shanghai   Taipei   Toronto

With offices in
Argentina   Austria   Brazil   Chile   Czech Republic   France   Greece
Guatemala   Hungary   Italy   Japan   Poland   Portugal   Singapore
South Korea   Switzerland   Thailand   Turkey   Ukraine   Vietnam

Copyright © 2008 by Oxford University Press, Inc.

Published by Oxford University Press, Inc.
198 Madison Avenue, New York, New York 10016

www.oup.com   /005478711

Oxford is a registered trademark of Oxford University Press.

Library of Congress Cataloging-in-Publication Data
Weber, Wendell W.
Pharmacogenetics / Wendell W. Weber.—2nd ed.
   p. ; cm.
Includes bibliographical references and index.
ISBN 978-0-19-534151-5
1.   Pharmacogenetics.
[DNLM: 1. Pharmacogenetics.   QV 38 W376p 2008]
I. Title.
RM301.3.G45W42 2008
615'.7—dc22
2007033606

9 8 7 6 5 4 3 2 1
Printed in the United States of America
on acid-free paper

To LaDonna and our two children, Jane and Theodore

Preface

The first edition of this book published in 1997 was written with the purpose of showing how the convergence of pharmacology and genetics in the new hybrid field of pharmacogenetics is complementary and how individuals more or less susceptible to a given chemical differ from each other by describing the genetics and molecular basis of specific traits of pharmacogenetic importance. In the 10 or so years since that edition was published, much new pharmacogenetic information has been gathered and many conceptual and technological advances have occurred. To accommodate these changes, the current edition was divided into four sections: Foundations, Fundamentals, Futures, and Synthesis. Foundations describes the origins and defining features of the field. Fundamentals expands on the principles of pharmacogenetics with detailed discussions of the pharmacologic and genetic profiling of human drug response, the molecular aspects of pharmacogenetics, the tools available for pharmacogenomic research and testing, ethnicity in pharmacogenetics, and the modeling of human drug response in experimental systems. Futures discusses the prospects of pharmacogenetics relevant to drug discovery and predictive biology. Synthesis concludes the book with a brief overview of the field.

Acknowledgments

For the past three decades, lectures on pharmacogenetics have been given in various courses at the University of Michigan to graduate students in pharmacology, toxicology, and public health, and to medical students, pharmacy students, and nursing students. Over the years, I have given the bulk of those lectures, but more recently Gerry Levy and Jerry Stitzel have performed that task as well. The notes of our lectures are well designed as a brief introduction to pharmacogenetics, and I have combined parts of their lectures with my own as a basis for Chapter 2, Defining Pharmacogenetics. I thank Gerry and Jerry for their contributions.

Numerous colleagues have also contributed directly or indirectly to this book. I express my sincere thanks to all, and especially to Bill Pratt, David Burke, Patrick A. Murphy, Harvey Kaplan, Namandje Bumpus, Ray Ruddon, and Jimmy Rae for their comments and criticisms. I also thank Harvey Kaplan for providing a version of Table 10.1 that I have updated and Faye Bradbury for providing Figure 10.3.

WWW

Contents

III. FUTURES

FOUNDATIONS

1

Beginnings

We hear almost every day about the unwanted effects of prescription drugs and over-the-counter nostrums, of unsafe substances in foods, and of the perils of tobacco smoking and drinking alcohol. We cannot help but wonder why such effects occur in only a fraction of persons exposed, or why a drug that is therapeutic in one person may be ineffective, or even toxic, in another. This is the province of pharmacology. During the period in and around the 1950s, pharmacologists demonstrated, contrary to common belief, that adverse responses accompanying exposure to exogenous substances were closely tied to a person's genetic makeup (Figure 1.1). When this concept was proposed, it was not entirely new because biologists had long understood that the capacity of organisms to respond differently to the environment was genetically determined. Even so, demonstrating that heredity exerted important effects on human drug responsiveness was an innovative step that cast doubt on the notion that the drug recipient was merely a passive bystander in this process.

Before 1950, few specifics were known about the effects of heredity on such responses, but then the potential significance of genetic differences to the safe, effective use of drugs and the unusual hazards posed by other environmental chemicals began to attract more and more attention from the biomedical community. Recently, the flourishing of genomics has changed the focus of pharmacogenetics from the effects of single genes, addressed one at a time, to the effects of a rich variety of functional elements that affect variation in the expression of many genes.

The periods in and around the 1950s and the year 2000, capped by the discovery of the DNA double helix and the maturation of the human genome initiative, respectively, were periods of remarkable achievement in the quest for knowledge of heredity. These periods tend to overshadow the time of earlier discoveries that led to the inception of modern genetics and pharmacogenetics. For a more balanced perspective on the evolution of pharmacogenetics, we turn to the middle of the nineteenth century, from which time the foundations of pharmacology and

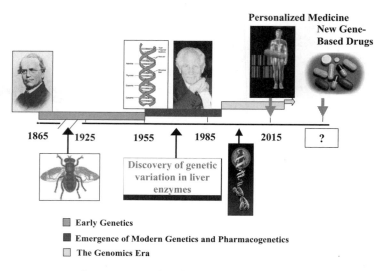

Figure 1.1 Landmarks in pharmacogenetics.

genetics, stretching to the present, can be divided into roughly four periods (Table 1.1). The first two periods, which extend from 1850 through the end of the second period to about 1960, define the cellular and molecular foundations of early pharmacology and genetics, while the last two periods address events from about 1960 to the present and define the informational and genomic foundations of modern biology and pharmacogenetics.

CELLULAR FOUNDATIONS OF EARLY PHARMACOLOGY AND GENETICS

The first period spanned some 60 years, closely tracking the rise of organic chemistry in Western Europe in the early 1800s. Between 1850 and 1910, physiological chemists, primarily in Germany and Switzerland, intrigued by the fate of foreign compounds in humans, discovered that humans could transform most drugs they ingested to relatively harmless products prior to excreting them. Gregor Mendel's (1822–1884) discovery in 1865 of the fundamental laws of inheritance also occurred during this period, as well as the inference during the 1870s of "drug receptor" molecules by Charles Langley in England and Paul Ehrlich in Germany. The cytopharmacological studies of Langley and Ehrlich were notable for clarifying why the actions of drugs and other chemicals were localized to specific tissues.

Table 1.1 Foundations of Pharmacogenetics

1850–1910 Cellular foundations	1910–1960s Molecular foundations	1960s–1990s Informational foundations	1990s–to date Genomics foundations
Mendel's laws discovered, lost, and rediscovered	DNA identified as the hereditary material	DNA–RNA hybrid helix discovered	Large-scale, high-throughput techniques developed
Biotransformation of chemicals discovered in humans	DNA double helix described	Genetic code for nuclear genes determined	Maturation of the human genome initiative
Drug receptors inferred	Central dogma of molecular biology formulated	Readout of nuclear genes worked out	Toxicogenomics applied to drug discovery
Chromosomes defined as locus of heredity	Protein polymorphism established	Recombinant DNA technologies invented	Construction of risk profiles for drug susceptibility (www.hapmap.org)
Chemical individuality of humans defined	Human chromosomes enumerated	Mitochondrial genome sequence determined	Epigenomics
	Disease associated with chromosomal aberrations	Mitochondrial genetic code determined	
	Experimental pharmacogenetics emerges	PCR invented	
		Genomics tools developed	
		DNA polymorphisms identified	
		Human genome initiative started	
		Epigenetics modifies gene expression	

MOLECULAR FOUNDATIONS OF EARLY PHARMACOLOGY AND GENETICS

The implications of Mendel's discoveries did not dawn on anyone until the turn of the twentieth century when their revival prompted an intense flurry of research. Lucien Cuenot in France was investigating the genetics of coat color in mice while Archibald Garrod and William Bateson in England were investigating various inborn traits in human subjects. Cuenot, Garrod, and Bateson suggested that the genetic material played an essential role in directing chemical transformations within organisms, and that enzymes, which were termed "diastases" or "ferments" at that time, were related in some unknown manner to the genetic material.

In 1902, Garrod proposed the concept of "chemical individuality" to explain the predisposition of certain individuals to alcaptonuria, and he concluded that alcaptonuria was an inherited condition. On Garrod's consultation with Bateson, the latter appears to have given the first suggestion of gene action in terms of "ferments," and of a recessive condition whose features depended on the absence of a particular "ferment" (enzyme). Stemming from earlier interest on a case of porphyria accompanying the ingestion of the hypnotic drug sulfonal, and observations on urinary pigments, Garrod extended his idea of chemical individuality to include the transformation of drugs into nontoxic conjugates such as hippurates and glycuronates. He said the formation of conjugates protected individuals from the poisonous effects of these agents.

Applying Bateson's suggestion to exogenous chemicals, Garrod proposed that the noxious effects these substances produce in some persons might be due to failure of their enzymes to detoxify them. In the course of these and later studies, Garrod came to believe that "substances in foods, drugs and in exhalations of particular animals and plants may produce in some people effects wholly out of proportion to any they bring about in most persons, and that such effects were due to derangement of metabolic factors." He also pointed out that "the ultimate toxic agent could be a product of normal metabolism formed in undue amount, or it could be an intermediate product that escaped the further changes it normally undergoes, or possibly an abnormal product formed by way of derangement of normal metabolic processes," and because metabolic deviations from the average were less obvious than variations in form, he believed "they would attract little attention and the great majority of them would most likely escape observation." Garrod spoke out firmly about these ideas until his life ended in 1936, yet they are as fresh and true today as when he first stated them nearly 100 years ago.[1,2]

Several studies on *Drosophila* (fruit fly) by Thomas Hunt Morgan and his students also contributed major advances to an understanding of heredity and hereditary mechanisms during the early years of this period. In 1913, Sturtevant constructed the first genetic map and showed that genes are arranged in a linear order. In 1914 and 1916, Bridges provided the first proof that chromosomes contained genes, ruling out the possibility that genes and chromosomes were separate hereditary elements.

Eventually, a few biologists began to take note of Garrod's keen foresight regarding the chemical individuality of humans (Figure 1.2). In 1918, Marshall and co-workers reported that black soldiers were much more resistant than whites to the blistering of skin from exposure to mustard gas, a substance introduced as a chemical warfare agent in the first World War.[3] In 1919, Hirschfeld and Hirschfeld, building on Landsteiner's analysis of isoagglutinins in human blood, were the first to describe serological differences between the blood of Europeans, Middle Easterners, and Asians by examining 500–1000 persons of each of 10 racial groups, finding remarkable racial differences in the proportions of blood groups A and B.[4] By 1929, reports on racial differences in ophthalmic effects of cocaine, euphthalmine, ephedrine, and atropine had appeared,[5] and during the 1920s and 1930s hereditary deficits in two modalities of sensory perception, "odor

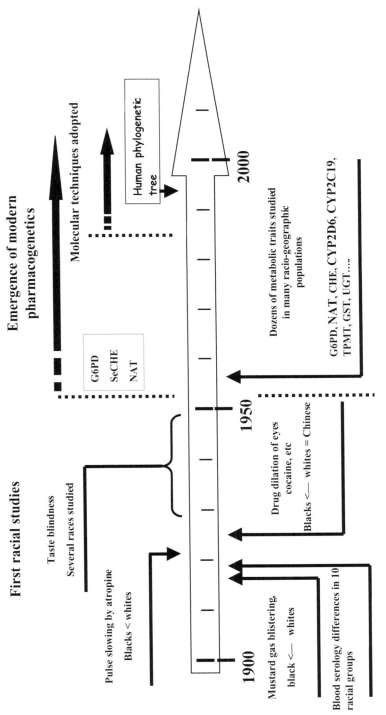

Figure 1.2 Timeline of the pharmacogenetics of raciogeographic variation.

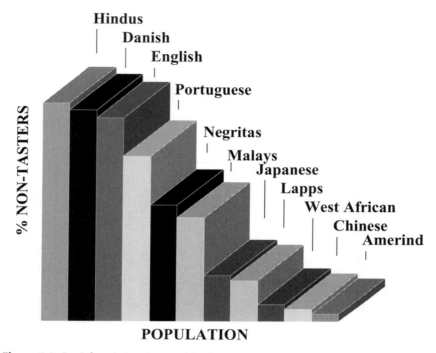

Figure 1.3 Racial variation in taste blindness, the first systematic study of ethnicity.

blindness"[6,7] and "taste blindness,"[8] were identified. Human family studies of "taste blindness" revealed the heritability of the trait as a feature that came to be accepted as characteristic of human responsiveness to exogenous chemicals.[9]

"Odor blindness" and "taste blindness" were among the first traits to reveal the high specificity and sensitivity of the human response to chemicals. Figure 1.2 shows a timeline of these ethnogeographic observations. Additional studies performed in several populations and subpopulations in different parts of the world revealed that taste blindness varied by more than 15-fold from one population to another, and showed that the frequency of "nontasters" in Europeans of 35–40% was appreciably greater than the 2–6% found in Africans, Chinese, Japanese, South Amerinds (Brazil), and Lapps (Figure 1.3). These population studies were the first systematic documentation of the association of race or ethnicity to the human response to chemicals. Since then, investigation of ethnogeographic variation has been regarded as an important part of pharmacogenetics.

EMERGENCE OF MODERN GENETICS
AND EXPERIMENTAL PHARMACOGENETICS

Throughout the decade prior to 1950, much of the world had been engaged in and was recovering from World War II, and many scientists had participated in behind-the-scenes efforts to defend the Allied cause against the impending threat of warfare by radiological, biological, and chemical weapons. Scientific progress on a broad front had slowed, but from another perspective, the period in and around 1950 was a time of renewed scientific optimism in which scientists turned their efforts from nationalistic to more humanitarian goals.

In 1948, hemoglobins S and C were identified, and their mode of inheritance was determined. Of these, the first hereditary protein variant to be identified was hemoglobin S, and a few years later it was also the first variant protein in which replacement of a single amino acid residue within the protein molecule was associated unequivocally with a change in the functional effect of the protein. In 1953, the double helix of DNA, the molecular basis of heredity, was described. Within another 2–3 years, the chromosomes of human cells were visualized and the normal diploid number was established as 46. Soon thereafter, the chromosomal bases of several pathological states were identified with aberrations in normal chromosome number (e.g., aberrant numbers of X chromosomes in Klinefelter syndrome and trisomy 21 in Down syndrome) or structure (e.g., the chimeric Philadelphia chromosome associated with chronic myeloid leukemia). Following closely on the demonstration of polymorphic forms of hemoglobin S and hemoglobin C by electrophoresis, application of this technique to plasma proteins showed that protein polymorphism, initially associated with enzymes that occur in multiple forms and used mainly for diagnostic purposes, was recognized as a phenomenon of much broader significance that would engage the interest of many investigators.

Working with various chromatographic technologies that became available in the 1950s, and drawing on various pharmacological and biochemical studies performed on patients and members of their families, pharmacologists disclosed new relationships between genetically conditioned differences in drug response and their metabolic fate. "Primaquine sensitivity," "succinylcholine sensitivity," and isoniazid-induced neuropathy were the drug-related traits first to be intensely scrutinized in this fashion. Primaquine, an antimalarial drug that was used in the South Pacific during World War II, caused hemolysis of red blood cells in a large fraction of black Africans; succinylcholine (also called suxamethonium), a muscle relaxant drug used as an adjunct in general anesthesia, caused prolonged paralysis and apnea ("succinylcholine or suxamethonium sensitivity") in Caucasian subjects; and isoniazid (isonicotinyl hydrazide), a new, highly effective drug in trial for treatment of tuberculosis, caused peripheral nerve damage in a large fraction of patients administered the drug. Primaquine sensitivity was found to be due to a genetically deficient variant of the housekeeping enzyme, glucose-6-phosphate dehydrogenase (G6PD), succinylcholine sensitivity was attributed to an atypical variant of serum cholinesterase, and isoniazid-induced nerve damage was attributed to "slow acetylation," later shown to be a functionally impaired acetyltransferase variant.

In 1962, Werner Kalow (Figure 1.1) published the first systematic account of pharmacogenetics. His monograph revealed the potential significance of genetic variation to responses of a host of organisms including bacteria, insects, and numerous vertebrates including humans, to environmental chemicals. By the mid-1980s, dozens of additional traits had been added to the list of drug-metabolizing enzymes and other enzymes of physiological importance in support of this view. We also learned that such sensitivities might also extend to food-stuffs as well as to sporadic disorders associated with exposures to hazardous chemicals in the workplace. This was no great surprise because pharmacologists and toxicologists had demonstrated that the biotransformation of dietary components and other exogenous chemicals involved the same enzymes as those that biotransform drugs. Because certain drug-metabolizing enzymes were also capable of metabolizing certain hormones and other endogenous messengers, variation in hormonal response was another potential hallmark of pharmacogenetics.

Most of the well-studied, metabolic traits attributed to the drug-metabolizing enzymes appeared to be monogenic (i.e., in a particular family, only one gene locus is thought to be variant) and exhibited heterogeneity (i.e., might involve variants of different genes in different families). Like other hereditary traits, pharmacogenetic traits might be due to new mutations, their demographic features might also vary, and at times they might cause devastating illness and death. An overview of these studies revealed that the frequency of polymorphisms that are responsible for many metabolic traits was often much greater than that of human disease genes, and further, in the absence of exposure to drugs, these metabolic polymorphisms were, unlike other genes implicated in human disease, usually latent, having no perceptible effect on the health of predisposed persons.

Thus, the predictions of Garrod and Bateson regarding the role of heredity and the importance of enzymes in the transformation of exogenous chemicals including drugs were affirmed again and again during this period. Hence, the years from 1950 to about 1990 may be thought of as the period when the functional variation of human drug-metabolizing genes was established and the field of pharmacogenetics emerged as an experimental science.

INFORMATIONAL FOUNDATIONS OF MODERN GENETICS

The informational foundations of modern genetics were established during the 1960s and 1970s. Early in this period, the genetic code was deciphered as were the rules by which cells read the information encoded in the gene. A flood of new gene discoveries, the development of new approaches to the discovery and scoring of drug susceptibility loci, and advances in pharmacogenomics and toxicogenomic strategies to facilitate drug discovery and development that followed in short order have continued to the present. Technical advances, described briefly below and more extensively in Chapter 7 and charted in Table 1.2, led the way in transforming the nature of biomedical research, and greatly increased the pace and scope of investigation.

Beginning in 1975, a variety of techniques were invented for sequencing and scanning or scoring all manner of lesions in DNA relevant to human disease and pharmacogenetics. In 1979, a consensus was reached and an award was made enabling the creation of an international database for the collection, storage, and

Table 1.2 Charting the Evolution of Genomics Tools

Technology	1975	1985	1995	2005
Conventional DNA technologies	Southern blots; Sanger sequencing; Northern blots; RFLPs	DNA fingerprinting; PCR; Dot blots, slot blots	Reverse blots	
Computational biology	GenBank established	FASTA developed; NCBI established; BLAST developed		PHRED/PHRAP/CON-SET developed
Automated DNA sequencing		First automated sequencer commercialized	First CE sequencer; Human genome project begins	Yeast genome sequenced; Worm genome sequenced; Fruit fly genome sequenced; Human genome draft complete
Microarray analysis		Microarray analysis applied to DNA	Genomic DNA analysis; Gene expression profiling of cancer	Genome-wide DNA analysis
MALDI-TOF mass spectrometry		Analysis of proteins	Analysis of DNA	High-resolution analysis of DNA; Primer extension applied to DNA analysis
Y2H system			Y2H system invented	Yeast interactome mapped; Fruit fly interactome mapped; Worm interactome mapped

processing of molecular sequences of DNA and proteins at the National Institutes of Health. As the collection of sequences of proteins and nucleic acids expanded, and the demand for efficient, rapid, and economical methods to perform searches on these molecules increased throughout the 1980s, older, computationally intensive, and costlier methods were replaced by new approaches to sequence comparisons that were much faster and more accessible than existing search tools for DNA and protein sequences, motifs, and gene identification. The invention of fluorescent detection systems made it possible to automate DNA sequencing and by 1986 the first automated sequencers became commercially available. Since then, the speed of DNA sequencing has increased by several orders of magnitude through the development of simpler chemistry and more sensitive dyes for DNA labeling, more powerful computers, and improved optical systems. Alternative sequencing methodologies have led to further increases in the speed, sensitivity, and accuracy of sequencing at reduced cost.

During the 1980s, as the density of information derived from sequencing, mapping, and identifying human genes increased, so did the demand for analytical tools capable of exploiting this information. In a sequence of events reminiscent of the evolution of conventional techniques for sequencing DNA, a means was developed of generating probe arrays on solid supports for highly parallel hybridization analysis of DNA. These probe arrays, termed "DNA microarrays," have come to occupy niches in nearly every area of basic biological and biomedical science, including genome mapping, genotyping and reference-based sequence checking (resequencing), and gene expression profiling. Later, the technology was transferred to the development of proteomic, glycomic, tissue arrays, and G-protein-coupled microarrays, and to the assessment of RNA and protein alterations as diagnostic markers, particularly in oncology. The dramatic increase in information that could be gathered from a single profiling experiment with DNA microarray technology and its ready adaptability to interdisciplinary research were highly advantageous.

Toward the end of the 1980s, the introduction of matrix-assisted laser desorption (MALDI) time of flight (TOF) mass spectrometry revolutionized the analysis of large biomolecules. Using this technique, proteins with masses of up to several hundred thousand could be analyzed. By combining improved signal resolution with less expensive, more efficient lasers to increase sequencing fidelity, large DNA biomolecules could also be analyzed. The simplicity of MALDI-TOF mass spectrometry increased its popularity and substantially expanded its range of applications to the discovery and identification of SNPs, sizing of nucleotide repeats, estimation of allele frequencies, and the quantitative analysis of gene expression and DNA methylation patterns. And finally, the invention of the yeast-two-hybrid (Y2H) system in 1989 provided a strategy for identifying interactions of pairs of proteins. With the aid of the Y2H system, partial maps of protein–protein interactions ("interactomes") have been determined for the yeast, worm, and fruit fly genomes. The Y2H approach, a unique facility to target protein–protein interactions in model organisms, set the stage for the determination of human interactomes.

THE GENOMICS ERA

The genomics era overlaps somewhat with the preceding period and extends from about 1985 to the present. The chart of benchmarks relevant to pharmacogenetic polymorphisms (Figure 1.4) helps us visualize this overlap and how the emergence and growth of experimental pharmacogenetics from the 1950s through the 1980s foreshadowed the trend toward genomics in and around the 1990s. It is clear that a large number of pharmacogenetic traits were identified by classical genetic methods before recombinant DNA sequencing techniques were invented during the 1970s and 1980s (Table 1.2). Whereas allelic variants could be inferred by classical genetics only one gene at a time, they could be identified and directly visualized after molecular techniques became available and were widely adopted.

Additionally, Figure 1.4 reveals that enzymatic polymorphisms of the drug-metabolizing enzymes (pharmacokinetic variability) and enzymes of physiological importance preceded the identification of receptor variants by nearly three decades, supporting the view that the former were almost entirely responsible for setting the research agenda of pharmacogenetics and shaping the initial development of the field. The fact that genetic heterogeneity of receptors (and transporters) could not be defined adequately by pharmacological approaches alone explains the relative lag in progress of receptor-mediated pharmacogenetics (pharmacodynamic variability), but the cloning and sequencing of receptor genes quickly demonstrated their heterogeneity and enabled well-defined receptor and transporter proteins to be expressed in amounts sufficient for biochemical and pharmacological characterization. The rhodopsin receptor was cloned in 1984 and within 5 years the cloning of the receptors for insulin, glucocorticoids, estrogen, mineralocorticoids, retinoic acid, β-adrenergic agonists, and vitamin D quickly followed.

The extensive legacy of pharmacogenetic polymorphisms makes a strong case for structural and functional analyses aimed at producing a complete catalog of human genetic diversity (chromosome structural and copy number polymorphisms, SNPs, deletions, insertions, repeats, and rearrangements). Molecular studies suggest that pharmacogenetic polymorphisms are usually associated with only a limited number of important variants, raising the prospect that their genotypes and related haplotypes might be cataloged relatively quickly for many populations.[10,11] By establishing associations between the unique genetic makeup of individuals as described by pharmacogenetic polymorphisms, and their responsiveness to drugs, foods, and other exogenous substances, we hope to design better therapies and improve prospects for individualized medicine.

THE EFFECT OF MOLECULAR BIOLOGY
ON PHARMACOGENETICS

The central dogma of molecular biology as formulated in the 1950s asserted that the cardinal function of gene action was protein synthesis. Protein synthesis

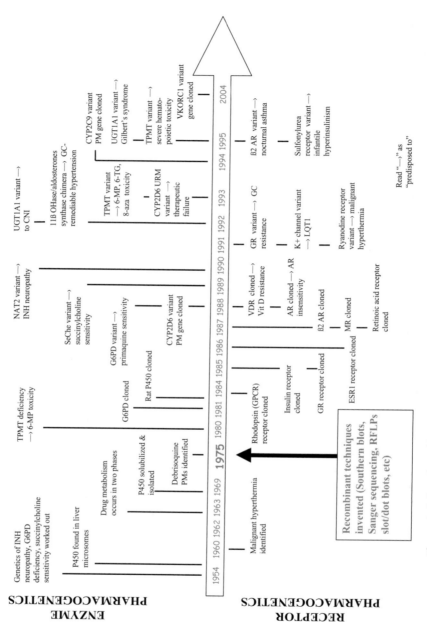

Figure 1.4 Benchmarks in human enzyme and receptor pharmacogenetics.

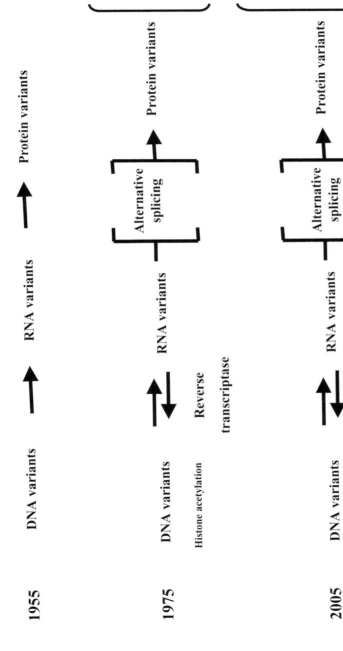

1955

DNA variants → RNA variants → Protein variants

1975

DNA variants
Histone acetylation

Reverse transcriptase

RNA variants

Alternative splicing

Protein variants

Phosphorylation
Glycosylation
Acetylation

Other

2005

DNA variants
DNA methylation
Histone acetylation methylation, phosphorylation

Reverse transcriptase

RNA variants
RNAi

Alternative splicing

Protein variants

Phosphorylation
Glycosylation
Acetylation

Editing

Other

Figure 1.5 Expanding the central dogma of molecular biology. With permission from *The Scientist.*

proceeded according to a well-defined program of instructions encoded in the DNA that was transcribed into RNA and subsequently translated into the primary protein sequence. Hence, the gene was deterministic of unidirectional gene expression. For more than 50 years, genomic research has been guided by this model of genetic inheritance. The insights into human development, physiology, medicine, and evolution gained through the maturation of this work constitute a signal achievement in modern biology, but recent discoveries have revealed that such a simplistic model of the gene–protein relationship was no longer tenable. The idea of a unidirectional nature gene expression was negated by reverse transcriptase; posttranslational protein modifications added another twist, and more recently, the predictive value of the genotype was confounded when it became apparent that some genes encoded just one protein, while other genes encoded more than one protein, and still others did not encode any protein. The complexity of cellular events was illustrated by the identification of previously unknown pathway components, and the recognition that gene expression could be altered at the translational, transcriptional, and posttranslational levels by a host of factors has necessitated wider views of phenotypic expression and expansion of the basic principles of gene expression as originally formulated (Figure 1.5).[12]

Advances in molecular biology were brought into sharper focus during the 1980s and 1990s by cloning and sequencing genes predictive of disease, expression of the proteins they encode, and fixing their chromosomal location in the human genome. Allelic variants that could be inferred only from familial inheritance patterns prior to the advent of molecular genetics could now be demonstrated by direct evidence. The polymerase chain reaction (PCR) combined with gene expression systems increased the availability of well-defined recombinant proteins in quantities sufficient for biochemical and pharmacological characterization. Strategies to target and modify genes in a predictable manner could be created in animal and cell models possessing knockout, overexpressed, and "humanized" alleles in specific tissues and at specific developmental stages. In short, molecular biological approaches in many forms permeated and dominated biological research, setting the stage for the convergence of basic research and clinical medicine. The changing scene surrounding these events solidified the foundations of genetics by providing novel insights into the multiplicity of factors affecting gene expression, and invigorating and redefining pharmacogenetics.

REFERENCES

1. Garrod AE. Medicine from the chemical standpoint. Lancet 1914; ii:281–289.
2. Garrod AE. The Inborn Factors in Disease. An Essay. London: Oxford at the Clarendon Press, 1931.
3. Marshall EK, Lynch V, Smith HW. On dichloroethylsulfide (Mustard gas). II. Variation in susceptibility of the skin to dichloroethylsulfide. JPET 1918; 12:291–301.
4. Hirschfeld L, Hirschfeld H. Serological differences between the blood of different races. Lancet 1919; 2(Oct 18):675–679.

5. Chen KK, Poth EJ. Racial differences as illustrated by the mydriatic action of co-caine, eupthalmine, and ephedrine. JPET 1929; 36:429–445.
6. Blakeslee AF. Unlike reaction of different individuals to fragrance in verbena flowers. Science 1918; XLVIII:298–299.
7. Blakeslee AF, Salmon MR. Odor and taste blindness. Eugen News 1935; 105–110.
8. Fox AL. The relationship between chemical constitution and taste. Proc Natl Acad Sci USA 1932; 18(1):115–120.
9. Snyder LH. Studies in human inheritance. IX. The inheritance of taste deficiency in man. Ohio J Sci 1932; 32:436–440.
10. Stephens JC. Single-nucleotide polymorphisms, haplotype, and their relevance to pharmacogenetics. Mol Diagnosis 1999; 4(4):309–317.
11. Drysdale CM, McGraw DW, Stack CB, Stephens JC, Judson RS, Nandabalan K, et al. Complex promoter and coding region beta 2-adrenergic receptor haplotypes alter receptor expression and predict in vivo responsiveness. Proc Natl Acad Sci USA 2000; 97(19):10483–10488.
12. Silverman PH. Rethinking genetic determinism. Scientist 2004; 18(10):32–33.

2
Defining Pharmacogenetics

In an address on "Medicine from The Chemical Standpoint" before the British Medical Association in 1914,[1] Archibald Garrod spoke of the difficulty in covering the foundations and recent progress in the field of medicine that should treat the subject in any of its wider aspects. About a third of his presentation dealt with drugs as toxic substances, foreign to the organism, and that enzymes were agents of detoxication of these substances. He cautioned that drugs often produced the effect aimed at, along with side effects that could not be fully estimated, and stressed the importance of pharmacology in teaching how drugs act, the nature of their active principles and their limitations, and how they might be best employed. In this way, he believed that "blunderbuss prescription would be replaced by single drugs of known efficiency," and that "the discoveries of empirical therapeutics would be placed on a scientific footing."

Today, as in Garrod's time, the goal of drug therapy is to provide effective treatment without toxicity. Ideally a drug is delivered so that it achieves a blood concentration that is within the therapeutic range. A drug concentration that is too low is ineffective while one that is too high is frequently toxic. No drugs are effective for 100% of patients, as the following data for a number of commonly used classes of drugs show.

Class of drug	Effectiveness (therapeutic failure or adverse drug reactions)
Selective serotonin reuptake inhibitors (SSRIs)	10–25%
ACE inhibitors	10–30%
β_2-Adrenergic receptor blockers	15–25%
Tricyclic antidepressants	15–25%
Statins (HMG-CoA reductase inhibitors)	30–70%
β_2-Adrenergic receptor agonists	40–70%

THE GENETIC PROFILE OF HUMAN DRUG RESPONSE

Responses that we associate with a particular drug are actually due to physiological and biochemical properties of cells targeted by receptors of the recipient.
They are determined by interactions between physiological, pathophysiological,
environmental, and genetic factors. Patient physiology, pathophysiology, and
environment are usually considered when prescribing a drug, but genetic variation,
which may be the single most significant contributor to the drug effectiveness and
toxicity, is often given short shrift.

	Pathophysiology	Environment	Genetics
Age	Liver function	Drug therapy	Drug-metabolizing enzymes
Sex	Kidney function	Smoking status	Drug transporters
Weight	Cardiovascular functon	Alcohol consumption	Drug receptors
BMI	Lung function	Nutrition	Ion channels
	Other diseases	Pollutants	Target enzymes
		Occupation	Signal transduction

By dividing these factors into two groups, pharmacologists have reconstructed
a picture of drug response that is somewhat idealized but more accessible to
analysis. Pharmacokinetic factors include the absorption, distribution, metabolism, and excretion of drugs and determine the time course of drug disposition, while pharmacodynamic factors are receptor mediated and determine the
response.

$$\text{Drug response} = \sum \text{pharmacokinetics} + \sum \text{pharmacodynamics}$$

Absorption	Receptor mediated
Distribution	
Metabolism	
Excretion	

Because the free drug concentration in tissue water bathing drug-receptor (DR)
complexes is in rapid equilibrium with plasma water, changes in the concentration of DR complexes, and hence response, parallel changes in plasma drug
concentration as schematized in the following diagram.

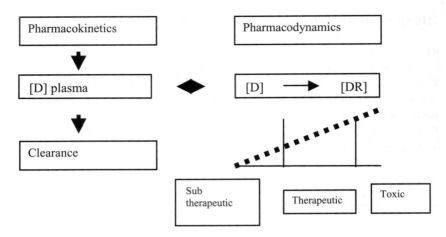

However, the factors that determine the plasma drug level vary from person to person. When the "between-persons" differences are greater than "within-person" differences, genetic factors may be largely responsible for the variation.

How do genes influence drug response? Genes contain information that determines the amino acid sequence of proteins: proteins are vital to virtually every process of biological importance including drug response. The DNA of genes consists of several basic elements: enhancers, a promoter that regulates the expression of the gene, 5′ and 3′ untranslated regions (UTRs), exons that encode the protein, and introns. The net result of gene action is the synthesis of proteins and the transport of these proteins to their characteristic sites in cells and tissues of the individual. If the DNA has sequence variations (mutations), the proteins may not be expressed properly, or not function properly, or not reach the appropriate site, as follows:

DNA Mutation	Protein Defect
Open reading frame (ORF coding region)	
Start codon	No protein
Stop codon	Improper size protein, altered
Other codons	function, poor binding, poor stability
Promoter/enhancer	improper expression, failure to respond to normal control signals
3′ UTR-polyadenylation signal	Increase/decrease in stability, improper expression

DNA mutations that occur at a frequency of 1% or greater are termed polymorphisms. DNA polymorphisms include copy number, insertions, deletions, duplications, inversions, and single nucleotide polymorphisms (SNPs). Polymorphisms in any of the basic gene elements may affect either the function or expression of the gene product.

How can pharmacokinetics alter drug response?

Absorption: To enter the body, drugs must cross membranes either by diffusion or active transport. Mutations in membrane proteins or transporter proteins can alter the drug absorption.

Distribution: Drug distribution, like absorption, depends on the drug's ability to cross membranes and/or be transported by carrier proteins. Variation in these proteins can influence the distribution of drugs.

Metabolism: Once in the bloodstream, drugs are metabolized. The majority of pharmacogenetic studies have been conducted on metabolism of drugs, and one of the main applications of pharmacogenetic principles concerns genetic variation in drug-metabolizing enzymes.

Oxidation–reduction–hydrolysis (Phase 1) and conjugation (Phase 2) reactions are catalyzed by many enzymes. Phase 1 metabolism may lead to active (synergistic, complementary, or antagonistic), inactive, or toxic products. Some important examples of genetic variation (polymorphism) in human drug metabolism are as follows:

Phase 1	Aldehyde dehydrogenase (ALDH2)
	Cytochrome P450 2C9 (CYP2C9)
	Cytochrome P450 2C19 (CYP2C19)
	Cytochrome P450 2D6 (CYP2D6)
Phase 2	*N*-Acetyltransferases (NAT1, NAT2)
	Glutathione-*S*-transferases (GSTM1, GSTP1, GSTT1)
	Thiopurine methyltransferase (TPMT)

Excretion: Drug excretion is intricately linked to metabolism. Many drugs must be metabolized to more water-soluble forms before they can be excreted efficiently. Some drugs are eliminated via active transport processes.

How can pharmacodynamics alter drug response? The therapeutic potential of many drugs depends upon their interaction with receptors, ion channels, transporters, etc. Drug–receptor interactions can produce a direct effect on the body or initiate a cascade of changes in several proteins that causes the effect (asthma, blood coagulation, arachidonic acid metabolism, blood pressure regulation, etc.). The structural diversity that has emerged from molecular studies of receptors is enormous, and the contribution of these proteins to genetic variation in drug response is steadily coming into view. Genetic differences in pharmacodynamics are often found to produce significant consequences during drug therapy.

Any genetic variation that affects the absorption, distribution, metabolism, excretion, or target of the drugs will likely affect the therapeutic potential of the drug. Most pharmacologically relevant genetic variants that have been identified are in genes that encode drug-metabolizing enzymes. The variants that have been identified may affect the expression or function of a variety of both Phase 1 and Phase 2 enzymes (Figure 2.1).[2]

Common genetic variants of drug-metabolizing enzymes lead to either an increase or decrease in the rate of metabolism of the drug. The effect of altered

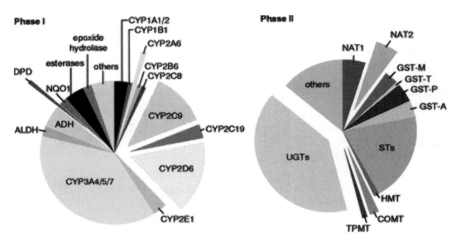

Figure 2.1 Pie chart. Most drug-metabolizing enzymes exhibit clinically relevant genetic polymorphisms. Essentially all of the major human enzymes responsible for modification of functional groups [classified as Phase I reactions (*left*)] or conjugation with endogenous substituents [classified as Phase II reactions (*right*)] exhibit common polymorphisms at the genomic level; those enzyme polymorphisms that have already been associated with changes in drug effects are separated from the corresponding pie charts. The percentage of Phase I and Phase II metabolism of drugs that each enzyme contributes is estimated by the relative size of each section of the corresponding chart.[2] With permission from the American Association for the Advancement of Science.

metabolism on the predicted therapeutic outcome of a drug depends upon whether the drug is delivered in its active form or in an inactive prodrug form that requires metabolism for activation.

Drug responses that are influenced by genetic factors can often be identified by phenotypic or genotypic analysis. (1) Phenotypic analysis: drug responses that exhibit a multimodal distribution pattern (nonnormal distribution) are indicative of genetic influences on the drug response in the test population. (2) Drug response phenotype exhibits significant heritability in family pedigrees. Knowledge of genotype/phenotype allows for a more informed decision in managing pharmacogenetic disorders.

Conceptually, pharmacogenetics may be regarded as the third leg in the triad of factors that determine drug response (see Figure 2.2).

Physiological changes that accompany normal growth and development of infants and children and of aging persons add another level of variability to drug responses that must be considered in making clinical and therapeutic decisions. During the first months and years after birth, changes in body composition and organ function are cyclic or periodic and may be discordant in different tissues. During the middle years of life, these changes abate and homeostatic mechanisms maintain a functional equilibrium. In the elderly, person-to-person variability in drug response increases owing to a series of age-related asynchronous morphological and functional changes that occur in many organs and tissues. The prin-

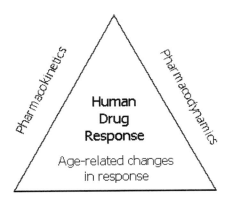

Pharmacogenomics

Figure 2.2 Pharmacogenetics may be regarded as the third leg in the triad of factors that determine drug response.

ciples underlying age-appropriate adjustments in drug dosing to provide safe and effective pharmacotherapy are considered separately below.

Examples of Phase 1 and Phase 2 drug-metabolizing enzyme variants and their effect on response to exogenous chemicals are shown in the following.

Phase	Enzyme	Phenotype	Drugs/chemicals	Response
Phase 1	CYP2D6	Ultrarapid metabolizer (URM)	Debrisoquine, codeine, nortryptyline, dextromethorphan	URM: therapeutic failure
		Extensive metabolizer (EM)		PM: drug toxicity, therapeutic failure
		Poor metabolizer (PM)		
	CYP2C9	Reduced activity	Warfarin, tolbutamide, NSAIDs, phenytoin, ACE inhibitors	Bleeding from warfarin
	CYP2C19	Extensive metabolizer (EM) Poor metabolizer (PM)	Proguanil, barbiturates	PM: drug toxicity
Phase 2	NAT2	Slow acetylator	Isoniazid, hydralazine, procainamide, sulfasalazine, aromatic amine carcinogens	Peripheral neuropathy, lupus, CNS toxicity
	TPMT	Slow methylator	6-MP, 6-TG, azathioprine, maxlactam, cefatoxim	Bone marrow toxicity
	GST M1 GST T1 GST P1	Reduced activity	GST M1: aflatoxin B1 GST T1: haloalkanes GST P1: electrophilic carcinogens, pesticides	Associated with prostate, colon, and lung carcinogens

EVIDENCE FOR INDIVIDUAL VARIATION IN DRUG RESPONSE

Most pharmacologically relevant genetic variants result in dramatic differences in gene product function or expression (complete loss of function, substantial increase in expression, etc). As a consequence, they have a major effect on the pharmacokinetic or pharmacodynamic properties of a drug. This is illustrated by

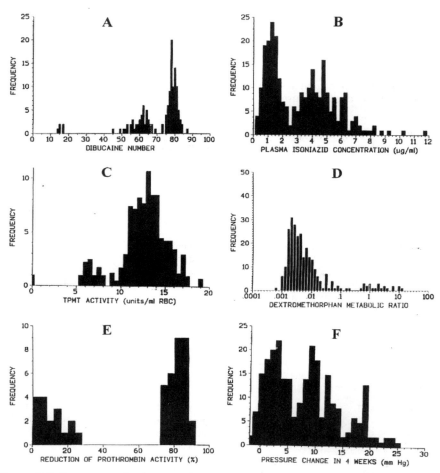

Figure 2.3 Frequency distributions for genetically heterogeneous drug responder populations. (*A*) Succinylcholine sensitivity: dibucaine number; (*B*) acetylation (NAT2 polymorphism: plasma isoniazid concentrations; (*C*) TPMT deficiency: TPMT activity in red blood cells; (*D*) CYP2D6 polymorphism: dextromethorphan/dextrorphan metabolic ratio; (*E*) warfarin resistance: reduction of prothrombin-complex activity after a single dose of warfarin; (*F*) steroid-induced glaucoma: applanation pressure change in 4 weeks after intraocular administration of dexamethasone.

the bimodal and trimodal frequency distributions of drug response phenotypes in populations as shown in Figure 2.3.

EVIDENCE THAT VARIATION IN DRUG RESPONSE IS INHERITED

Twin Studies

Identical (monozygotic) twins have identical DNA sequences, but fraternal (dizygotic, nonidentical) twins do not; they are no more closely related than other full siblings. If a response is studied in sets of identical and fraternal twins, the response will be much more concordant (similar) in the identical twins than in the fraternal twins if the response is hereditary as shown below for the urinary elimination of isoniazid.

Urinary elimination of isoniazid (INH)			
Identical (monozygotic) twins		Fraternal (dizygotic) twins	
Sex	INH eliminated (% dose ingested)	Sex	INH eliminated (% dose ingested)
M	8.8	F	12.1
M	8.3	F	13.7
F	26.0	F	10.9
F	25.2	F	4.6
M	11.8	M	11.0
M	12.4	M	8.5
F	12.2	F	3.9
F	11.5	F	15.2
F	4.1	M	10.5
F	4.1	M	15.6

Family Studies

The drug response phenotype exhibits significant heritability in family pedigrees. Inheritance of pharmacogenetically relevant traits follows the basic (Mendelian) laws of genetics. All standard patterns of inheritance including autosomal dominant, autosomal recessive (codominant), sex-linked, and maternally inherited mitochondrial traits have been identified from analysis of such traits in family pedigrees.

Clinically, it may be important to understand the mechanism of inheritance of a trait since other family members may be affected, and this knowledge can be vital to predict the response in the patient or members of the patient's family. Inheritance patterns of some pharmacogenetic traits are listed in the following.

Inheritance patterns of some pharmacogenetic traits

Autosomal dominant traits
  Aldehyde dehydrogenase (ALDH2) ethanol metabolism
  Glucocorticoid remediable hypertension
  Insulin resistance due to the insulin receptor gene
  LQT syndrome
  Malignant hyperthermia
  Thrombophilia

Autosomal (codominant) recessive traits
  Acetylation (NAT2) polymorphism
  α_1-Antitrypsin deficiency
  CYP2C9 polymorphism
  CYP2C19 (mephenytoin) polymorphism
  CYP2D6 (debrisoquine/sparteine) polymorphism
  Dihydropyrimidine dehydrogenase (DPD) deficiency
  Fish malodor syndrome (FM03 deficiency)
  Fructose intolerance
  Glutathione-S-transferase polymorphism
  Thiopurine methyltransferase deficiency

Sex-linked recessive traits
  G6PD deficiency
  Pyridoxine responsive deficiency
  Vasopressin resistance

Mitochondrial traits—maternally transmitted
  Aminoglycoside antibiotic–induced deafness

Population Studies

Frequencies of phenotypes and genotypes that characterize a trait in populations at large are determined from studies of biologically unrelated persons by plotting the frequency distribution of the response. Ethnogeographic variation is regarded as an important facet of any comprehensive pharmacogenetic study. Ethnic differences for some human drug metabolizing enzymes are shown in the following.

Ethnic differences in human drug metabolizing enzymes

Trait	Population frequency (%)
CYP2C19 PMs	Caucasian (4%)
CYP2C19 PMs	Asian (13–23%)
CYP2D6 PMs	Caucasian (5–10%)
CYP2D6 PMs	Japanese (<1%)
CYP2D6(L)URMs	Swedish (1–2%)
CYP2D6(L)URMs	Hispanic (7%)
CYP2D6(L)URMs	Zimbabwean (13%)
NAT2	Caucasian, black (40–65%)
NAT2	Asian (10–20%)
GST M1 (null)	Blacks (35%)
GST M1 (null)	Caucasian (49%)
GST M1 (null)	Indian (5%)

INTERACTION WITH OTHER FIELDS EMPOWERS PHARMACOGENETICS

Pharmacogenetic studies are frequently jump-started by isolated observations of unexpected drug responses or anecdotal accounts of esoteric epidemiological findings, but they ultimately involve in-depth studies at all levels of gene action from the genotypic properties of the gene itself to its phenotypic effects in individuals and populations. The essence of pharmacogenetics lies in the application of the principles of pharmacology and genetics to variation of human drug response, but the expertise and technical know-how available in other fields, biochemistry, toxicology, epidemiology, and computational biology, are usually called upon to attain a comprehensive understanding of the root causes of pharmacogenetic traits. And while the discussion here centers on the investigation of human subjects, studies of knockout, transgenic animals and other eukaryotic models can often provide new insight into the biological basis of pharmacogenetic traits as well as the mechanisms that underpin them. Study designs that exclude such systems may thus sacrifice an invaluable alternative to the strategy and tactics of human pharmacogenetic investigations.

PHARMACOGENETICS IS A COMPONENT OF ECOGENETICS

Hereditary differences in toxicity or efficacy that result from exposure to therapeutic agents are obviously relevant to *pharmacogenetics,* but if the unexpected response results from exposure to other chemicals, or to physical, climatic, or atmospheric agents, it may be classified as *ecogenetic.* Ecogenetics encompasses genetically conditioned responses to exogenous substances from any source, and as such, includes the pharmacogenetics of drugs used in medical practice. Despite this distinction, the literature does not always adhere to this convention. When it is of interest to assess the characteristics of a given response, the criteria to be met in designing and executing a proper study to determine the heritability of the response in twins and families, and the distribution and incidence of genotypes and phenotypes in larger populations, are, in fact, identical for pharmacogenetics and ecogenetics.

THE SCOPE OF PHARMACOGENETICS

The development of pharmacogenetics from 1950 to 2000 is charted in Table 2.1. Xenobiotic targets relevant to pharmacogenetics include drug-metabolizing enzymes, non-drug-metabolizing enzymes, receptors, ion channels, and other proteins, some of whose functions may be unknown or not well defined. Human sensitivities to nutritional and dietary components, occupational pollutants, or industrial chemicals, and to personal life-style habits such as smoking or drinking alcohol, may also be hallmarks of pharmacogenetic phenomena. Historically, the drug-metabolizing enzyme polymorphisms are foremost in pharmacogenetics.

Table 2.1 Charting the Growth of Human Enzyme and Receptor Pharmacogenetics

Enzyme Traits	Receptor Traits	
1950		1950
1952 Crigler–Najjar syndrome (nonhemolytic jaundice) identified		
1953 Slow acetylation predisposes to INH-induced nerve toxicity		
1956 G6PD deficiency explains primaquine sensitivity		
1956 Fructose intolerance identified		
1957 Succinylcholine sensitivity is due to a serum ChE variant		
1957 Gilbert's syndrome is due to glucuronosyltransferase deficiency		
1958 G6PD deficiency is a sex-linked recessive trait		
1960 Slow acetylation is a recessive autosomal trait	Malignant hyperthermia identified	1960
1962 P450 identified in liver microsomes		
1963 Drug metabolism occurs in two phases		
1964 Phenytoin slow hydroxylators identified	Anticoagulant resistance may be due to an altered "receptor"	1964
1964 Slow acetylation is due to a variant N-acetyltransferase		
1966 Dexamethasone-suppressible hypertension identified		
1967 Slow acetophenetidin dealkylators identified		
1969 Crigler–Najjar syndromes 1 and 2 differentiated		
1970 Fish malodor syndrome (trimethylaminuria) identified		1970
1971 α_1-Antitrypsin deficiency is a biomarker for emphysema		
1973 Paraoxonase polymorphism identified		
1973 Lactose intolerance attributed to lactase polymorphism		
1975 Poor metabolizers of debrisoquine and sparteine identified		
1977 COMT activity a genetic marker for levodopa response	APL attributed to balanced translocation t(15;17)	1977
1978 Slow tolbutamide metabolizers identified		
1978 Chlorpropamide flushing is due to ALDH deficiency		
1978 α_1-Antitrypsin Pittsburg predisposes to a bleeding disorder		
1980 High and low thiopurine inactivators identified		1980
1981 G6PD gene cloned		
1982 α_1-Antitrypsin variant predisposes to premature emphysema		

Year	Event	Year	Event
1982	cDNA sequence of rat P450 determined	1984	G-protein-coupled (rhodopsin) receptor isolated and cloned
1983	α_1-Antitrypsin Pittsburg variant identified	1985	Insulin receptor cloned and mapped to chromosome 19p13.2–13.3
1984	ALDH2 variant protects against alcoholism	1985	Glucocorticoid receptor cloned
1984	Slow mephenytoin metabolizers identified	1986	Estrogen receptor ESR1 cloned and mapped to chromosome 196q25.1
1984	Aldolase B cloned, sequenced, and mapped to chromosome 9	1987	β_2-Adrenergic receptor cloned and mapped to chromosome 5q31–32
1985	DPD deficiency is a biomarker for fluorouracil toxicity	1987	Mineralocorticoid receptor cloned
		1987	Retinoic acid receptor cloned
1987	Serum ChE amino acid sequence determined	1988	Vitamin D receptor cloned and sequenced
		1988	Vitamin D receptor variant predisposes to Vitamin D-resistant rickets
1988	CYP2D6 gene cloned and sequenced	1988	ESR1 genomic structure determined
1988	GST M1 cloned and null variant identified	1988	Androgen receptor cloned; AR variant predisposes to androgen insensitivity
1988	ALDH2 variant protects against aversive effects of alcohol		
1988	Aldolase B variant is a biomarker for fructose intolerance	1988	Insulin receptor variant predisposes to insulin resistance
1988	G6PD variant is a biomarker for primaquine sensitivity	1988	Retinoic acid receptor localized to chromosome 17q21
1989	Atypical serum ChE gene and variant cloned and sequenced	1990	FcεRI receptor (α chain) mapped to chromosome 1q23
1990	NAT1 and NAT2 cloned, sequenced and mapped to chromosome 8; NAT2 explains the INH acetylation polymorphism	1991	Ryanodine receptor variant associated with malignant hyperthermia
1991	Diverse allelic variants characterize acetylation polymorphism	1991	GCR variant allele predisposes to GC resistance
		1991	Potassium ion channel variant predisposes to LQT1
		1991	APL is associated with ATRA responsive chimera PML-RAR α
1992	UGT1A1 variant predisposes to Crigler–Najjar I syndrome	1992	X-linked AVPR2 variant is a biomarker for vasopressin resistance
1992	Chimeric 11β-hydroxylase/aldosterone synthase predisposes to dexamethasone-remediable aldosteronism and hypertension	1992	FcεRI β-chain mapped to chromosome 11q13
1992	δ-Aminolevulinate synthase variants predispose to X-linked sideroblastic anemia	1992	Angiotensin II type 1 receptor cloned, sequenced, and mapped to chromosome 11q13

(continued)

Table 2.1 (*continued*)

Enzyme Traits	Receptor Traits	
	β₂-Adrenoceptor variants identified	1993
1993 UGT1A1 variant associated with Crigler–Najjar 2		
1993 TPMT cloned and sequenced from colon cancer cell line		
1993 NAT1 cloned, sequenced, and variants identified		
1993 CYP2D6 URM variant identified		
	AH receptor mapped to chromosome 7p21–15	1994
	CAG repeats of androgen receptor are tied to paradoxic responses of antiandrogens	1994
	Estrogen receptor null variant is a biomarker for severe estrogen resistance	1994
	Vitamin D receptor mapped to chromosome 12.12–q22	1994
	LQT3 mapped to chromosome 3p21–24	1994
1995 UGT1A1 variant is a biomarker for Gilbert's syndrome	β₂ AR polymorphism is a biomarker for nocturnal asthma	1995
1995 TPMT variant is a biomarker for severe hematopoietic toxicity	Sulfonylurea receptor is cloned and is a biomarker for infantile hyperinsulinism and is mapped to chromosome 11p15.1	1995
1995 Unidentified cis-acting element controls lactase persistence/nonpersistence polymorphism	FcεRI β subunit variant is a biomarker for an asthmatic phenotype	1996
	CCR5Δ32 variant is a biomarker for resistance to HIV-induced infection in adults	1996
1997 FMO3 variant is a biomarker for fish malodor syndrome	Vitamin D receptor gene genomic structure determined	1997
1997 DPD genomic structure determined	AH receptor polymorphism is a biomarker for high CYP1A1 activity	1997
	Mineralocorticoid receptor variant is a biomarker for mineralocorticoid resistance	1997
	Tlr4 receptor variant is a biomarker for Gram-negative (LPS) shock	1997
	ESR2 cloned and mapped to chromosome 14q22–24	1997
	Vitamin D receptor mapped to chromosome 12cenq12	1999
2000 DPD gene promoter cloned and sequenced	CCR2-64I variant is a biomarker for resistance to HIV-induced infection in children, but not in adults	2000
2003 DPD is a biomarker for lethal 5-fluorotoxicity, but there is a complex relationship of genotype to phenotype		

They are recognized as the cornerstone of the field. Most well-studied polymorphisms derive from investigations of therapeutic agents, because they can be administered safely to individuals of all ages in defined amounts and their disposition patterns can be measured. The enzymes that metabolize exogenous substances may also metabolize hormones and other endogenous messengers that regulate cell signaling, and mutations that affect those pathways may also cause differences in individual responses. The range of such phenomena is virtually without limit.

By the time of Garrod's address in 1914, physiological chemists had already identified most kinds of metabolic reactions of drugs and other exogenous chemicals that we know today. Most of those reactions were identified between 1850 and 1910,[3] but the precise dates of their discovery are less relevant to the emergence of modern pharmacogenetics than that they set the stage for unraveling the nature of the enzymes involved in those reactions. In the 1950s, Julius Axelrod at the National Institutes of Health in the United States discovered the subcellular localization of the prime oxidative enzymes and showed them to be responsible for a wide variety of oxidative reactions. These enzymes, now known as the P450 enzymes,[4,5] are situated in the endoplasmic reticulum of liver and other tissues. In a much broader look at metabolism, R. Tecwyn Williams, at St. Mary's Medical School in London, authored a compendium of metabolic reactions and proposed the distinction between types of reactions that he termed Phase 1 (oxidation, reduction, and hydrolysis) and Phase 2 (conjugation).[6] The designation of Phase 1 and Phase 2 pathways has been widely adopted and is eminently suited for discussions of the biochemical and pharmacological mechanisms of human variation in drug responses.

Enzymes, Transporters, Receptors, and Other Protein Targets

Drug-metabolizing enzymes and drug transporters play an important role in the pharmacokinetics of many drugs of clinical importance. A total of 57 CYP450 (Phase 1) enzymes in human cells are contained in the human genome[7,8] (http://drnelson.utmem.edu/CytochromeP450.html); at least a dozen members of three families, CYP1, CYP2, and CYP3, are responsible for oxidation of the bulk of environmental chemicals, including drugs. Among these, CYP1A2, 2A6, 2B6, 2C8, 2C9, 2C19, 2D6, 2E1, 3A4, and 3A5 are most prominent. Phase 2 reactions include the glucuronosyltransferases (UDPGTs), N-acetyltransferases (NATs), glutathione-S-transferases (GSTs), sulfotransferases (STs), and thiopurine methyltransferases (TPMTs). Characterization of the enzyme variants isolated from tissues or expressed in heterologous systems revealed them as high or low (or null) variants that might alter the susceptibility of individuals to adverse reactions to drugs or other exogenous chemicals.

The following websites contain information about human drug-metabolizing enzyme traits. <http://www.imm.ki.se/CYPalleles/> is a database of variant isoforms of these enzymes and <http://medicine.iupui.edu/flockhart/p450ref3.html #2C9sub> is a database of drug substrates, inducers, and inhibitors of these enzymes. GeneCards (http://www.genecards.org/index.shtml) is another valuable resource on human genes. Genetic polymorphisms of drug-metabolizing enzymes can result in individual differences in pharmacokinetics and there is a growing appreciation that genetic polymorphisms of drug transporters can also exert a significant effect on pharmacodynamics. A wide variety of transporters capable of drug efflux and drug uptake have been identified. Efflux transporters are mainly represented by the ABC cassette (ABC) family that utilizes energy derived from the hydrolysis of ATP to move substrates out of cells. Efflux transporters include the multidrug resistance proteins (MDR), the multidrug resistance-related protein (MRP), the bile salt export pump (BSEP), and the breast cancer resistance protein (BCRP). Uptake transporters, on the other hand, facilitate the translocation of drugs into cells by exchange or cotransport of intracellular and/or extracellular ions (Na^+, H^+, HCO_3^-). Members of this class include organic anion transporters (OATP), organic cation transporters (OCT, OCTN), and peptide transporters (PepT).[9]

Characterization of transporters expressed in intestine, liver, kidney, and brain indicates that genetic heterogeneity contributes not only to individual variations in drug disposition and elimination, but also to drug response. It is also increasingly recognized that because of the overlap between transporters and P450 drug-metabolizing enzymes in liver and intestine, genetically determined differences in transport can affect the metabolism of shared substrate drugs. Hence, it is reasonable to expect that drug transporter pharmacogenetics and drug-metabolizing enzyme pharmacogenetics taken together may be a better predictor of individual variation in drug efficacy and toxicity than either one alone.

Rapid advances in the structural and functional analysis of receptor genes have occurred since the classical pharmacological approaches to drug receptor identification were combined with molecular technologies during the 1980s. Many altered drug responses that are associated with genetically aberrant forms of receptors and functional modifications in the abundance, affinity, or stability of these molecules explain much of the variation in drug response they express.

The CYP2D6 polymorphism, variant forms of the multidrug-resistance transporter, and the mineralocorticoid receptor are described below. Supplementary information on additional polymorphic traits is presented in Table 2.2 (see also Appendix A at the end of this volume). These accounts emphasize the *genetics,* the *molecular basis,* and the *medical or biological significance (clinical outcome)* of specific traits as keys to the organization and retention of vital information about a trait, but they are not intended as exhaustive treatments of the traits described. This sample of traits is meant to illustrate the range and forms of hereditary variations of proteins that may be encountered in response to drugs and other environmental chemicals but it does not define the limits of such variations. Any polypeptide or protein that exerts a significant influence on the response of cells or individuals to these agents is of pharmacogenetic interest.

Drugs and other substances that have been found to be useful as selective probe substrates for phenotyping drug-metabolizing enzyme traits are listed in Appendix B at the end of this volume.

Table 2.2 Range of Pharmacogenetic Traits: Structural and Functional Correlates

Trait	Variant protein	Structural correlate	Functional correlate
Drug-metabolizing enzyme targets			
CYP2D6(L)	Phase 1 enzyme	2- to 13-fold multiplication of gene	Failure to respond to nortryptyline; toxicity to codeine
CYP2C19	Phase 1 enzyme	SNP truncates gene	Failure to respond to proton inhibitors and proguanil
CYP2C9	Phase 1 enzyme	Two major SNPs (Arg-144-Cys) (Ile-359-Leu) impair metabolic efficiency	Toxicity to warfarin and phenytoin
VKROC1	Enzyme–drug receptor complex	Promoter variants impair or enhance vitamin K reductase efficiency	Toxicity to, or lack of efficacy of, warfarin
ALDH2	Phase 1 enzyme	SNP (Glu-487-Lys)	Impaired metabolism of ethanol that protects against aversive effects of ethanol
Succinylcholine sensitivity	Phase 1 enzyme	Atypical SeChE (Asp-70-Gly)	Prolonged apnea to succinylcholine
Acetylation polymorphism	Phase 2 enzyme	Multiple SNPs impair metabolic efficiency of NAT2	INH-induced peripheral neuropathy; susceptibility to bladder cancer from aromatic amine carcinogens
TPMT deficiency	Phase 2 enzyme	SNP (Pro-238-Ala)	Drug-induced (6-MP, 6-TG, azathioprine) bone marrow toxicity
Dihydropyrimidine (DPYD, DPD) polymorphism	Phase 1 enzyme	Splice site mutation IVS14 + 1G > A	Severe 5-fluorouracil toxicity
Glucuronosyltransferase polymorphism	Phase 2 enzyme	Mutated promoter $(TA)_7TAA$ polymorphism	Severe irinotecan toxicity
Fish malodor syndrome	Phase 1 enzyme FMO3	SNP (Pro-153-Leu)	Psychosocial disorders resulting from inability to metabolize trimethylamine in foods
Multidrug resistance transporter (MDR1)	Drug (efflux) transporter	MDR1 (C3435T)	Enhances therapeutic effect of antiretroviral (efavirenz, nelfinavir) drugs in HIV-infected patients
Multidrug resistance-related protein (MRP2)	Drug (efflux) transporter	Absence of functional MRP2	Dubin–Johnson syndrome

(*continued*)

Table 2.2 (*continued*)

Trait	Variant protein	Structural correlate	Functional correlate
Organic anion transporter (OATP-C)	Drug (uptake) transporter	Functional loss associated with the OATP-C*15 haplotype is related to the V174A polymorphism	Altered uptake of many organic anionic drugs
Drug receptor targets			
Mineralocorticoid receptor polymorphism	Cytoplasmic receptor	SNP (Ser-810-Leu)	Early onset hypertension; exacerbation of hypertension in pregnancy
Malignant hyperthermia (RYR1)	Calcium release channel of skeletal muscle	SNP (Arg-615-Cys) impairs calcium release from skeletal muscle	Elevated temperature, hypermetabolism, muscle rigidity
CCR5 polymorphism	HIV-1 entry receptor	32 base pair deletion mutant	Protects against and slows progression of HIV-1 infection
Toll receptor (TLR4)	Cell surface receptor	Sequence polymorphism (Asp-299-Gly)	Hyporesponsive endotoxin (LPS) phenotype
Other drug target proteins			
Glucose-6-phosphate dehydrogenase deficiency	Housekeeping enzyme	Many coding region SNPs	Drug-induced red blood cell hemolysis
α_1-Antitrypsin deficiency	Nondrug enzyme inhibitor	SNP (Glu-342-Lys substitution)	Smoking-induced emphysema
Hereditary fructose intolerance (aldolase B)	Lyase	SNP (Ala-149-Pro)	Marked aversion to foods that contain fructose resulting in abdominal and liver disorders
Long QT syndrome	Ion channel receptor	Potassium and sodium channel SNPs	Spontaneous and drug-induced ventricular arrhythmias
Retinoic acid resistance and acute promyelocytic leukemia	Chimeric PML-RARα gene	Chromosomal translocation (q15;17) (q22;q11.2–12)	Acute promyelocytic leukemia
Aminoglycoside antibiotic-induced deafness	Protein undefined	SNP (A > G at nt 1555) in mitochondrial DNA	Streptomycin-induced nonsyndromic hearing loss
Thrombophilia	Coagulation Factor V	SNP (Arg-506-Glu)	Deep vein thrombosis; candidate for lifelong anticoagulation
MHC ancestral haplotype	Proteins undefined	Ancestral haplotype *HLA-B*5701*, *HLA-DR7*, and *HLA-DQ3*	Hypersensitivity among abacavir-treated AIDS patients

CYP2D6 Debrisoquine/Sparteine Polymorphism

Polymorphic CYP2D6 was one of the first and most important drug-metabolizing enzyme pharmacogenetic traits to be characterized at the molecular (DNA) level. Polymorphisms of the CYP2D6 gene affect the metabolism of some 25% of frequently used drugs. CYP2D6 was originally named for the test drugs debrisoquine (an antihypertensive) and sparteine (an antiarrhythmic), but now dextromethorphan (an antitussive), a drug with fewer side effects, is favored to test for this polymorphism. The metabolic ratio of dextromethorphan/dextrorphan (the product of oxidative demethylation) is the marker of CYP2D6 activity. Four phenotypes can be separated by this method: poor metabolizers (PMs) with high ratios, homozygous and heterozygous extensive metabolizers (EMs) with lower ratios, and ultrarapid metabolizers (URMs) with extremely low ratios.

More than 80 CYP2D6 SNP variants have been identified, but five or six of these variants account for at least 95% of the variation in worldwide populations. In URMs the mutated allele is duplicated 2–13 times. The duplication (multiplication) results in 2–13 extra copies of the gene that is responsible for the increased activity.

PMs are at increased risk of toxicity from CYP2D6 substrate drugs and are more likely to have drug interactions between drugs that are metabolized by CYP2D6. URMs may not reach therapeutic levels on usual doses and may require several times the usual dose to achieve a response. Prodrugs such as codeine (which must be converted to their active form—morphine, in the case of codeine) are ineffective in PMs and may cause toxicity in URMs.

Some drug substrates of CYP2D6	
Antiarrhythmics	Amiodarone, encainide, flecainide, mexiletine, procainamide, sparteine
Antidepressants	Imipramine, clomipramine, desipramine, amitriptyline, nortryptyline, maprotiline
β_2-Adrenergic receptor blockers	Alprenolol, propranolol, timolol, bufuralol, metoprolol, bunitrolol
Neuroleptics	Bisperidone, perphenazine, thioridazine, zuclopenthixol
Other drugs	Codeine, 4-methoxyamphetamine, paroxetine, fluoxetine, phenformin

Multidrug Resistance P-Glycoprotein MDR1 (ABCB1)

The multidrug-resistance transporter gene *MDR1* (HUGO nomenclature, ATP-binding cassette gene *ABCB1*) that codes for P-glycoprotein is the most extensively studied efflux transporter. The P-glycoprotein gene, identified in 1987 by Ueda and co-workers, has an important role in transportation of many different substrates (e.g., digoxin, verapamil, cyclosporine A, colchicine, and vinblastine) at compartmental and cellular levels. The protein is specifically localized to several normal human tissues (liver, pancreas, kidney, colon, jejunum) and diffusely distributed over the surface of cells of the adrenal cortex and medulla. In the intestine, MDR1 restricts drug entry into the body. The protein is abundant in the apical membrane of many epithelial barriers, such as the blood–brain, blood–nerve, blood–testis, and maternal–fetal barriers, and it is expressed in hematopoietic progenitor cells, lymphocytes, and macrophages in development-specific and differentiation-specific manners.[9]

P-glycoprotein is colocalized with the drug-metabolizing enzyme CYP3A4 in the small intestine and liver, suggesting that this transporter is implicated in the absorption and elimination of drugs. Evidence obtained in genetic knockout mice deficient in *mdr1a* supporting such a role demonstrated altered disposition of cyclosporine and increased neurotoxicity to the antiparacidal drug ivermectin.

HIV-infected patients vary considerably in response to treatment with antiretroviral drugs, and antiretroviral drugs such as efavirenz and nelfinavir are substrates of MDR1. To date, more than 50 single nucleotide polymorphisms (SNPs) have been reported for MDR1. One of these, a synonymous SNP in exon 26 (C3435T), has been associated with altered (decreased) MDR1 function when it appears in a haplotype. In a study by Fellay and co-workers who conducted pharmacogenetic studies with efavirenz and nelfinavir in HIV-infected persons with the MDR1 3435 TT, CT, and CC genotypes, nelfinavir plasma concentrations were found to be two or three times lower, while CD-4 cell recovery was 2- to 3-fold higher and the viral load was decreased in patients with the TT genotype compared to those with CT and CC genotypes. These findings suggested that MDR1 C3435T has an important effect on the admittance of antiretroviral drugs to restricted compartments *in vivo*, but the mechanism of the effect was unclear because the synonymous SNP was presumed to be silent. However, a number of studies have demonstrated linkage disequilibrium between the synonymous polymorphism in exon 26 and other SNPs in MDR1 including the exon 21 G2677T/A and exon 12 C1236T, suggesting that the functional effect may be haplotype dependent.[9]

In support of a role for haplotype dependency, the study by Kimchi-Sarfaty and co-workers[10] provides evidence that naturally occurring, silent SNPs alter *in vivo* protein folding and, consequently, affect function.[11] They demonstrated that three known SNPs for the MDR1 gene (C1236T, G2677T, and C3435T) alter MDR1 activity that can change chemotherapy treatments. The MDR1 inhibitors, cyclosporine A and verapamil, were less inhibitory against proteins that were produced from haplotypes that consisted of the polymorphic double (C1236T–G2677T, C1236T–C3435T, G2677–C3435T) and triple (C1236T–G2677T–C3435T) variant combinations. They also showed that it was not the presence of the nonsynonymous polymorphic G2677T that changed the phenotype, but rather the presence of C3435T in combination with one or two of the other "silent" polymorphisms.

This study is one of the first to demonstrate that naturally occurring variations in synonymous codons can give rise to a protein product with the same amino acid sequence but different structural and functional features. It will, no doubt, open a new avenue of research to unravel the causes and progression of genetic disorders, including pharmacogenetic disorders.

Mineralocorticoid Receptor (MR)

The mineralocorticoid receptor (MR) mediates the sodium-retaining effects of aldosterone in the kidney, salivary glands, sweat glands, and colon. The human *MR* gene was cloned in 1987 and bears structural and functional kinships to the glucocorticoid receptor.[12] The gene encoding the receptor spans 60–90 kb on chromosome 4q31.2,[13,14] and contains 10 exons including two exons (1α and 1β) that encode different 5′ untranslated sequences whose expression is controlled by two different promoters.[15] A missense mutation (MRS810L) in the ligand-binding domain of the mineralocorticoid receptor causes an autosomal dominant form of early onset hypertension.[16,17] This mutation was discovered in a 15-year-old boy with severe hypertension and tests of his family revealed 11 of 23 relatives had the mutation, all of whom had been diagnosed with severe hypertension before they were 20 years old. The mutation results in constitutive MR receptor activity in the absence of added steroid, but normal activation by aldosterone, while progesterone and other clinically used corticocoid antagonists, such as spironolactone lacking 21-hydroxyl groups, become agonists. Since progesterone levels are usually elevated by as much as 100-fold during pregnancy, reaching concentrations of 500 nM, the investigators thought that pregnant females with the S810L variant isoform of the MR receptor might develop severe hypertension. Two MR carriers of the family mentioned above had undergone five pregnancies, all of which were complicated by exacerbation of hypertension. The absence of proteinuria, edema, or neurological changes excluded preeclampsia.

Molecular modeling and site-directed mutagenesis demonstrated that the leucine (L810) residue in the 5 helix of the ligand-binding *MR* domain makes a new van der Waals interaction with asparagine (A773) in helix 3. This interaction eliminates the requirement for the 21-hydroxy group of aldosterone to interact with N770 in helix 3. An effective therapy to correct this disorder has not been developed, but since every other steroid hormone receptor as well as several other nuclear hormone receptors has leucine–alanine or methionine–glycine pairs at homologous positions in helix 5 and helix 3, molecular modeling suggests a general approach to the creation of a steroid receptor antagonist.[18]

STRATEGIES FOR GENE IDENTIFICATION

From the dozens of pharmacogenetic traits identified between the 1960s and the mid-1980s, it was evident that genetically determined differences in drug response were not an uncommon occurrence in human subjects. But since all of these studies were performed before the invention of recombinant DNA techniques, the presence of the responsible gene could only be inferred. Knowledge of the basic biological defect extended this inference to a specific metabolic defect, or provided evidence of the pathway or the protein involved. In some cases, unusual catalytic properties suggested a defective form of the putative enzyme, as for the association of "succinylcholine sensitivity" with a defective form of serum cholinesterase; in other cases, a particular biochemical pathway was affected as shown by the association of isoniazid-induced peripheral nerve damage with "slow acetylation" of isoniazid. The strategy that pharmacogeneticists generally adopted for the identification of a hereditary component was referred to as "forward" or "functional genetics." Forward genetics usually begins with the collection of susceptible responders and members of their families. It relies on the detection of differences between the physiological and biochemical properties of the protein variant isolated from susceptible responders to establish the biological defect that distinguishes them from nonsusceptible responders.

After the invention and adoption of conventional recombinant technologies for gene cloning and sequencing, hundreds of disease genes including many of interest to pharmacogenetics had been cloned and analyzed by the 1990s. In addition to determining the clinical significance of specific traits, the common goal of those studies was to relate the susceptibility phenotype to the responsible gene(s) and the spectrum of mutations that conferred the susceptibility. But even with the benefit of these new technologies, the process of gene identification was slow, laborious, and expensive, and could, at first, be performed on only one gene at a time.

The strategies for gene identification derived directly from conventional technologies generally fall into two groups referred to as "functional cloning" and "positional cloning." Functional cloning, as described above, could be supplemented with information about the particular target gene, by assignment of the target gene to a specific chromosomal region, and by previous studies in animals or other model systems. It might also include information about the protein product (such as a partial amino acid sequence obtained from the purified protein and/or from antibodies to the protein or regions of the protein) or its function (such as obtained by a selective protein marker or specific receptor ligand).[19,20]

Positional cloning of the responsible gene, on the other hand, depended on knowledge of its genetic or physical location on a chromosome or in the genome. The technique of positional cloning was invented by Bender and colleagues who used it to isolate the bithorax complex in *Drosophila*.[21] The usual scheme for gene identification according to this approach began with the collection of pedigrees in which the responsible gene was segregating, iterative rounds of fine mapping with polymorphic markers associated with the trait to localize the responsible gene to a restricted region of the genome, and finally searches through all transcripts of the region in affected individuals to identify DNA mutations specific for the trait.[19] This process was originally referred to as "reverse genetics" (Figure 2.4), but previously this term referred to the analysis of function by creating mutations and assessing their effects. As Collins notes, gene identification by mapping is not "reverse," but rather genetics unadulterated by physiology, biochemistry, or cell biology.[19] Positional cloning grew steadily for a while and was successful for the identification of several disease genes, including some of the more common single gene disorders[19] [such as the transmembrane conductance receptor (CFTR) gene for cystic fibrosis[22–24]]. By 1997, close to 100 disease-gene loci had been identified by means of this approach. But as this is a brute force strategy that requires laborious chromosome walking and might incur the identification of a large number of expressed transcripts,[19,20] its popularity waned.

The "candidate gene" approach presents another avenue to gene identification. This approach has some features in common with functional cloning but it differs from the latter by employing information available from previously isolated genes. The candidate gene approach has succeeded in identifying variations in genes in pathways of drug disposition, in pharmacological targets, and in homeostatic pathways as shown in Table 2.3. If, however, knowledge of previously isolated genes or of the biological basis of the trait under study is incomplete, the candidate gene approach may fail to identify every important genetic determinant in the genome as shown in the upper panel of Figure 2.5.

More recently, completion of the human genome initiative and the availability of new tools for genome-wide mapping have prompted investigators to look for ways to improve gene identification. Risch and Merakangas suggested that a genome-wide map of simple nucleotide polymorphisms combined with the candidate gene approach to search for associations would be superior to this approach alone, or to linkage analysis, to find major genes.[25] Collins and colleagues proposed that a genome-wide, high-density map of SNPs, evenly spaced throughout the entire genome, could be used to track gene loci.[26] The strategy proposed

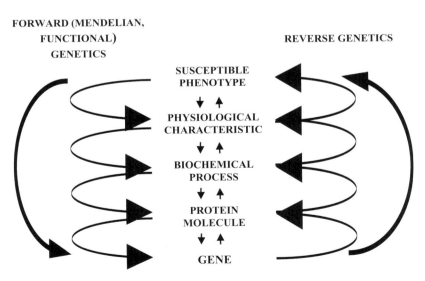

Figure 2.4 Gene identification strategies 1: forward genetics compared to reverse genetics.

Table 2.3 Gene Identification Strategies in Pharmacogenetics[a]

Gene cloned	Year	Cloning method	Strategy to identify the human gene	References[b]
Human enzymes				
Aldolase B	1984	Functional-candidate gene	Used probes from previously cloned human aldolase A sequence to identify the gene	1
ALDH2	1985	Functional-candidate gene	Used probes designed from tryptic peptides isolated from purified enzyme to identify the gene	2
Serum cholinesterase	1987	Functional-candidate gene	Used probes designed from tryptic peptides isolated from purified enzyme to identify the gene	3
CYP2D6	1988	Functional-candidate gene	Used probes obtained from screening human liver RNA with rat antibody to identify the gene	4, 5
GSTM1	1988	Functional-candidate gene	Used probes isolated from human mRNA to identify the gene	6
NAT1 and NAT2	1990	Functional-candidate gene	Used probes designed from tryptic peptides isolated from animal (rabbit) model NAT to identify the gene	7, 8
NAT2	1991	Functional-candidate gene	Used probes from previously cloned human NAT2 to identify the gene	9, 10
GR aldosteronism	1992	Functional-candidate gene	Used probes from previously cloned human CYP11B1 and human CYP11B2 to identify the chimeric gene	11–13
FMO3	1992	Functional-candidate gene	Used probes from previously cloned animal (pig liver, rabbit liver) FMO to identify the gene	14, 15
δ-ALAS	1992	Positional-functional	Used probes from VNTR in exon 7 of the δ-ALAS gene locus previously assigned to the X chromosome to identify the gene	16
DPD promoter	2000	Functional-candidate gene	Used probes from the previously cloned human DPD sequence to extend it to include 5′ region	17

Table 2.3 (*continued*)

Gene cloned	Year	Cloning method	Strategy to identify the human gene	References[b]
Human receptors				
Rhodopsin	1984	Functional-candidate gene	Used probes from a previously cloned animal model (bovine) gene sequence to identify the human gene	18
Insulin	1985	Functional-candidate gene	Used probes designed from peptides obtained from purified α and β subunits to screen a cDNA library prepared from human placental membranes to identify the gene	19
Glucocorticoid	1985	Functional-candidate gene	Used GR-specific antiserum to screen libraries of cDNA clones from human lymphoid and fibroblast cells to isolate clones containing GR cDNA inserts to identify the gene	20
Estrogen	1986	Functional-candidate gene	Used probes synthesized from peptide ER sequences to isolate an ER cDNA clone from MCF-7 cell lines to identify the gene	21
β_2-Adrenergic	1987	Functional-candidate gene	Used probes from a previously cloned animal model (hamster) gene sequence to identify the gene	22
Mineralocorticoid	1987	Functional-candidate gene	Used probes from a previously cloned human GR to isolate MR clones from a kidney library to identify the gene	23
Retinoic acid	1987	Functional-candidate gene	Used a probe synthesized from the immunogenic region (region C) of the ER consensus sequence to screen breast cancer cells known to contain retinoid binding proteins. Since region C is conserved in GR, ER, and progesterone receptors, clones to these receptor genes were eliminated from plaques giving positive signals with this probe to identify the gene	24

(*continued*)

Table 2.3 (*continued*)

Gene cloned	Year	Cloning method	Strategy to identify the human gene	References[b]
Vitamin D	1988	Functional-candidate gene	Used probes from a previously cloned animal (chicken) cVDR to screen a human library to identify the gene	25
Androgen	1988	Functional-candidate gene	Used probes from a previously cloned human GR to isolate an AR clone from a human prostate library to identify the gene	26
Ryanodine	1989	Positional-functional-candidate gene	Used probes from a previously cloned animal (rabbit) cDNA to identify the human gene that had been previously assigned to human chromosome 11p to identify the gene	27
Potassium channel	1991	Functional-candidate gene	Used probes from a previously cloned rat K^+ channels complemented by data on linkage to the ras-1 locus on chromosome 11 to identify the K^+ channel gene	28–30
Antidiuretic (AVPR2)	1992	Functional-candidate gene	Lolait et al. used a probe from a previously cloned rat V1a receptor for homology screening of rat kidney cDNA to identify the rat AVPR2. Birnbaumer et al. constructed a cDNA library from transformed cells expressing the ADH receptor; they probed this library with a *Bam*HI restriction fragment (known to contain the human V2R gene) to identify the gene	31, 32
Type 1 angiotensin II	1992	Functional-candidate gene	Used previously cloned rat and bovine AT1 cDNA sequences for homology screening of human total adrenal RNA to identify the AT II gene	33
Factor V Leiden (APC resistance)	1994	Gene association	Used probes from the region of previously cloned human Factor V that contained the APC cleavage site	34–37

Table 2.3 (*continued*)

Gene cloned	Year	Cloning method	Strategy to identify the human gene	References[b]
Sulfonylurea	1995	Functional-candidate gene	Used V8 protease peptides from the N-terminal sequence of the purified hamster sulfonylurea receptor to design primers to probe a random human cDNA library	38
CCR5	1996	Gene association	Used probes from a previously cloned human CCR5	39–42

[a]As defined in Collins[43] and Ballabio.[44]

[b]**References**

1. Rottmann WH, Tolan DR, Penhoet EE. Complete amino acid sequence for human aldolase B derived from cDNA and genomic clones. Proc Natl Acad Sci USA 1984; 81(9):2738–2742.
2. Hsu LC, Tani K, Fujiyoshi T, Kurachi K, Yoshida A. Cloning of cDNAs for human aldehyde dehydrogenases 1 and 2. Proc Natl Acad Sci USA 1985; 82(11):3771–3775.
3. Lockridge O, Bartels CF, Vaughan TA, Wong CK, Norton SE, Johnson LL. Complete amino acid sequence of human serum cholinesterase. J Biol Chem 1987; 262(2):549–557.
4. Gonzalez FJ, Skoda RC, Kimura S, Umeno M, Zanger UM, Nebert DW, et al. Characterization of the common genetic defect in humans deficient in debrisoquine metabolism. Nature 1988; 331(6155): 442–446.
5. Kimura S, Umeno M, Skoda RC, Meyer UA, Gonzalez FJ. The human debrisoquine 4-hydroxylase (CYP2D) locus: Sequence and identification of the polymorphic CYP2D6 gene, a related gene, and a pseudogene. Am J Hum Genet 1989; 45(6):889–904.
6. Seidegard J, Vorachek WR, Pero RW, Pearson WR. Hereditary differences in the expression of the human glutathione transferase active on trans-stilbene oxide are due to a gene deletion. Proc Natl Acad Sci USA 1988; 85(19):7293–7297.
7. Andres HH, Vogel RS, Tarr GE, Johnson L, Weber WW. Purification, physicochemical, and kinetic properties of liver acetyl-CoA:arylamine N-acetyltransferase from rapid acetylator rabbits. Mol Pharmacol 1987; 31(4):446–456.
8. Blum M, Grant DM, McBride W, Heim M, Meyer UA. Human arylamine N-acetyltransferase genes: Isolation, chromosomal localization, and functional expression. DNA Cell Biol 1990; 9(3):193–203.
9. Blum M, Demierre A, Grant DM, Heim M, Meyer UA. Molecular mechanism of slow acetylation of drugs and carcinogens in humans. Proc Natl Acad Sci USA 1991; 88(12):5237–5241.
10. Vatsis KP, Martell KJ, Weber WW. Diverse point mutations in the human gene for polymorphic N-acetyltransferase. Proc Natl Acad Sci USA 1991; 88(14):6333–6337.
11. Mornet E, Dupont J, Vitek A, White PC. Characterization of two genes encoding human steroid 11 beta-hydroxylase (P-450(11) beta). J Biol Chem 1989; 264(35):20961–20967.
12. Pascoe L, Curnow KM, Slutsker L, Connell JMC, Speiser PW, New MI, et al. Glucocorticoid-suppressible hyperaldosteronism results from hybrid genes created by unequal crossovers between CYP11B1 and CYP11B2. Proc Natl Acad Sci USA 1992; 89:8327–8331.
13. Lifton RP, Dluhy RG, Powers M, Rich GM, Cook S, Ulick S, et al. A chimaeric 11 beta-hydroxylase/aldosterone synthase gene causes glucocorticoid-remediable aldosteronism and human hypertension. Nature 1992; 355:262–265.
14. Lomri N, Gu Q, Cashman JR. Molecular cloning of the flavin-containing monooxygenase (form II) cDNA from adult human liver. Proc Natl Acad Sci USA 1992; 89(5):1685–1689.
15. Phillips IR, Dolphin CT, Clair P, Hadley MR, Hutt AJ, McCombie RR, et al. The molecular biology of the flavin-containing monooxygenases of man. Chem Biol Interact 1995; 96(1):17–32.

(*continued*)

Table 2.3 (continued)

16. Cotter PD, Baumann M, Bishop DF. Enzymatic defect in "X-linked" sideroblastic anemia: Molecular evidence for erythroid delta-aminolevulinate synthase deficiency. Proc Natl Acad Sci USA 1992; 89(9):4028–4032.
17. Shestopal SA, Johnson MR, Diasio RB. Molecular cloning and characterization of the human dihydropyrimidine dehydrogenase promoter. Biochim Biophys Acta 2000; 1494(1–2):162–169.
18. Nathans J, Hogness DS. Isolation and nucleotide sequence of the gene encoding human rhodopsin. Proc Natl Acad Sci USA 1984; 81(15):4851–4855.
19. Ullrich A, Bell JR, Chen EY, Herrera R, Petruzzelli LM, Dull TJ, et al. Human insulin receptor and its relationship to the tyrosine kinase family of oncogenes. Nature 1985; 313(6005):756–761.
20. Hollenberg SM, Weinberger C, Ong ES, Cerelli G, Oro A, Lebo R, et al. Primary structure and expression of a functional human glucocorticoid receptor cDNA. Nature 1985; 318(6047):635–641.
21. Green S, Walter P, Kumar V, Krust A, Bornert JM, Argos P, et al. Human oestrogen receptor cDNA: Sequence, expression and homology to v-erb-A. Nature 1986; 320(6058):134–139.
22. Kobilka BK, Dixon RA, Frielle T, Dohlman HG, Bolanowski MA, Sigal IS, et al. cDNA for the human beta 2-adrenergic receptor: A protein with multiple membrane-spanning domains and encoded by a gene whose chromosomal location is shared with that of the receptor for platelet-derived growth factor. Proc Natl Acad Sci USA 1987; 84(1):46–50.
23. Arriza JL, Weinberger C, Cerelli G, Glaser TM, Handelin BL, Housman DE, et al. Cloning of human mineralocorticoid receptor complementary DNA: Structural and functional kinship with the glucocorticoid receptor. Science 1987; 237(4812):268–275.
24. Petkovich M, Brand NJ, Krust A, Chambon P. A human retinoic acid receptor which belongs to the family of nuclear receptors. Nature 1987; 330(6147):444–450.
25. Baker AR, McDonnell DP, Hughes M, Crisp TM, Mangelsdorf DJ, Haussler MR, et al. Cloning and expression of full-length cDNA encoding human vitamin D receptor. Proc Natl Acad Sci USA 1988; 85(10):3294–3298.
26. Chang CS, Kokontis J, Liao ST. Structural analysis of complementary DNA and amino acid sequences of human and rat androgen receptors. Proc Natl Acad Sci USA 1988; 85(19):7211–7215.
27. Takeshima H, Nishimura S, Matsumoto T, Ishida H, Kangawa K, Minamino N, et al. Primary structure and expression from complementary DNA of skeletal muscle ryanodine receptor. Nature 1989; 339(6224):439–445.
28. Tamkun MM, Knoth KM, Walbridge JA, Kroemer H, Roden DM, Glover DM. Molecular cloning and characterization of two voltage-gated K+ channel cDNAs from human ventricle. FASEB J 1991; 5(3):331–337.
29. Keating M, Atkinson D, Dunn C, Timothy K, Vincent GM, Leppert M. Linkage of a cardiac arrhythmia, the long QT syndrome, and the Harvey ras-1 gene. Science 1991; 252(5006):704–706.
30. Keating M, Dunn C, Atkinson D, Timothy K, Vincent GM, Leppert M. Consistent linkage of the long-QT syndrome to the Harvey ras-1 locus on chromosome 11. Am J Hum Genet 1991; 49(6): 1335–1339.
31. Lolait SJ, O'Carroll A, McBride OW, Konig M, Morel A, Brownstein MJ. Cloning and characterization of a vasopressin V2 receptor and possible link to nephrogenic diabetes insipidus. Nature 1992; 357:336–339.
32. Birnbaumer M, Seibold A, Gilbert S, Ishido M, Barberis C, Antaramian A, et al. Molecular cloning of the receptor for human antidiuretic hormone. Nature 1992; 357(6376):333–335.
33. Curnow KM, Pascoe L, White PC. Genetic analysis of the human type-1 angiotensin II receptor. Mol Endocrinol 1992; 6(7):1113–1118.
34. Bertina RM, Koeleman BP, Koster T, Rosendaal FR, Dirven RJ, de Ronde H, et al. Mutation in blood coagulation factor V associated with resistance to activated protein C. Nature 1994; 369(6475): 64–67.
35. Voorberg J, Roelse J, Koopman R, Buller H, Berends F, ten Cate JW, et al. Association of idiopathic venous thromboembolism with single point-mutation at Arg506 of factor V. Lancet 1994; 343(8912): 1535–1536.
36. Zoller B, Dahlback B. Linkage between inherited resistance to activated protein C and factor V gene mutation in venous thrombosis. Lancet 1994; 343(8912):1536–1538.

Table 2.3 (*continued*)

37. Zoller B, Svensson PJ, He X, Dahlback B. Identification of the same factor V gene mutation in 47 out of 50 thrombosis-prone families with inherited resistance to activated protein C. J Clin Invest 1994; 94(6):2521–2524.
38. Glaser B, Chiu KC, Liu L, Anker R, Nestorowicz A, Cox NJ, et al. Recombinant mapping of the familial hyperinsulinism gene to an 0.8 cM region on chromosome 11p15.1 and demonstration of a founder effect in Ashkenazi Jews. Hum Mol Genet 1995; 4(5):879–886.
39. Samson M, Labbe O, Mollereau C, Vassart G, Parmentier M. Molecular cloning and functional expression of a new human CC-chemokine receptor gene. Biochemistry 1996; 35(11):3362–3367.
40. Liu R, Paxton WA, Choe S, Ceradini D, Martin SR, Horuk R, et al. Homozygous defect in HIV-1 coreceptor accounts for resistance of some multiply-exposed individuals to HIV-1 infection. Cell 1996; 86(3):367–377.
41. Samson M, Libert F, Doranz BJ, Rucker J, Liesnard C, Farber CM, et al. Resistance to HIV-1 infection in caucasian individuals bearing mutant alleles of the CCR-5 chemokine receptor gene. Nature 1996; 382(6593):722–725.
42. Dean M, Carrington M, Winkler C, Huttley GA, Smith MW, Allikmets R, et al. Genetic restriction of HIV-1 infection and progression to AIDS by a deletion allele of the CKR5 structural gene. Hemophilia Growth and Development Study, Multicenter AIDS Cohort Study, Multicenter Hemophilia Cohort Study, San Francisco City Cohort, ALIVE Study. Science 1996; 273(5283):1856–1862.
43. Collins FS. Positional cloning: Let's not call it reverse anymore. Nature Genet 1992; 1(Apr):3–6.
44. Ballabio A. The rise and fall of positional cloning. Nature Genet 1993; 3(Apr):277–279.

for gene identification by "candidate gene association" studies would determine the frequency of SNP markers in populations of affected individuals versus those in unaffected individuals. Comparing the frequencies of markers in these two populations should reveal the identity of each genetic determinant as schematized in the lower panel of Figure 2.5.

So far, gene association studies have not yielded many clinical successes. In their comprehensive review, Hirschhorn and colleagues find over 600 reports of positive associations between common gene variants and diseases including disorders of pharmacogenetic interest, but of the 166 putative associations that had been studied three or more times, they identify only six that had been consistently replicated.[27] They concluded that most reported associations are not robust. However, among those with consistently high reproducibility (>75% positive results) were two of pharmacogenetic relevance as noted in the tabular summary (Table 2.3): the polymorphism in factor V (Leiden) that is associated with a predisposition to deep vein thrombosis (also known as APC resistance) and the Δ32 base pair deletion polymorphism in the CCR5 receptor that affords protection from, and slows the progression, of HIV-1 infection (AIDS) in adults.

LINKING PHARMACOGENETICS TO CLINICAL APPLICATIONS

Pharmacogenetics in Drug Interactions

When two or more drugs are given that are metabolized by the same enzyme they will compete with each other for that enzyme. If the enzyme is present in sufficient amount or high enough activity, no additional problems from the drug

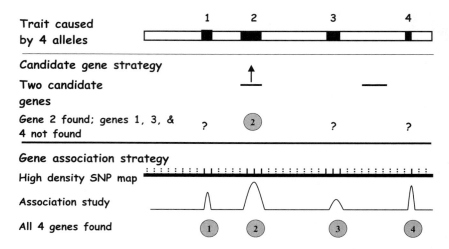

Figure 2.5 Gene identification strategies 2: candidate gene strategy (*upper panel*); candidate gene association study (*lower panel*).

combination should occur. However, if the amount or activity of the enzyme is decreased, such as by genetic variation, the drug concentration may well reach a toxic level. Knowing the route of drug metabolism and any relevant phenotype of the drug-metabolizing enzymes can help prevent this type of drug interaction.

A drug that is not a substrate for a particular drug-metabolizing enzyme may still be an inhibitor of that enzyme; the inhibition of CYP2D6 by quinidine is such an example. Individuals with normal activity for metabolism and elimination of a drug may behave as though they were defective metabolizers in the presence of an inhibitor. In this way, a mimic of a genetic trait, called a "phenocopy," may be produced. Genetically poor metabolizers would show even less metabolism under this circumstance.

Note: The term "drug" as used here is defined in the broadest possible sense to include prescriptions and over-the-counter medications as well as foods and "alternative medicines." Many of the herbal supplements that are marketed over-the-counter contain substrates, inhibitors, or inducers of drug-metabolizing enzymes.

Pharmacogenetics as Risk Factors for Cancer and Other Diseases

Many pharmacogenetic polymorphisms are being studied as possible risk factors for cancer. Most environmental chemical carcinogens require metabolic activation before they can damage DNA and cause somatic mutations that lead to initiation of cancer. Since many of the enzymes known to be involved in the activation and detoxification of carcinogens are polymorphic, it is reasonable to expect an association of the activity of these enzymes with risk of cancer. Drug-metabolizing enzymes that may be related to altered susceptibility to chemical carcinogenesis include P450s, epoxide hydrolases, glutathione-S-transferases, and N-acetyltransferases among others.[28,29]

Some polymorphisms of drug-metabolizing enzymes, ion channels, and other proteins have been identified as causative (or preventive) factors of certain diseases. These are traits that when present together with the appropriate environmental element alter the normal pharmacokinetics or pharmacodynamics in such a manner that the pathological condition will occur. Examples include G6PD deficiency, α_1-antitrypsin deficiency, fructose intolerance, long QT syndrome, and Gilbert's syndrome. The CCR5Δ32 polymorphism is an example of a polymorphism that can prevent or slow the progression of AIDS in adults infected with HIV-1.

Options for Treating Pharmacogenetic Disorders

The care of patients with genetic disorders involves approaches to diagnosis and treatment that are commonly used in medical practice, but the focus in medical genetics is more on prevention or avoidance of the disorder. Presymptomatic (including prenatal) diagnosis, genetic screening programs, and genetic counseling are concepts central to this approach.

Options for the treatment of genetic disorders at the environmental level routinely involve a combination of restriction, replacement, and removal of the toxic agents. Restriction of potentially toxic environmental substances could, for example, involve restriction of certain foods or other dietary constituents. Fructose is one of the major components of human diets, and fructose intolerance is represented by a polymorphism in the gene for aldolase B. The wide distribution of fructose and its congeners places genetically susceptible persons at constant risk from a serious but avoidable nutritional disorder. Fish malodor syndrome (trimethylaminuria), a trait that confers the smell of rotting fish on affected persons, with devastating educational, economic, and social consequences, is another example of a variation in the human response to foods. A polymorphism in the gene for flavin monooxygenase 3 (FM03) that results in impaired FM03 activity accounts for some cases of this disorder. Management of trimethylaminuria remains empirical, but the main recourse for affected persons is dietary restriction to reduce trimethylamine precursors. This may require avoidance of foods rich in choline, such as eggs, liver, soya beans, and marine fish.

Restriction of certain therapeutic agents is an option that is usually applied by physicians to avoid adverse drug reactions in genetically susceptible persons. Individuals with a deficiency in G6PD avoid oxidant stresses such as those that accompany ingestion of antimalarials, sulfonamides, and an extensive list of other drugs; exposure to these drugs can result in drug-induced hemolysis of red blood cells. Individuals with TPMT deficiency must be treated with much smaller (up to 15-fold) doses of 6-mercaptopurine, 6-thioguanine, and 8-azathioprine, to avoid bone marrow suppression by those agents. Persons with TPMT deficiency are intolerant of those agents and may suffer delayed responses that can be life threatening.

Toxicity can result from exposure to cigarette smoke in persons afflicted with α_1-antitrypsin deficiency. The destructive effects on lungs that result in premature emphysema and chronic obstructive pulmonary disease can be prevented or slowed if they avoid cigarette smoking.

The option to remove iron from the environment of persons is taken in hemochromatosis, a disorder of iron metabolism that affects one in 300 people of northern European descent. Most cases of hereditary hemochromatosis are due to a polymorphism of the HFE gene that results in substitution of tyrosine for cysteine at codon 282. Untreated, the disorder leads to early death from liver cirrhosis, heart failure, or diabetes; phlebotomy to remove excess iron allows affected persons to live a normal life span.

SUMMARY

Pharmacogenetics has taught us that single gene polymorphisms are excellent prognosticators of unwanted responses to xenobiotics, but as we learn more about these patterns of response, few, if any, phenotypic outcomes appear to be reliably predicted from analyses at a single gene locus. Only when the capacity for genotyping/phenotyping, as well as bioinformatics methods to analyze large data sets, is fully developed, and the rich legacy of pharmacogenetics provides a starting point from which to develop profiles more suitable for medical practice, will the full potential of pharmacogenetics be realized. The participation and cataloging of the effects of variant proteins in pathways and networks that determine individual responsiveness to drugs and other exogenous substances are the next great challenges for pharmacogenetics.

With completion of the human genome initiative and the continuing development of tools to explore the human genome and those of other organisms,

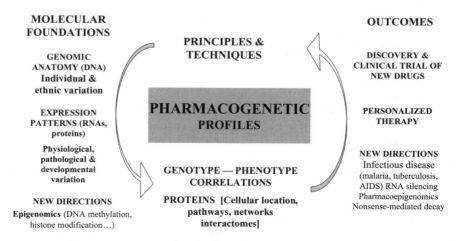

Figure 2.6 From molecular foundations to clinical outcomes.

pharmacogenetics is experiencing a period of rapid growth and redefinition. We often hear pharmacogenetics and pharmacogenomics used interchangeably, but whichever term is used, the main question before us is how best to accommodate the major shift in the scale of operations entailed in going from genetics to genomics.

Physicians have learned to cope with adverse reactions to drugs and other substances by replacing the offending substance or removing it from the patients' environment. If treatment were to be guided by "pharmacogenetic profiles" individualized for susceptibility to these agents, therapeutic failure and drug toxicity would be greatly reduced or avoided in genetically susceptible persons. These profiles would serve as stepping-stones from the molecular foundations to the long-term objectives of pharmacogenetics (Figure 2.6).

REFERENCES

1. Garrod AE. Medicine from the chemical standpoint. Lancet 1914; ii:281–289.
2. Evans WE, Relling MV. Pharmacogenomics: Translating functional genomics into rational therapeutics. Science 1999; 286(5439):487–491.
3. Murphy PJ. Xenobiotic metabolism: A look from the past to the future. Drug Metabol Dispos 2001; 29(6):779–780.
4. Omura T, Sato R. A new cytochrome in liver microsomes. J Biol Chem 1962; 237:1375–1376.
5. Omura T, Sato R, Cooper DY, Rosenthal O, Estabrook RW. Function of cytochrome P-450 of microsomes. Fed Proc 1965; 24(5):1181–1189.
6. Williams RT. The biogenesis of conjugation and detoxication products. Biogenesis Natural Compounds 1963; 1–48.
7. Nelson DR, Zeldin DC, Hoffman SM, Maltais LJ, Wain HM, Nebert DW. Comparison of cytochrome P450 (CYP) genes from the mouse and human genomes, including nomenclature recommendations for genes, pseudogenes and alternative-splice variants. Pharmacogenetics 2004; 14(1):1–18.
8. Guengerich FP. Human cytochrome P450 enzymes. In: Ortiz de Montellano PR, editor. Cytochrome P450. Structure, Mechanism, and Biochemistry. New York: Kluwer Academic/Plenum, 2005: 377.
9. Marzolini C, Tirona RG, Kim RB. Pharmacogenetics of drug transporters. In: Kalow W, Meyer UA, Tyndale RF, editors. Pharmacogenomics. Boca Raton: Taylor & Francis, 2005: 109–155.
10. Kimchi-Sarfaty C, Oh JM, Kim IW, Sauna ZE, Calcagno AM, Ambudkar SV, et al. A "silent" polymorphism in the MDR1 gene changes substrate specificity. Science 2007; 315(5811):525–528.
11. Komar AA. Genetics. SNPs, silent but not invisible. Science 2007; 315(5811): 466–467.
12. Arriza JL, Weinberger C, Cerelli G, Glaser TM, Handelin BL, Housman DE, et al. Cloning of human mineralocorticoid receptor complementary DNA: Structural and functional kinship with the glucocorticoid receptor. Science 1987; 237(4812):268–275.
13. Morrison N, Harrap SB, Arriza JL, Boyd E, Connor JM. Regional chromosomal assignment of the human mineralocorticoid receptor gene to 4q31.1. Hum Genet 1990; 85(1):130–132.

14. Fan YS, Eddy RL, Byers MG, Haley LL, Henry WM, Nowak NJ, et al. The human mineralocorticoid receptor gene (MLR) is located on chromosome 4 at q31.2. Cytogenet Cell Genet 1989; 52(1–2):83–84.

15. Zennaro MC, Keightley MC, Kotelevtsev Y, Conway GS, Soubrier F, Fuller PJ. Human mineralocorticoid receptor genomic structure and identification of expressed isoforms. J Biol Chem 1995; 270(36):21016–21020.

16. Geller DS, Farhi A, Pinkerton N, Fradley M, Moritz M, Spitzer A, et al. Activating mineralocorticoid receptor mutation in hypertension exacerbated by pregnancy. Science 2000; 289(5476):119–123.

17. Geller DS, Rodriguez-Soriano J, Vallo BA, Schifter S, Bayer M, Chang SS, et al. Mutations in the mineralocorticoid receptor gene cause autosomal dominant pseudohypoaldosteronism type I. Nat Genet 1998; 19(3):279–281.

18. Lifton RP, Gharavi AG, Geller DS. Molecular mechanisms of human hypertension. Cell 2001; 104(4):545–556.

19. Collins FS. Positional cloning: Let's not call it reverse anymore. Nature Genet 1992; 1(Apr):3–6.

20. Ballabio A. The rise and fall of positional cloning. Nature Genet 1993; 3(Apr):277–279.

21. Bender W, Akam M, Karch F, Beachy PA, Peifer M, Speirer P, et al. Molecular genetics of the Bithorax complex in Drosophila melanogaster. Science 1983; 221 (1 Jul):23–29.

22. Riordan JR, Rommens JM, Kerem B, Alon N, Rozmahel R, Grzelczak Z, et al. Identification of the cystic fibrosis gene: Cloning and characterization of complementary DNA. Science 1989; 245(4922):1066–1073.

23. Rommens JM, Iannuzzi MC, Kerem B, Drumm ML, Melmer G, Dean M, et al. Identification of the cystic fibrosis gene: Chromosome walking and jumping. Science 1989; 245(4922):1059–1065.

24. Kerem B, Rommens JM, Buchanan JA, Markiewicz D, Cox TK, Chakravarti A, et al. Identification of the cystic fibrosis gene: Genetic analysis. Science 1989; 245(4922): 1073–1080.

25. Axelrod J. The enzymatic deamination of amphetamine (benzedrine). J Biol Chem 1955; 214(2):753–763.

26. Collins FS, Guyer MS, Chakravarti A. Variations on a theme: Cataloging human DNA sequence variation. Science 1997; 278:1580–1581.

27. Hirschhorn JN, Lohmueller K, Byrne E, Hirschhorn K. A comprehensive review of genetic association studies. Genet Med 2002; 4(2):45–61.

II

FUNDAMENTALS

3

Pharmacology of Human
Drug Response

Drugs and other exogenous substances may be viewed as agents that exert characteristic effects on cells and tissues, but they may also be regarded as agents on which individuals exert important differential effects. To develop explanatory and predictive insights relevant to pharmacogenetics, pharmacologists are more likely to view the effects of a specific drug from the former perspective, while geneticists are more likely to see them from the latter.

PHARMACOLOGY AND GENETICS OF HUMAN
DRUG RESPONSE ARE COMPLEMENTARY

From a pharmacological viewpoint, individual responsiveness depends on the intrinsic properties of the drug at hand and can be analyzed from observations of its pharmacokinetic and the pharmacodynamic properties. Often the plasma drug concentration or pattern of drug metabolites correlates with an unusual therapeutic effect or an adverse drug reaction, and observations of parameters such as peak and steady-state levels of the drug in plasma, half-lives of drugs in plasma, the ratio of parent drug to metabolite, or the urinary pattern of drug metabolites are successfully employed to study the dose–response and dynamics of the response. Other indices may be examined, depending on the intrinsic properties of the drug, such as red blood cell counts, white blood cell counts, hormone levels, blood pressure, enzyme inhibition, clotting factor activity, intraocular pressure, respiratory air flow, and so on. Using observations such as these, the pharmacologist would determine whether an unusual drug response was a consequence of a defect in the absorption, distribution, or elimination of the drug, or of a receptor or another protein targeted by the drug.

Geneticists, on the other hand, are attuned to look for differences that discriminate one person from another, and would regard person-to-person differences in drug response as a sign of a possible inborn difference between the responders. In many populations, phenotypic criteria enable individuals to be classified into two, or more, types of responders. The geneticist would draw on information about the affected person and about the biological relatives of the affected person to explain the differential response. The relative roles of heredity and environment would be gauged from studies in identical and fraternal twins; from family studies it would be determined whether the response was monogenic or polygenic and what the mode of transmission of the trait from parents to offspring is. Comparative studies in different populations would turn up differences in response due to new mutations and differences in etiology and prevalence of ethnic and geographic origin. Studies of biologically unrelated persons would provide the raw material from which differences in the frequency of phenotypes and genotypes of individuals and populations could be determined.

Consider first the framework for dissecting the basis of variations in drug response from a pharmacological perspective. The framework for identifying the sources of genetic variation will be considered later.

DOSE–RESPONSE RELATIONSHIPS

The relationship between the dose of a drug administered and the response evoked is a pillar of pharmacology that is central to quantitative analysis of intersubject variability in human drug responses. Traditionally, two models have been used in pharmacogenetics to describe the dose–response relationship. One model involves the measurement of the *frequency* of the response relative to the drug concentrations (or doses) to produce a quantal dose–response relationship. Applications of this model are represented by the frequency distributions in Figure 2.1. The second model involves the measurement of the *intensity* of a specified response relative to the concentration (or dose) of the drug to produce a graded dose–response relationship as shown in Figure 3.1. This model assumes there is no safe level of exposure and is represented by a linear (or no-threshold) relation between dose and response. A third model, the *hormetic dose–response* relationship, challenges these traditional models. Hormetic dose–responses are biphasic, displaying either a U-shape, or inverted U-shape, depending on the endpoint measured (Figure 3.2).

Strictly speaking, the concentrations used in any of these models should be those present at receptor sites, but because they are technically so difficult to measure, the concentration of the drug in blood (or plasma or serum), or the drug dosage (amount administered), is usually substituted for them in these relationships, as explained later (see p. 58). Quantal and graded relationships are used to search for different pharmacogenetic phenotypes that may be present within drug responder populations, but they are applied in different ways.

Quantal Dose-Response Relationships

The need for quantal measurements is particularly acute in pharmacogenetics because the effects of Mendelian characters are "all-or-none" phenomena. Such responses cannot be graduated because the determinant allele is either present or

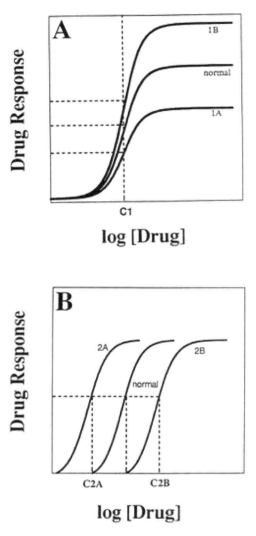

Figure 3.1 Theoretical graded dose–response curves for different types of pharmacogenetic variation. The normal dose–response curve is labeled in each panel. (*A*) In one type of variation, the maximal response is deficient (1A) or supranormal (1B) at all concentrations of the drug, but the concentration required for half-maximal response is normal. (*B*) In the other type of variation, the maximal response is normal at elevated (C2B), or decreased (C2A), drug concentrations.

not. Likewise, for a monogenic drug-induced disorder, the response specified is observed as "occurring" or "not occurring," or as "present" or "not present."

The presence of distinct subgroups of drug responders within populations is evidence for a difference that may be a consequence of true genetic differences (metabolic phenotypes, receptor phenotypes, gender differences, etc.) or of

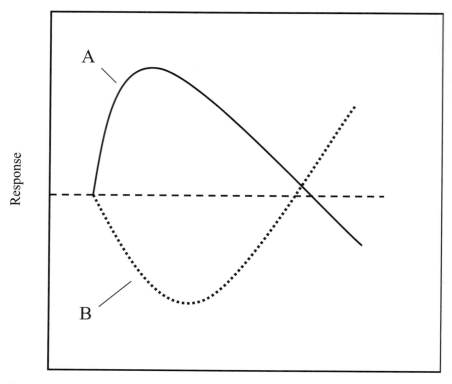

Figure 3.2 Hormetic dose–response curves. (*A*) A low-dose stimulatory and high-dose inhibitory response. (*B*) A low-dose inhibitory and high-dose stimulatory response. (*A*) Endpoints include growth, fecundity, and longevity, and (*B*) endpoints include carcinogenesis, mutagenesis, and disease incidence. (*Source:* Drawn from Calabrese.[5])

environmental effects (ill vs. healthy persons, smokers vs. nonsmokers, particular occupational groups vs. the general population, etc.). Frequency distributions for such populations may be unimodal or multimodal. Multimodal distributions may be more readily interpreted because each mode may correspond to a particular phenotype or genotype, and different modes may represent susceptible and non-susceptible subpopulations that are separable. Several examples of genetically heterogeneous populations in which individuals have been classified according to pharmacological criteria into two or more distinct phenotypes of responders are represented by the frequency distributions shown in Figure 2.1.

Unimodal frequency distributions, in contrast to multimodal distributions, may be difficult to interpret because genetic heterogeneity may be hidden within them. Such a distribution is more likely to occur when the measurement of the variability in response is quantitative rather than qualitative. Quantitative

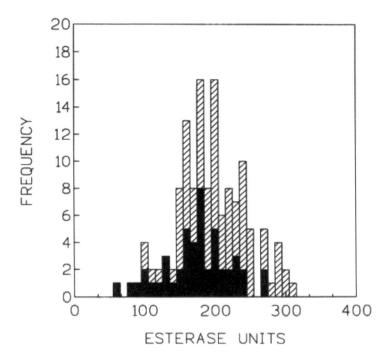

Figure 3.3 Frequency distributions for serum cholinesterase activity levels among 135 members of seven families. The black bars indicate esterase levels of sera with dibucaine numbers below 70.[1] With permission from the NRC Research Press.

responses of several genetic phenotypes may overlap, and the overlap may be increased by environmental factors that contribute to the variability within a phenotype. Consequently, genetically heterogeneous populations may appear to be distributed normally, or near normally, with large variability about the average. The distribution of serum cholinesterase activities of individuals provides an example of a unimodal distribution of a quantitative variable that contains hidden genetic modes (Figure 3.3).[1] In this case, even though the average of the serum cholinesterase activities of succinylcholine-sensitive persons (dibucaine numbers below 70) is shifted to a lower value, the shift is not great enough to separate normal from abnormal responders. This distribution of enzyme activities is to be contrasted with the distribution of dibucaine numbers that divides the same individuals into three distinct modes (see Figure 2.1A). The dibucaine number, which denotes the sensitivity of serum cholinesterase to dibucaine inhibition, measures a qualitative difference between usual and atypical cholinesterase variants. The modes with average dibucaine numbers of approximately 16, 60, and 80 correspond to succinylcholine-sensitive responders, heterozygous carriers of this trait, and homozygous normal responders to succinylcholine, respectively.

Graded Dose–Response Relationships

The graded response relationship affords an experimental approach that may shed light on the pharmacodynamic mechanism responsible for a modified drug response. Graded measurements are often preferred to quantal measurements for this reason. When a direct relationship exists between the receptor binding of the xenobiotic and the response, changes in the dose–response relationship for the drug would be expected if either the abundance (i.e., the number of receptor sites) or the affinity of the receptor sites is altered (Figure 3.1); the abundance and affinity of receptor proteins are, like half-lives and K_ms, individual characteristics that may exhibit considerable person-to-person variation. If the abundance of receptors is decreased, elementary receptor theory predicts that the maximum response that could be attained would be decreased, while the concentration of the drug at which a half-maximal response is attained would be unchanged; conversely, if the abundance increased, the maximal response would theoretically increase without a change in the drug concentration at the half-maximal response. On the other hand, if the affinity of the receptor for the xenobiotic is increased, the maximal response would theoretically not increase, but the concentration of the drug needed to attain that response would decrease, and vice versa.

The application of these concepts to a real situation is illustrated in the analysis of the pharmacological mechanism for hereditary resistance to coumarin anticoagulant drugs such as warfarin. In this case, the absorption, distribution, and elimination of the drug as well as other pharmacokinetic mechanisms were not found to be aberrant in warfarin-resistant individuals. A comparison of the dose–response relations of the normal responder to that of the resistant responder showed that the slopes of the dose–response lines are nearly identical, but the line for the resistant subject is shifted to the right. This observation indicates that the resistant responder requires a larger amount of the drug than the normal responder to achieve a given anticoagulant response (Figure 3.4). The study revealed the affinity of the receptor for warfarin in resistant subjects is much lower, some 20 times lower than that in normal responders. This trait was described by O'Reilly and colleagues in the 1960s prior to the advent of recombinant DNA technology, and the molecular basis of a putative receptor was not defined.[2]

Hormetic Dose-Response Relationships

Hormesis refers to a biphasic dose–response phenomenon characterized by low-dose stimulation and high-dose inhibition, resulting in a U- or inverted U-shaped dose–response (Figure 3.2). The term hormesis associated with this relationship was coined in 1943 by investigators who were apparently unaware that biphasic dose–response relationships had been characterized well over a century earlier. Historically, researchers, including pharmacogenetic researchers, have placed a strong emphasis on high-dose evaluation, as these doses are more definitive for establishing and reporting the drug level of NOAEL (no observed adverse effect level). Additionally there is the long-standing belief that responses below the NOAEL are, because of their modest nature, not reproducible effects but are most

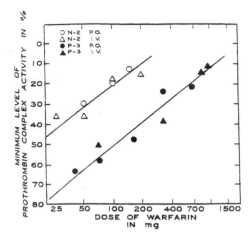

Figure 3.4 Human dose–response relationships for resistant (solid symbols) and nonresistant (open symbols) responders to warfarin.[2]

likely due to normal variation. For this reason, only a small fraction of studies has the appropriate dosage design necessary to assess this controversial hypothesis.[3–5]

Some of the concerns and limitations of this concept are addressed by Calabrese and Baldwin who find in assessing the frequency of U-shaped dose–responses in the toxicological literature that hormetic responses are commonly encountered if the study design is appropriate.[6] Features that are important and necessary to more properly determine the dose–response in the low-dose zone include multiple and carefully spaced doses below the NOAEL, and possibly a temporal component within the study design if the hormetic mechanism represents an overcompensation response. For assessments of endpoints such as mutagenicity, carcinogenicity, and teratogenicity within a hormetic framework, models with zero or negligible background/control incidence cannot be used.

Most of the prior investigations have focused on toxicologically derived data. Even so, sufficient data exist to suggest that biphasic dose–response relationships are quite common in toxicology and pharmacology, and for a large number of endpoints, including cancer risks, longevity, growth, and more, are common across the spectrum of biological, pharmacological, and biomedical disciplines.[7] It seems reasonable to suggest that future modeling of biological responses, including pharmacogenetic study designs, should consider incorporating features for detecting hormetic dose–responses.

Analyzing Dose-Response Relationships

Plots of quantal or graded data, i.e., a plot of frequencies, or intensities, of responses (y-axis) vs. log concentration or dose (x-axis) for normally distributed data, resemble the bell-shaped (Gaussian) curve. These data can also be graphed as cumulative plots because a high dose of drug affects less responsive individuals (or cells) as well as more susceptible individuals for whom a lower dose would have been sufficient. Cumulative plots are sigmoidal for normally distributed measurements.[8-10]

The probit (probability) plot provides a simpler approach to the graphic analysis of dose–response data. Table 3.1 shows that probit values correspond to "normal equivalent deviate" (NED) values plus 5, and the relation of percent response, NED, and probit values. Probits were originally introduced to simplify numerical calculation by eliminating negative numbers for NED values.

Certain advantages accrue to probit plots in pharmacogenetics. First, for a set of normally distributed data that has been transformed to probits, a graph of probits vs. dose (log dose) is linear; second, the greater the variability (standard deviation), the lesser the slope of the probit plot; and third, the occurrence of nonlinearity in probit plots indicates there is heterogeneity in the population sample of responders tested.

Although probit plots may clearly reveal heterogeneity among responders, they may be inefficient for this purpose, particularly if the fraction of unusual responders is small, say a few percent or less, of the total sample tested. This point is evident from the distribution of thiopurine methyltransferase activity in human red blood cells (see Figure 2.1C). The red cells with very low or undetectable activity comprise only about 1 in 300 individuals, or about 0.3% of the population; the nonlinearity would hardly be evident in a probit plot. The differential plot shown in Figure 2.1C is better to demonstrate such a small fraction of unusual responders.

PHARMACOKINETICS IN PHARMACOGENETICS

A fundamental premise of pharmacology holds that a drug must be present at receptor sites to produce its responses. For a drug that binds reversibly to its receptor, the magnitude and characteristics of its responses are directly dependent on the concentration of complexes between the drug and the receptor, and the concentration of these complexes, in turn, depends on the concentration of the

Table 3.1 The Relation of Percent Response, Normal Equivalent Deviate, and the Probits for Normally Distributed Data

Percent response	Normal equivalent deviate	Probit
0.1	−3	2
2.3	−2	3
15.9	−1	4
50.0	0	5
84.1	+1	6
97.7	+2	7
99.9	+3	8

drug at the receptor sites. Technically, it is quite difficult to obtain a reliable measure of the concentration of drug–receptor complexes or of the free drug at those sites, but the formation and breakdown of those complexes are rapid and obey the law of mass action for drugs that bind reversibly. Hence, changes in the tissue concentration of the drug–receptor complexes would be expected to parallel changes in the concentration of free drugs in the tissue water bathing them, and because the tissue water and plasma water are in rapid equilibrium, changes in the complex concentration, and hence in response, would parallel changes in the drug concentration in plasma.

To elucidate relationships between the levels of a given drug and its characteristic effects, measurements of the drug are made of peak (or trough) levels of the drug in the plasma of individuals, of changes in the plasma levels of the drug with time expressed as the elimination half-life ($t_{1/2}$), and of plasma levels that have reached a steady state (c_{ss}). Since most drugs are eliminated by the kidneys, valuable information on the pharmacokinetics is provided by rates of urinary drug elimination and by the patterns of urinary drug metabolites.

The concentration of a drug in plasma at a steady state (c_{ss}) is directly related to the dose of the drug, the half-life ($t_{1/2}$), the dosing interval (τ), and the distribution volume (V_d) by Equation 3.1. This equation is valid for drugs that are eliminated by first-order kinetic processes and it can be derived from first principles of pharmacokinetics.*

$$c_{ss} = (1.44\,F\,[\text{Dose}]\,[t_{1/2}])/\tau V_d \qquad (3.1)$$

Thus for a given drug, the c_{ss} would be expected to change directly with the dose, the bioavailability (F), and the half-life ($t_{1/2}$), and indirectly with the dosing interval (τ) and apparent distribution volume (V_d). For a given dose and dosing interval, c_{ss} depends on three parameters that are determined experimentally in individual subjects—the bioavailability, the plasma half-life, and the apparent distribution volume of the drug. The values obtained for c_{ss} should reflect the interindividual variability for each of these parameters, but among these, the plasma half-life exhibits the greatest interindividual variability (see p. 62).

---

*The rate of change of a drug in the body = {rate of drug absorption} – {rate of drug elimination}. When the "rate in" equals the "rate out," the drug concentration approaches a plateau. This elementary principle of pharmacology is usually referred to as the *plateau principle*.

Under steady-state conditions c_{ss} = {rate of drug in}/{rate of drug out}. The numerator equals the dose divided by the dosing interval, $\tau(\text{dose}/\tau)$ multiplied by the bioavailability, which is the fractional rate of absorption, F, gives {F×Dose}/τ. The denominator is the drug clearance, which equals the volume of blood cleared of drug per unit time, usually expressed as liters/hour. But the clearance can be substituted by its dimensional equivalent, V_d (liters) $\times k$ (hour^{-1}), where V_d is the distribution volume and k is the first order elimination rate constant. The k, in turn, is substituted by ln $2/t_{1/2}$, from which the expression for drug clearance becomes {0.693 V_d}/ $t_{1/2}$, where 0.693 is the numerical value for ln 2. Substituting the expressions for the numerator and denominator of the ratio for c_{ss} and rearranging terms yields the final expression for c_{ss} (Equation 3.1).

Equation 3.1 applies only to drugs that are eliminated by first-order processes, but this is a technical point that does not invalidate the well-defined relationship between the rate of drug elimination and the plasma drug concentration. The elimination of many drugs exhibits saturation kinetic behavior (also called Michaelis–Menten kinetics) in human subjects, and the equation for c_{ss} that applies under those circumstances is

$$c_{ss} = (R_O K_m)/(V_{max} - R_O) \qquad (3.2)$$

in which R_O (milligrams/day) represents the rate of drug administration and the K_m (milligrams/liter) represents the steady-state plasma drug concentration at which the rate of drug elimination is one-half the maximum rate, V_{max}. For drugs that exhibit such kinetics, a relatively small increase in the plasma drug dose may be accompanied by a disproportionately large increase in c_{ss}. Consequently, a small change in dose at or near saturation could increase the c_{ss} from the therapeutic range to the toxic range. Since the K_m is a characteristic of the individual that varies remarkably in different subjects, the value of c_{ss} will vary accordingly. The antiepileptic drug phenytoin, for instance, displays saturation kinetics and its K_m in humans may vary at least 16-fold (1.5–25.2 mg/liter) between individuals.[11] Equation 3.2 has been used primarily as a tool for optimizing drug dosage regimens, but it can also be used to assess pharmacogenetic phenotypic individuality.

The majority of xenobiotics act reversibly at receptor sites, but some xenobiotics act nonreversibly. They attach covalently, or bind noncovalently tightly, to receptors or other macromolecules and remain fixed to those sites even after the drug is undetectable in plasma. The biological effects of these substances persist for prolonged periods and recovery depends on regeneration or repair of receptor sites. Since the effects of nonreversible xenobiotics may be cumulative in the absence of the xenobiotic, plasma levels do not serve as a guide to the responses.

Existing Pools of Pharmacokinetic Data

Extensive tabulations of human pharmacokinetic data are available that contain quantitative information about the bioavailability, binding, distribution, and clearance, renal and metabolic, for therapeutic agents, and clinical pharmacological data on the absorption, distribution, and elimination of these agents. These resources contain a vast amount of drug data, especially for preliminary design of dosage regimens, but they may not represent patients whose pharmacokinetics are different from the average. The values tabulated have usually been measured on healthy adults, or on patients with specified diseases, but they have not usually been obtained with a view toward specifying particular phenotypic differences in genetically or ethnogeographically distinct subjects. Occasionally, the effect of a particular metabolic phenotype on the disposition of a drug may be specified as it is for isoniazid in Table 3.2. The alternative is to consult recent reviews, primary

Table 3.2 Variation in Plasma Elimination Half-Life Values for Several Agents Widely Used in Medical Therapy

Drug	Half-life Variation	Fold variation
Antipyrine	5–15 hours	3
Carbamazepine	18–55 hours	3
Dicumarol	7–74 hours	10
Indomethacin	9–53 hours	6
Isoniazid[a]	0.5–7.5 hours	>10
Rapid acetylators	0.5–1.8 hours	>3
Slow acetylators	1.8–7.5 hours	>4
6-Mercaptopurine	< 0.5–>1.6 hours	>3
Nortriptyline	15–90 hours	6
Phenylbutazone	1.2–7.3 days	6
Phenytoin	10–42 hours	4
Primidone	3.3–12.5 days	4
Tolbutamide	4–10 hours	2.5
Warfarin	15–70 hours	>4

[a]Data for rapid and slow acetylators are summarized from Table 4.4, Weber.[12]

research papers, and proceedings of conferences for this information, but even those sources may be insufficient for pharmacogenetic analysis.

Intersubject variability in the pharmacokinetics of a given drug is revealed by drug half-lives of several drugs in Table 3.2; 4- to 6-fold individual variability is common for many drugs widely used in medical therapy. Other pharmacokinetic parameters including those mentioned above also exhibit interindividual variability of a similar magnitude.

A pharmacokinetic variability of this magnitude is of clinical significance. For example, in a clinical trial involving Indian tuberculosis patients who had been treated with isoniazid for 1 year, genetically rapid acetylators responded much less satisfactorily than slow acetylators (60% of rapids vs. 82% of slows) by remaining bacteriologically positive longer, and relapsing more frequently because the rate of isoniazid inactivation by acetylation became important to its effectiveness. An impaired therapeutic effectiveness of the vasodilator drug hydralazine, observed in rapid acetylators, was found to be due to the same mechanism as for isoniazid, i.e., lower systemic bioavailability resulting from greater first pass metabolism by phenotypically rapid acetylators compared to slow acetylators; doses of hydralazine for rapid acetylators were up to 15 times larger than those required to achieve comparable effects in slow acetylators.[12] Additional examples of pharmacokinetic variations that result in severe toxicity include the dramatic fall in blood pressure described for the poor debrisoquine metabolizer and the bone marrow suppression that occurs in slow methylators of thiopurines in leukemic children treated with 6-mercaptopurine.

PHARMACOGENETIC MECHANISMS OF HUMAN DRUG RESPONSE

Mechanistic variations in response to drugs and other exogenous chemicals are grouped in Table 3.3 according to pharmacokinetic and pharmacodynamic criteria.

Mechanisms of variation of genetically altered human drug responses include the following: (1) Modification of the absorption of the xenobiotic as could result from increased "first pass metabolism" by a rapid metabolizer enzyme, from decreased abundance of a transporter protein, or from enhanced excretion by the multidrug resistance receptor protein. Pharmacokinetic as well as pharmacodynamic mechanisms are represented by these examples. (2) Modification of the metabolism that results in modification of the rate or the pattern of elimination, detoxification, or activation of a given xenobiotic. If the main metabolic pathway leading to a harmless metabolite is blocked, the parent drug could accumulate and cause toxicity, or if the metabolism is shunted from the harmless to a toxic pathway, metabolites could cause toxic manifestations. An example of the first possibility is represented by the dramatic fall in blood pressure experienced by the poor metabolizer of debrisoquine after a single dose of that drug, while the latter is exemplified by acetophenetidin-induced methemoglobinemia. (3) Modification of the abundance, affinity, or function of a target enzyme or receptor. Enzymatic mechanisms that exemplify these possibilities include the "silent" variants of serum cholinesterase associated with succinylcholine sensitivity and the poor metabolizer variants associated with polymorphisms of CYP2C9, CYP2C19, and CYP2D6 enzymes; those that exemplify receptor-related mechanisms include several hormone-resistant states such as insulin-resistant diabetes mellitus, vasopressin-resistant diabetes insipidus, and resistance to glucocorticoids, estrogens, and androgens.

Several entries listed in Table 3.3 will be recognized as relevant to pharmacogenetics: they include (1) modification in the repair capacity of a drug-induced effect, (2) modification of an immune responsive protein, and (3) modification of interactions between a given xenobiotic and inhibitors or antagonists, competitive substrates, and diastereoisomers. Among the various mechanisms listed, those that involve a competition between xenobiotics for a common enzyme or receptor or an interaction between the xenobiotic and a specific protein (enzyme, receptor, immune response, etc.) targeted by the xenobiotic are of primary interest in pharmacogenetics.

TESTING PHARMACOGENETIC HYPOTHESES

No hard and fast rules can be quoted to guide the investigator who wishes to explore human drug responsiveness for altered pharmacogenetic mechanisms. There are, however, some general principles that are widely applicable as E. Bright Wilson explains in his book *An Introduction to Scientific Research* (1952). First, an experiment is almost inevitably based on a main hypothesis, and one or more auxiliary hypotheses, that the experimenter attempts to disprove; the novice investigator may, in fact, proceed with only a vague notion of the hypothesis

Table 3.3 Pharmacologic Mechanisms Responsible for Human Pharmacogenetic Traits

Pharmacologic mechanism	Drug or other substance	Comment
Altered pharmacokinetic mechanisms		
Drug entry		
Increased first pass metabolism	Hydralazine, isoniazid	Rapid acetylator phenotype predisposes to drug failure
Drug inactivation		
Increased	Isoniazid	Rapid acetylator phenotype predisposes to drug failure
Increased	Many drugs	CYP2D6 ultra rapid metabolizer phenotype predisposes to drug failure
Decreased	Nicotine	CYP2A6 poor metabolizer phenotype protects against cigarette smoking
Decreased	Many drugs	CYP2C19 and CYP2D6 poor metabolizer phenotype predisposes to drug toxicity
Decreased	6-Mercaptopurine, 6-thioguanine, 8-azathioprine	Thiopurine methyltransferase deficient variants predispose to neutropenia
Decreased	Methotrexate	Amplification of dihydrofolate gene protects against methotrexate therapy
Decreased	5-Fluorouracil	Pyrimidine dehydrogenase deficiency predisposes to drug toxicity
Drug conversion		
Increased	Isoniazid	Slow acetylator phenotype predisposes to isoniazid hepatitis
Increased	Benzidine and other carcinogenic arylamines	Slow acetylator phenotype predisposes to bladder urinary cancer
Increased	Cooked food mutagens (heterocyclic amines)	Polymorphic acetylator variants may predispose to colorectal cancer
Decreased	Acetophenetidin	Decreased CYP catalyzed O-dealkylation predisposes to methemoglobinemia
Drug interaction		
Decreased enzyme activity	Drugs that compete for the same drug-metabolizing enzyme	CYP2D6, CYP2C19, CYP2C9 poor metabolizer variants and other polymorphic drug metabolizing enzyme targets predispose to interactions
Drug targeted enzyme		
Increased abundance	Many drugs	CYP2D6 and CYP2C19 ultra rapid metabolizer phenotype predispose to drug failure
Increased abundance	Succinylcholine	Cynthiana serum cholinesterase variant predisposes to drug failure

(*continued*)

Table 3.3 (*continued*)

Pharmacologic mechanism	Drug or other substance	Comment
Increased abundance	Aldosterone	Ectopic overexpression of chimeric aldosterone synthase variant causes early-onset, dexamethasone-remediable hypertension
Decreased activity	Succinylcholine	Silent serum cholinesterases predispose to prolonged apnea
Decreased activity	Many oxidant drugs	G6PD deficiency predisposes to spontaneous and drug-induced hemolysis
Decreased activity	Many drugs	CYP2C19, CYP2C9 and CYP2D6 poor metabolizer phenotypes predispose to drug toxicity
Decreased activity	Smoking	α1-Antitrypsin null variants predispose smokers (and non-smokers to a lesser degree) to premature emphysema
Decreased activity	Parathion	Low-activity paraoxonase variant predisposes to parathion toxicity
Decreased activity	Fructose	Low-activity aldolase B variant predisposes to fructose intolerance
Decreased activity	Epoxides of benzopyrene, aflatoxin, and styrene	Glutathione-S-transferase null mutants predispose to cancer of various tissues
Decreased activity	Trimethylamine	Fish malodor syndrome due to an FMO3 variant predisposes to odor of rotting fish
Decreased activity	Licorice (glycyrrhentic acid)	Licorice ingestion pseudoaldosterone causes state with hypertension attributed to β-hydroxylase deficiency or a glycrrhentic acid-induced inhibition
Decreased affinity	Succinylcholine	Atypical serum cholinesterase predisposes to prolonged apnea
Decreased affinity	Vitamin B_6	Aminolevulinate synthase variant predisposes to anemia
Enzyme (CYP2C9) inhibition	Phenytoin/isoniazid	Slow acetylator phenotype predisposes to phenytoin toxicity from phenytoin/isoniazid interaction
Enzyme (CYP2D6) inhibition	Quinidine/propafenone	Quinidine inhibition of CYP2D6 EM variants produces PM phenocopies that may predispose to toxicity or therapeutic ineffectiveness of many CYP2D6 drug substrates
Enzyme (CYP2C19) substrate competition	R and S enantiomers	CYP2C19 PM variants

Table 3.3 (*continued*)

Pharmacologic mechanism	Drug or other substance	Comment
Altered pharmacodynamic mechanisms		
Drug entry		
Decreased uptake	Vitamin B$_{12}$	B12 transporter variant predisposes to B12 deficiency
Increased excretion	Alkylating agents	Multidrug resistance transporter predisposes to therapeutic ineffectiveness
Drug-targeted receptor		
Decreased abundance	Insulin	Insulin-resistant diabetes mellitus
Decreased abundance	Vasopressin	Vasopressin-resistant diabetes insipidus
Decreased abundance	Glucocorticoids, estrogen	Resistance to steroid hormones
Increased function	Cyproterone, hydroxyflutamide, nilutamide	Androgen receptor variant causes a paradoxical response to prostate cancer antiandrogens
Decreased function	All-*trans*-retinoic acid	Chimeric retinoic acid receptor blocks terminal differentiation of myeloid cells to cause retinoic acid resistance
Decreased function	Halothane/succinylcholine	Ryanodine-receptor variant of skeletal muscle predisposes to malignant hyperthermia
Decreased function	Not applicable	CCR5 coreceptor Δ32 variant protects against, and slows progression, of HIV-1 infection
Decreased function	Endotoxin (lipopolysaccharide, LPS)	TLR4 variant predisposes to endotoxin-mediated disorders such as asthma and septic shock
Decreased function	Quinidine, psychotropics, antihistamines	Ion channel variants predispose to spontaneous and drug-induced ventricular arrhythmias and sudden death
Decreased down-regulation	Albuterol	Nocturnal asthmatics with the Gly variant of the β2-adrenergic receptor (Arg16Gly) may be more resistant to albuterol treatment than those with the Arg isoform
Altered function	Spironolactone	Mineralocorticoid receptor variant predisposes to early-onset hypertension; progesterone and clinically used antagonists lacking 21-hydroxy groups such as spironolactone become agonists
Decreased affinity	Dicumarol/warfarin	VKORCI variants predisposes to anticoagulant resistance
Decreased affinity	Insulin	Insulin-resistant diabetes mellitus
Decreased affinity	Glucocorticoids	Glucocorticoid receptor variant predisposes to glucocorticoid resistance

being tested, but skilled investigators know that it is advantageous to have thought about it explicitly. Auxiliary hypotheses are set forth as reasonable alternatives in case the main hypothesis proves to be untrue. Second, investigators should keep in mind that for every discovery made with innovative approaches, many important advances are made simply by recognizing that an established method or familiar technique devised for one application can be employed for another. And third, in some cases, it is possible to design a single experiment that decides the fate of a given hypothesis.

An authentic example of pharmacogenetic variation may provide a more ready understanding of important principles. Consider an episode that took place in the 1970s at St. Mary's Medical School in London during a small trial with debrisoquine, a new therapeutic agent for treating high blood pressure. A number of healthy human volunteers were each given a small dose of the drug, and afterward one of the volunteers suddenly collapsed because of a drastic fall in his blood pressure. None of the other volunteers experienced anything out of the ordinary. After several days in the hospital the unusually sensitive man had fully recovered, but the reaction in a healthy person was so startling that more tests were run to find the reason for it. The hyperresponsive individual was found to process the drug in a way that turned a normal dose into a massive overdose because he did not make the normal enzyme required to hydroxylate the drug and eliminate it from his system. Further tests led to the discovery of two medical students at St. Mary's who also were unable to hydroxylate debrisoquine. The occurrence of such an unusual response in three individuals among so few persons tested raised the possibility that there could be many others who would respond similarly; indeed, larger studies revealed at least one person in ten in the British population at large possessed the same trait. Later, family studies demonstrated that persons who are sensitive to debrisoquine carry a double dose of the defective gene responsible for the trait. This dramatic discovery of the CYP2D6 polymorphism is described by Moyra Bremner in the *Sunday Times* (London), October 2, 1983.

Presumably, hyperresponsive individuals had developed an elevated concentration of the debrisoquine in plasma (i.e., at receptors) despite receiving only a therapeutic dose of the drug, but had reacted as though they had received an overdose. The investigators reasoned that a defect in the pharmacokinetics (absorption, distribution, or elimination) of debrisoquine would account for the excessive response; also, it was reasonable to propose auxiliary hypotheses that a defect in the receptor for debrisoquine, or a defect in the regulation (signal transduction) of the receptor, could be responsible if the main hypothesis proved untrue. Being experienced investigators, they knew that safe, noninvasive methods for characterizing the pharmacokinetics of debrisoquine in plasma and urine were available that could be used to obtain the information they sought and that values for most of the pharmacokinetic parameters that were necessary for their analysis could be determined by simple arithmetic or computer techniques.

The investigators had previously shown that debrisoquine was mainly converted to a single, biologically inactive metabolite, and they set out to disprove the main hypothesis by examining the urinary metabolite pattern. They found that debrisoquine hyperresponders excreted a much greater quantity of unmetabolized (active) debrisoquine as well as a much smaller quantity of the inactive metabolite than normal responders. From this observation, they could conclude that their main hypothesis was substantially correct, namely that one of the pharmacokinetic mechanisms for disposing of debrisoquine was defective in the hyperresponder. The next step, to get a more fundamental explanation of this trait, was carried out by other investigators more than 10 years later when techniques for identifying, cloning, and sequencing genes were available.[13] The defect was demonstrated to be a variant form of the enzyme that failed to convert debrisoquine to the main biologically inactive product (see CYP2D6, also known as the debrisoquine/sparteine oxidation polymorphism) confirming the main hypothesis.[†]

Suppose, on the other hand, that a normal pattern of urinary metabolites for debrisoquine had been found in the hypersensitive responder instead of the abnormal pattern. This finding would strongly suggest that a pharmacokinetic defect was unlikely, and that the main hypothesis proposed was false. The alternative possibility speaks to a functional change in the receptor that might be responsible, as proposed in the auxiliary hypothesis. How might the investigators test for such a change in the debrisoquine receptor? Two possibilities might be proposed: there might be an altered receptor with an increased affinity for debrisoquine, or an overabundance of the unaltered debrisoquine receptor. To test the validity of these hypotheses, investigations would assume a direction similar to that taken to investigate the mechanism of warfarin resistance described in connection with graded dose–response relationships. If the affinity of the receptor was increased, the concentration of debrisoquine needed to attain a given response would be decreased; if a more complete graded dose–response curve were obtained, theoretically the curve would be shifted to the left as shown in Figure 3.1B (curve 2A). In that case, an ordinary dose would produce a hyperresponse. If the abundance of unaltered receptors was increased, a therapeutic dose would result in a hyperresponse, as shown in Figure 3.1A (curve 1B). Determination of graded dose–response curves for abnormal and normal responders to debrisoquine would thus help the investigators decide whether a change in the abundance or in the affinity of the debrisoquine receptor had occurred.

If an increased affinity or an overabundance of debrisoquine receptors were found in abnormal responders compared to normal responders, additional studies would be undertaken to obtain a more detailed view of the receptor. They would probably include the isolation, cloning, sequencing, and expression of the genes

[†]Many years may elapse between the observation of a phenomenon and its explanation. Mendel singled out the seven contrasting characters for his study of inheritance in pea plants—one of them being seed shape, either round (the dominant form) or wrinkled. Plant scientists in England showed with recombinant DNA techniques that the wrinkling of peas is due to a deficiency of starch branching enzyme I, which results in a high sucrose content and, consequently, a high osmotic pressure. This leads to the accumulation of water, but when the seed dries out, the skin collapses into a mass of wrinkles. Peas homozygous for the defective "wrinkled" gene completely lack the starch branching enzyme, whereas the normal enzyme is active in peas with the "round" gene.[14]

for the receptor from both responder phenotypes. The goals of these studies would include a search for structural and regulatory differences of receptor synthesis, stability, and targeting (to ascertain the mechanism for overabundance), and a search for overexpression of the receptor gene and for structural change in the receptor molecules (to determine the mechanism for increased affinity). Quite possibly, the abundance of receptors, or the receptor affinity, for debrisoquine for hyperresponsive subjects might not be found to differ from those of normal responders. Although these findings would disprove the auxiliary hypothesis, they would not preclude the possibility of other, associated alterations that could overamplify the signal from debrisoquine and generate intracellular changes resulting in the dramatic fall in blood pressure in abnormal responders. These include (1) an altered signal transduction system such that the coupling between the drug–receptor complex and stimulation of an effector protein (e.g., adenylyl cyclase) is enhanced; (2) an altered effector protein that overamplifies the signal generated by the coupling (e.g., overactive adenylyl cyclase or underactive phosphodiesterase); and (3) an altered protein kinase or substrate for the kinase that mediates the drug effects, and so on.

The precise nature of the receptor-related defect responsible for the hyperresponse to therapeutic concentrations of debrisoquine could then be sought by correlating the molecular characteristics with the functional properties of the expressed receptors within each phenotype, and then by comparing the receptors, or the signal transduction systems, for normal responders and the abnormal responders.

SUMMARY

The characteristic pharmacological profile associated with a specific drug is due to the physiological and biochemical makeup of cells targeted by specific drug receptors, but extrinsic and intrinsic influences that impinge on targeted cells can cause a remarkable degree of variation in response. Variations are best considered in the light of the drug's pharmacokinetics and pharmacodynamics, mechanisms that define the disposition and actions of drugs in individuals. Mechanisms that involve interactions between the xenobiotic and specific enzymes or receptors targeted by the xenobiotic are usually pertinent to variations of interest. Identification of the pharmacological mechanism responsible for an unusual variation in drug response can be a formidable task, but performance of a pharmacokinetic analysis in susceptible persons can often yield preliminary insights into the relative importance of the pharmacokinetic and pharmacodynamic phases of the response.

REFERENCES

1. Kalow W, Staron N. On distribution and inheritance of atypical forms of human serum cholinesterase, as indicated by dibucaine numbers. Can J Med Sci 1957; 35(12): 1305–1320.

2. O'Reilly RA, Pool JG, Aggeler PM. Hereditary resistance to coumarin anticoagulant drugs in man and rat. Ann NY Acad Sci 1968; 151:913–931.

3. Calabrese EJ, Baldwin LA. Chemical hormesis: Its historical foundations as a biological hypothesis. Hum Exp Toxicol 2000; 19(1):2–31.

4. Calabrese EJ, Baldwin LA. Tales of two similar hypotheses: The rise and fall of chemical and radiation hormesis. Hum Exp Toxicol 2000; 19(1):85–97.

5. Calabrese EJ. Hormesis: From marginalization to mainstream: A case for hormesis as the default dose-response model in risk assessment. Toxicol Appl Pharmacol 2004; 197(2):125–136.

6. Calabrese EJ, Baldwin LA. The frequency of U-shaped dose responses in the toxicological literature. Toxicol Sci 2001; 62(2):330–338.

7. Calabrese EJ, Baldwin LA. Toxicology rethinks its central belief. Nature 2003; 421(13 Feb):691–692.

8. Kalow W. Dose-response relationships and genetic variation. Ann NY Acad Sci 1965; 123:212–218.

9. Hammonds RG Jr, Nicolas P, Li CH. Beta-endorphin-(1–27) is an antagonist of beta-endorphin analgesia. Proc Natl Acad Sci USA 1984; 81(5):1389–1390.

10. Nicolas P, Hammonds RG Jr, Li CH. Beta-endorphin-induced analgesia is inhibited by synthetic analogs of beta-endorphin. Proc Natl Acad Sci USA 1984; 81(10):3074–3077.

11. Ludden TM, Allen JP, Valutsky WA, Vicuna AV, Nappi JM, Hoffman SF, et al. Individualization of phenytoin dosage regimens. Clin Pharmacol Ther 1976; 21:287–292.

12. Weber WW. The Acetylator Genes and Drug Response. New York: Oxford University Press, 1987.

13. Gonzalez FJ, Skoda RC, Kimura S, Umeno M, Zanger UM, Nebert DW, et al. Characterization of the common genetic defect in humans deficient in debrisoquine metabolism. Nature 1988; 331(6155):442–446.

14. Bhattacharyya MK, Smith AM, Ellis TH, Hedley C, Martin C. The wrinkled-seed character of pea described by Mendel is caused by a transposon-like insertion in a gene encoding starch-branching enzyme. Cell 1990; 60(1):115–122.

4

Age-Related Pharmacology

Life in healthy individuals begins with a period of rapid growth and development followed by a prolonged period of maturity that slowly and progressively declines into senescence. For treatment of specific diseases, physicians strive to prescribe drugs appropriate for a patient's age and health on the premise that they will bring about favorable, reproducible responses. But young children and elderly persons differ in many ways from mature adults in their middle years, including their capacity to handle and respond to intrinsic and extrinsic stimuli. Aging dominates both the structure and function of cells and organs over a much lengthier period of life than processes involved in growing and development, but knowledge of the mechanisms associated with aging is still very limited and generally less well understood than those that regulate growth and functional advancement.

Nathan Shock, a pioneer of the physiology of aging, observed early that not all physiological functions change with age (e.g., blood volume, blood glucose, acid–base balance), but that many organ systems exhibit extremely wide age-related individual functional differences. He provided evidence that some age-related changes in physiological functions can be ascribed to loss of cells or functional tissue, while certain other cellular functions truly do change with age (e.g., renal plasma flow, tubular secretion, cardiac output, peripheral arterial resistance).[1] But representative biomarkers of aging that would allow a generalized definition of physiological age in humans have been difficult to identify, and no unifying explanation of the biology of aging that is applicable to cells and organ systems as well as to intact individuals has been proposed.

Technological advances that were introduced during the 1960s and 1970s have led to a better definition of ontogenic changes in organ and enzyme functions at the extremes of life. "Developmental pharmacology," the part of pediatric pharmacology that deals with age-related differences in drug response in neonates and children, underwent appreciable modification and amplification during that period.[2–5] At the same time, increases in elderly populations within developed countries directed attention to the biology of aging and stimulated interest in drug sensitivity in the elderly and the clinical aspects of therapeutic drug handling where ignorance was so marked.[6–11] Recently, a number of modern, noninvasive techniques have provided new approaches to investigate morphological and functional changes in the elderly.

If adult values in the middle years of life are taken as standards of reference, physiological variations at life's extremes, especially during infancy and childhood, are much greater than during the middle years, and provision of safe and effective pharmacotherapy must take account of the magnitude and timing of such variations in addition to genetic variation. This chapter attempts to describe the sources and most consistent patterns of constitutional variations observed in development and aging.

AGE-RELATED PHYSIOLOGICAL VARIATION

From gestation to maturity, the growth and development of individuals are marked by changes in shape and size resulting from cellular multiplication and by structural and functional maturation. No sharp distinction between these processes is possible, but together they make up a complex set of factors whose combined significance is greater than either process alone. For certain tissues, the rate of change is rapid, as it is between birth and 2 or 3 years of age for neural tissue, or for lymphoid tissue toward the end of the first decade. For other tissues, rates of change are more gradual. Thus, while the relative proportions of skeletal muscle and subcutaneous tissue change markedly toward the end of the first decade, there is little alteration in the weight and height of the individual. When variations are large, averages tend to lose their significance and norms are better expressed as a range of values. For certain attributes, separate norms are needed for males and females, and at certain stages of childhood, such as the onset of adolescence, a profusion of physiological changes occurs with such rapidity that the gross features of a person, such as age or body weight, are of little use as scales of reference. Such profound physiological differences that are inherent in infancy and childhood cannot be disregarded in therapeutic management.

As individuals approach maturity, structural and functional changes abate.[12] The problem of differentiating normal from abnormal development in the immature person is replaced later in life by the problem of sorting involutional from pathological change, especially at more advanced ages when morbidity is so common.[13] Furthermore, certain maturational changes may continue in some tissues while involutional processes have already commenced in others. For instance, while most individuals reach sexual maturity by 15 years of age, the ability for visual accommodation has already begun to decline. Maturation and involution may even occur simultaneously as shown by the coexistence of atrophy and hypertrophy in the gastric mucosa, and certain types of degenerative changes appear to exhibit aging at a chemical level without accompanying histological changes, while the opposite occurs in other situations. Loss of near vision with advancing age exemplifies the former and disseminated cerebral atrophy, in which cells disappear but vital function is maintained, exemplifies the latter.

Variations in physiological functions of living organisms imposed by changes of size and shape have been examined intensively.[14,15] The observation that certain functions may vary directly with body surface area was recognized and documented more than a century ago for numerous therapeutic and toxic agents.[16] A nomogram based on this principle has been applied to the adjustment of drug dosage between individuals of different sizes and different ages.[3] Its value in therapeutics stems from the observation that the extracellular water compartment, an important determinant of drug distribution, varies proportionately with its surface area. Consequently, drugs that are distributed in extracellular water would be expected to reach similar concentrations in persons of different sizes if they were dosed according to this principle. Dosages for drugs that are distributed in a space that exceeds the extracellular compartment cannot be estimated from the body area because the total body water, or any fraction in excess of extracellular water, does not vary in proportion to body area. The constitutional variability from one person to another suggests we adopt a conservative attitude toward extensions of this principle, particularly for extrapolations from mature individuals to infants and children.

Age-related changes in the time course of drug disposition (pharmacokinetics) and in the dynamics of drug responsiveness (pharmacodynamics) tend to occur in an orderly sequence at predictable stages in the life of individuals, but their onset and extent can vary widely from individual to individual. During infancy and childhood these changes are usually rapid and either periodic or cyclic, but throughout the adult years they are more gradual and progressive. With advancing age, a series of asynchronous anatomical and physiological effects occurs that results in increased interindividual variability. An accumulation of local effects at the molecular, cellular, and tissue levels impairs many regulatory processes that provide functional integration between cells and organs. The ability to maintain functional equilibrium through homeostatic mechanisms is reduced, which predisposes older persons to unusual or unexpected effects from several classes of drugs. Pharmacokinetic changes include a reduction in hepatic and renal clearance that prolongs drug elimination, while pharmacodynamic changes may alter the sensitivity to many drugs that are frequently used in older persons.

PHARMACOKINETIC VARIATION

Pharmacokinetics describes the time course of mechanisms that determine the level of drug (and its metabolites) in tissues and at receptor sites and terminate its biological actions (see pp. 18–50). Mathematical expressions that relate drug concentration to standard pharmacokinetic parameters (such as drug dose, dosing interval, bioavailability, rate of elimination, apparent volume of distribution, plasma half-life, and drug clearance) lend quantitative precision to estimates of the relative effects of absorption, distribution, and elimination on the response.

At the beginning of life, pharmacokinetic variations are related to maturational increases in liver and kidney function and to variations in gastrointestinal absorption, tissue distribution, plasma protein binding, and "drug extraction ratio" characteristics, but other physiological processes contribute to these variations.

Drug Absorption

In healthy infants and children, most of the physiological changes important for gastrointestinal absorption of drugs that are usually orally administered are quite variable and undergo continuous maturational changes. Gastrointestinal transit time, the area available for absorption from different segments of the gut, and the permeability and vascularity of different segments are some of the specific variables of concern during development. The gastric emptying time in the newborn is slower than at any other time in life. Many newborn infants require 8 hours for complete gastric emptying, and in some instances it may be much longer. In general, movements during the neonatal period are irregular and unpredictable, and are subject to various influences including nutritional status, diet, and feeding pattern. Changes in gastric acidity are cyclic, showing initially a low acidity that rises abruptly to adult levels on the first day of birth, and then declines to an achlorhydric state by about the tenth day after birth. Thereafter the acidity gradually rises again until it attains adult levels at approximately 3 years; later in life it may decline slowly. The relative achlorhydria may partially explain the higher bioavailability of acid-labile drugs such as several penicillins, and the reduced absorption of weakly acidic drugs such as phenobarbital, phenytoin, and naldixic acid. From the studies that have examined the absorption of drugs and nutrient molecules, both passive and active enteral absorptive transport processes are judged to be fully mature by approximately 4 months after birth. Additional developmental changes such as differences in intestinal drug-metabolizing enzymes and transporter mechanisms can also alter the bioavailability, but for the most part these are incompletely characterized.[7,17]

In elderly persons, a preponderance of information indicates that intestinal absorption of most drugs that cross the gastrointestinal barrier by diffusion, the primary process for absorption of orally administered drugs, is not altered to an extent that is clinically relevant. For drugs that cross the intestinal barrier by carrier-mediated transporter mechanisms, such as calcium, iron, vitamins, and possibly nucleoside drugs, absorption may occur at lower rates, although the data are limited. Because of a reduction in tissue blood perfusion associated with atrophy of the epidermis and dermis that occurs with advancing age, transdermal drug absorption may be diminished in the elderly. For the same reason, drug absorption from subcutaneous and muscular tissue sites may also occur at lower rates.[8,9,18]

Drug Distribution

Total body water, extracellular water, and intracellular water are functional compartments of pharmacological interest because the distribution of different classes of drugs within the body often corresponds to one of these spaces. The size of these body water compartments and the changes from birth to adulthood originally described by Friis-Hansen[19] have been reviewed in the present context by several authors.[7-9,20] Total body water is approximately 78% of body weight at birth, and decreases sharply to 60% at 1 year, which closely approximates that at maturity (Table 4.1 and Figure 4.1B). The extracellular water space is much greater in comparison to body weight in the newborn infant (45%) than in a 1-year-old child (27%), and subsequently decreases until it attains the adult standard at approximately 3 years (17%). This change is almost entirely due to changes in interstitial volume, because the size of the plasma water compartment, a component of extracellular water, is unaltered (4–5%) throughout life. The change in intracellular water space initially opposes that of total body and extracellular water, increasing from 34% of body weight at birth to 43% at 3 months and then decreasing to a value quite close to that at birth (40%). After 3 years of age, the size of all three compartments reaches their adult values. Person-to-person variations, especially at birth, are large but do not overlap those of older children or adults.

Differences in drug distribution can also be due to differences in the amount of binding protein, in the strength of protein–drug interaction, or a combination of these factors.[7] Levels of serum proteins have been studied at various ages from gestation through middle age into senescence. Albumin, the major drug-binding component of plasma, is present in fetal serum by 4 weeks of gestational age, increasing in proportion to gestational age and reaching an average of 1.8 g/100 ml of serum by 26–27 weeks gestation and 2.5 g/100 ml serum by 30–31 weeks gestation. Plasma albumin levels are sufficiently characteristic of fetal maturity that they can be used clinically to assess the gestational age of the newborn, and levels of less than 2.5 g/100 ml of serum, for example, are taken as evidence of immaturity. Levels do not appear to fluctuate appreciably during childhood, and in the adult they decline slowly with age. An average decrease of 20% occurs between the young adult and an elderly person of 60–70 years in one report,

Table 4.1 Variation in Body Water Compartments with Age[19]

	Average newborn	Average 1-year-old infant	Average adult
Body weight (g)	3,400	10,800	70,000
Total body water			
%	78	60	58
ml	2,650	6,500	41,000
Extracellular water			
%	45	27	17
ml	1,530	2,900	12,000
Intracellular water			
%	34	35	40
ml	1,160	3,800	28,000
Plasma water			
%	4–5	4–5	4–5
ml	140	430	3,000

With permission from Springer Verlag.

A

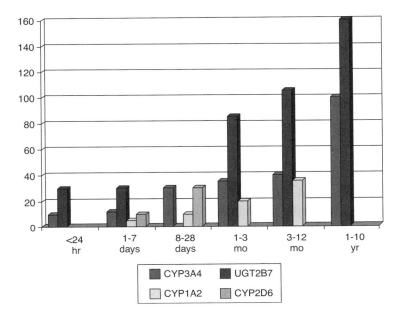

B

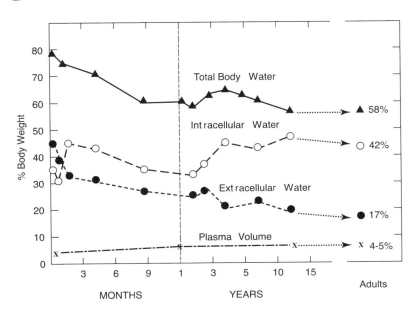

Figure 4.1 Age-related patterns of physiological change affecting drug disposition. (A) Changes in metabolic capacity. (B) Changes in body water compartments. (C) Changes in renal function. (*Source*: From Kearns et al.[17]) With permission from the *New England Journal of Medicine*.

C

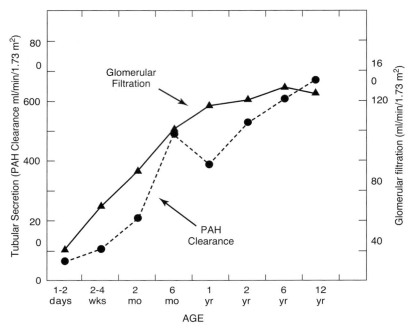

Figure 4.1 (*continued*)

although the extent of the decrease varies somewhat between reports. For younger age groups, binding affinity appears to be substrate specific. Thus, fetal serum albumin binds salicylate with lower avidity than adult serum albumin (association constants are $1.7–2.9 \times 10^5$ M^{-1} vs. 4.0×10^5 M^{-1}), whereas it binds bilirubin more strongly (association constants 5.2×10^7 M^{-1} vs. 2.4×10^7 M^{-1}).

For healthy elderly persons, in contrast to infants of age 1 year or younger, there is little conclusive evidence that dosage regimens of orally administered drugs, as recommended by Thummel and colleagues,[21] need be altered for expected changes in plasma protein binding associated with advancing age.[22]

Drug Metabolism

During the 1950s, a series of therapeutic disasters involving the administration of water-soluble preparations of vitamin K,[23] sulfonamides,[24] and chloramphenicol[25] to premature and newborn infants occurred at several pediatric centers. Careful study of these events prompted investigators to propose inefficient glucuronidation of vitamin K derivatives and chloramphenicol and inefficient acetylation of sulfonamides as factors responsible for these adverse drug reactions. From these studies, and additional studies in immature animals, the delayed development of drug-metabolizing enzymes during the perinatal period was suggested to be a phenomenon of general significance.[2] Since then, metabolic biotransformation has been amply demonstrated to be a major determinant of the pharmacokinetics of drugs (see pp. 18–50), usually by increasing the polarity of a drug to hasten its elimination through the action of Phase I enzymes that catalyze oxidation, reduction, and hydrolysis and Phase II enzymes that attach moieties such as glucuronic acid, acetate, sulfate, glutathione, and glycine to the drug molecule or its metabolites.

Hepatic Drug-Metabolizing Enzyme Capacity

A total of 57 cytochrome P450 genes distributed among nine gene families of the Phase I cytochrome P450 superfamily of genes have been identified in humans (see p. 31).[26,27] Among these, three families, *CYP1, CYP2,* and *CYP3,* as well as at least 24 individual enzymes they encode, dominate the biotransformation of therapeutic drugs and toxicants.[28] Studies of the content, activity, and, more recently, gene expression are beginning to provide insight into the complex patterns of developmental change of Phase I enzymes accompanying early growth and development.

Within the CYP3 family, CYP3A enzymes metabolize more therapeutics and toxicants than the CYP1 and CYP2 families. CYP3A4 and CYP3A5 gene products account for about 30–40% of the total cytochrome P450 in adult liver and intestine. CYP3A7, the predominant fetal form of CYP3A, is uniquely expressed in fetal liver as early as 50–60 days of gestation. CYP3A7 expression continues through the perinatal period after which it declines progressively, reaching undetectable levels by about 1 year of age. CYP3A7 has been considered a fetus-specific enzyme, but it has been shown more recently to be expressed in adult human livers carrying the CYP3A71C allele by Sim and colleagues.[29] CYP3A4/3A5 expression begins by about 1 week after birth, reaches 30% of adult levels by 1 month of age, and a maximum during childhood.[30,31] The clearance of the narcotic analgesic fentanyl is 11.5 ml/kg/min at 33 weeks gestation, about 30% of its value in term infants, provides a measure of developmental changes in CYP3A4[31] (Figure 4.1A).

Members of the CYP1 and CYP2 families of enzymes exhibit various maturational patterns. By 1–3 months after birth, CYP1A2 has reached full adult activity, while CYP2C9, CYP2C19, and CYP2D6 have reached less than 20% of adult activities. At 3–5 years of age, CYP1A2 has twice the adult activity, while CYP2C9 and CYP2C19 exceed 100% of adult activity by 50–60%. At puberty, activities of these three enzymes have decreased to adult levels.

The flavin-containing monoxygenases (FMOs), encoded by a six-member gene family, is a Phase I gene involved in oxidative metabolism of xenobiotics containing nitrogen, sulfur, selenium, and phosphorus. One member of this family, FM03, has been identified as genetically defective and causative of the fish malodor syndrome (see Appendix A). The human hepatic FMOs exhibit a developmental switch somewhat reminiscent of that seen in the CYP3A family.[28] FM01 was readily observed in two laboratories in hepatic tissue during gestation (at 14–17 weeks and 8–15 weeks), whereas FM03 was undetectable. FM01 expression declined during fetal development to undetectable levels at birth and was undetectable in adult tissues. In contrast, the onset of FM03 expression was highly variable. Most neonates failed to express FM03, but expression was evident by 1–2 years of age. Intermediate FM03 expression was observed until 11 years of age, after which a gender-independent increase was seen from 11 to 18 years. Because the decline in CYP3A7 expression is accompanied by a simultaneous increase in CYP3A4/3A5, CYP3A expression is relatively invariant. On the other hand, the absence of FM01 at birth and the delayed onset of FM03 result in a null hepatic FMO phenotype in the neonate. The developmental picture is not yet complete, however, because there is no information on the developmental expression of FMOs in extrahepatic tissues.

With respect to the ontogeny of Phase I enzymes in elderly persons, the bulk of evidence has not suggested any definitive relationship between age and change in hepatic microsomal protein content or activities of various cytochrome P450 enzymes including the common variants of CYP2D6.[11] Two laboratories observed an age-related decline in CYP3A and 2E1, but not in CYP1A2 or 2C; there were, however, also confounding factors including disease, drugs, and smoking that render these findings moot.[10]

Several decades have elapsed since the perinatal inefficiencies of glucuronidation and acetylation in infants were identified,[2] but knowledge of developmental changes is still far from complete, mainly because of ethical and technical difficulties that retard or prevent their systematic investigation. Nevertheless, there are indications that many drug-metabolizing enzymes are expressed early in development. For example, there is evidence for glutathione-S-transferases (GSTs) in fetal liver, lung, and kidney, for NAT1 in fetal tissues, for some isoforms of glucuronosyltranferases and sulfotransferases in fetal liver and other tissues, and for epoxide hydrolases 1 and 2 in fetal liver. However, nothing is known about human NAT2 developmental expression, the more important isoform of NAT to drug and toxicant metabolism in adults.[32]

Whether impairment of Phase I enzymes is associated with aging has, for some time, been a controversial issue. In their review of the literature, Le Couteur and McLean found no relationship between age and either the hepatic content or activity of various cytochrome P450 enzymes,[33] but by analyzing the results of published studies into in vivo clearance of drugs, they concluded that the effect of aging on hepatic drug metabolism was likely to be secondary to the reduction of blood flow and liver size, as stated in the following section.

With respect to the effects of aging on Phase II enzymes, data on human subjects are even more limited and spotty than for Phase I enzymes. One study found no change in paracetamol glucuronidation or sulfation in aging human liver preparations.[10]

Recently, three drug-metabolizing enzyme polymorphisms were examined to detect a relationship between them and longevity, but none was found.[34] The distribution of genotypes for CYP2D6, and two conjugating enzymes, NAT2 and GSTM1, but none of the phenotypes for CYP2D6 extensive or poor metabolizers, rapid or slow acetylators, and active or defective GSTM1 correlated with human longevity, alone or in combination. The expression or activity of drug transporters in liver, or of P-glycoprotein and multidrug resistance-associated protein, is of recent interest in drug clearance, but as yet no data are available that describe the effects of age on them.[10]

Hepatic Drug Clearance in Vivo

Bodily clearance of therapeutic drugs and other substrates is a function of both metabolic capacity and blood flow, and in some cases blood protein binding.[10,35] To interpret kinetic data at different stages of development and aging, it is important to distinguish between "high extraction" and "low extraction" drugs. The metabolic clearance of highly extracted drugs is primarily determined by hepatic blood flow, and is termed "flow-limited metabolism"; in contrast, the metabolic clearance of poorly extracted drugs is influenced mainly by intrinsic clearance (i.e., by the metabolizing capacity) of hepatic tissue, and is termed "capacity limited."

Studies in Infants and Children   A number of drugs that are substrates for Phase I metabolism have been classified as having high or low hepatic extraction from adult human pharmacokinetic data (Table 4.2). Antiepileptics and certain benzodiazepines that are frequently used therapeutically in infants are low extraction drugs. The half-life of these drugs depends primarily on drug-metabolizing activity and can serve as an approximate estimate of the capacity to metabolize the drug. Aminophylline and caffeine both have lengthy plasma half-lives compared to those in adults and both are substrates for CYP1A, which is consistent with the extremely low activity of CYP1A in fetal liver. On the other hand, the capacity to metabolize carbamazepine and phenytoin in newborns is well developed at birth. Carbamazepine is a substrate of CYP3A4/5 while phenytoin is a substrate of CYP2C9. Perhaps the enhanced capacity to metabolize these substrates in newborns is a result of intrauterine induction. The fact that the maximum velocity (V_{max}) for oxidation of phenytoin in children exceeds that in adults explains the recommendation of higher doses in children than adults.[35]

The half-life of drugs belonging to the high extraction group depends largely on hepatic blood flow, and only to a minor extent on metabolic capacity. All of the examples cited in Table 4.2 have longer elimination times after an intravenous dose in newborns than adults, but the drugs in this group are less commonly used in infants than adults.

Some drugs not classified with respect to hepatic clearance are also included in Table 4.2. Among these, the overall impression is that drug elimination in neonates is slower than in adults. Not only is there variation from drug to drug, but also from newborns to adults. This suggests that attempts to predict drug metabolic capacity for children from adult data would likely be unsuccessful.

The half-lives suggest that the metabolism of most drugs is reduced in the neonatal period, but many drugs do not conform to this trend. For certain drugs, alternative metabolic pathways may be quantitatively more significant during early life than later on, as acetaminophen, salicylic acid, and theophylline illustrate.[35] In the full-term neonate, acetaminophen and salicylic acid are eliminated primarily as the sulfate and glycine conjugates, respectively, while adults eliminate both drugs primarily as glucuronide conjugates. Theophylline, in contrast, is eliminated by premature and full-term neonates mainly by direct

Table 4.2 Half-Lives of Drugs with Low or High Hepatic Extraction and Drugs Unclassified with Respect to Hepatic Extraction[35]

Drug	Half-life (hours)	
	Newborns	Adults
Drugs with low hepatic clearance		
Aminophylline	24–36	3–9
Caffeine	103	6
Carbamazepine	8–28	21–36
Diazepam	25–100	15–25
Mepivacaine	8.7	3.2
Phenobarbitone	21–100	52–120
Phenytoin	21	11–29
Tolbutamide	10–40	4.4–9
Drugs with high hepatic clearance		
Meperidine	22	3–4
Nortriptyline	56	18–22
Morphine	2.7	0.9–4.3
Lidocaine	2.9–3.3	1.0–2.2
Propoxyphene	1.7–7.7	1.9–4.3
Drugs unclassified with respect to hepatic extraction		
Amikacin	2.8	2.9
Aminopyrine	30–40	2–4
Bupivacaine	25	1.3
Chloramphenicol	5.1	ND
Furosemide	7.7–19.9	0.5
Gentamicin	1.25	ND
Indomethacin	14–20	2–11
Oxazepam	21.9	6.5
Primidone	7–28.6	3.3–12.5
Phenylbutazone	21–34	12–30
Valproic acid	23–35	10–16

renal excretion with a small proportion being metabolized and excreted as 1,3-dimethyluric acid and 1-methyluric acid. In older children and adults, direct renal excretion of theophylline becomes less important as metabolic pathways mature, and an increasingly greater proportion is transformed and excreted as 1,3-dimethyluric acid, 1-methyluric acid, and 3-methylxanthine.

Studies in Aging Persons Studies of drug metabolism performed in aging rodent models suggest a decline in hepatic microsomal metabolism with age, but extrapolation of data generated in these models to humans is fraught with problems inherent in species differences. Clarification of the effects of aging on drug metabolism has also been sought by measuring several indices of hepatic function that might affect Phase I drug metabolism in human liver[36,37] and by analyzing studies of drug metabolism and drug clearance in elderly persons.[10,11,33,38] These investigations have led to multifarious observations, but no simple generalization: (1) A study of antipyrine, a drug that is metabolized by 10 cytochrome P450 enzymes, and is a general marker for oxidative capacity in all age groups, showed a reduction of *in vitro* and *in vivo* metabolism with age. Subjects could be divided into young, middle-aged, and elderly age groups, and a reduction of 30% was found after 70 years of age. (2) A review of the literature in 1998 found no relationship between old age and the activity or content of various Phase I enzymes in human liver preparations. (3) A close association between age and a reduction of about 40% in hepatic blood flow was found, and a consistent effect of age on the reduction of clearances of flow-limited drugs of about 30–40% was found that correlated well with the age-related reduction in blood flow. (4) Measurements of liver weight at autopsy and liver volume during life indicated that reduced liver volume was associated with old age.[33] (5) Reduced blood flow and reduced liver volume in the elderly permitted reconciliation of the *in vivo* clinical pharmacokinetic data indicative of reduced hepatic drug clearance in the absence of age-related declines in the amounts and activities of *in vitro* microsomal monooxygenases. The picture is complicated further by conflicting results reported in some studies, in that the clearance of some capacity-limited drugs such as phenytoin and warfarin is unrelated to age, and additionally, in that the clearances of many drugs metabolized via Phase I pathways (chlormethazole, diltiazem, propanolol, theophylline, imipramine, amitriptyline, verapamil, ibuprofen, and lignocaine), including flow-limited drugs as well as capacity-limited drugs (theophylline, antipyrine), are substantially reduced in old age. (6) Considerable interindividual variability reflecting the influence of a number of confounding factors (frailty, comorbidity, polypharmacy, smoking, and alcohol intake) was found in most of the studies that were analyzed. The increased variability was recognized as a feature that might obscure age-related differences. (7) Drug clearances assessed by various breath tests for cytochrome P450 activity reported conflicting results. Most of these studies failed to find an effect of age on activity, but one study showed that clearance of erythromycin was reduced in older people; another study that used the caffeine breath test showed that CYP1A2 was reduced in elderly humans.

While these observations reveal the complexities in understanding drug clearance in elderly persons, they do not provide a clear answer to the primary question of whether the clearance of drugs changes in a predictable manner as age increases. A comprehensive review of the CYP3A subfamily by Cotreau and colleagues[39] is especially noteworthy because this subfamily is involved in the metabolism of such a large fraction, some 50%, of all prescribed drugs. They find that CYP3A activity may vary, depending on its sensitivity to the route of drug administration and the contribution of hepatic blood flow to overall drug clearance. Since age may influence hepatic blood flow, it may, in turn, affect CYP3A activity. An overall evaluation of the literature supports the conclusion that many CYP3A substrates, including benzodiazepines, calcium channel antagonists and other cardiovascular agents, opioid analgesics, antidepressants, oncological agents, and various miscellaneous agents (atorvastatin, lovastatin, buspirone, clarithromycin, prednisolone, triilazad, and zolpidem), show reduced clearance in elderly persons. This review also finds that elderly men are more susceptible to age-related decrements in clearance than elderly women.

Additional evidence suggests that *in vivo* clearance of certain drugs that are eliminated by Phase I metabolism (in addition to CYP3A substrates) is likely to be reduced in elderly persons, particularly for highly extracted (flow-limited) drugs, and that a consistent effect of aging on the *in vivo* clearance of drugs eliminated by Phase II pathways is unlikely. However, the clearances of many important, widely used therapeutic drugs such as digitoxin, warfarin, phenytoin, salicylic acid, valproic acid, caffeine, isoniazid, paracetamol, and oxazepam do not conform to these simple generalizations.[10]

Renal Elimination

In general, the net functional capacity of the renal system controls the rate of drug elimination, but various intrinsic characteristics of drug molecules may alter the route by which a specific drug is excreted. During fetal life, anatomical and physiological features of the kidneys change with age, but after birth maturation of existing structures is the major factor responsible for age-related changes in renal function. In the newborn infant, glomerular filtration rates, as measured by mannitol or inulin clearance, may be as low as 3 ml/min compared to 130 ml/min in young adult men (Table 4.3 and Figure 4.1C). Infants generally achieve an adult glomerular filtration rate by 1 year of age,[40,41] although some infants have adult mannitol clearances by 10–20 weeks of age.[42] Glomerular filtration remains relatively constant up to about 20–25 years of age but then declines according to the relation $Cl_I = -0.96 \times Age \text{ (years)} + 153.2$.[43] The half-lives of kanamycin and gentamicin, which are aminoglycosides that are eliminated unchanged mainly by glomerular filtration, illustrate the pharmacological significance of these changes (Table 4.4).[44,45] In premature infants the half-life of these drugs is longer than in full-term infants, longer in young than older full-term infants, and longer in older full-term infants than adults. To be therapeutically beneficial, the serum concentration of kanamycin should remain at or slightly above 5 µg/ml. In healthy young adults, administration of 7.5 mg/kg every 6 hours yields therapeutic concentrations throughout the day, but for premature infants the drug is administered in 12 hourly doses of 7.5 mg/kg that are therapeutic and, with rare exceptions, avoid toxicity.

The secretory capacity of the renal tubules is very low in infancy (Figure 4.1C). In newborns, the clearance measured with *p*-aminohippuric acid (PAH) is 12 ml/min and peaks at the young adult level, 650 ml/min, by about 30 weeks after birth. By age 60–65 years, the clearance falls to about 30% of the peak level. Penicillin G and several semisynthetic penicillins such as methicillin, oxacillin, and ampicillin are secreted unchanged, mainly by tubular secretion at a very slow rate by newborn and premature infants.[46,47] Their elimination half-life and rate of urinary excretion both reach adult levels 3–4 weeks after birth. Consequently, the dose and time of administration are usually altered accordingly when these drugs are administered to infants during the first few weeks after birth.

In their review of clinical pharmacokinetics in newborns and infants, Morselli and colleagues compare the pharmacokinetic profiles and other kinetic data from the literature for a large number of drugs commonly used perinatally and in

Table 4.3 Drug Clearance and Elimination Half-Time for Drugs Distributed in Different Body Water Compartments in Newborn Infants and Adults Absent Protein Binding[a]

Renal clearance	Drug distributed in					
	Plasma water		Extracellular water		Total body water	
	Newborn (140 ml)	Adult (3000 ml)	Newborn (1530 ml)	Adult (12000 ml)	Newborn (2650 ml)	Adult (41,000 ml)
Tubular secretion						
PAH clearance (ml/min)	12	650	12	650	12	650
$t_{1/2}$ (minutes)	8.0	3.0	88.4	13	153	44
Glomerular filtration						
Inulin clearance (ml/min)	3	130	3	130	3	130
$t_{1/2}$ (minutes)	32	16	353	64	612	218

With permission from Springer Verlag.

[a]Half-life calculated from t½ (minutes) = 0.693 V_D /clearance which corresponds to the body water space.

infancy to those of adults.[20] Profiles for local anesthetics, narcotic analgesics, cardiorespiratory drugs, anticonvulsants, and aminoglycoside, macrolide, cephalosporin, penicillin, and miscellaneous antibiotics are included in their comparisons. These observations clearly generalize the effect of immaturity on the renal clearance of drugs.

Effect of Plasma Protein Binding on Distribution and Renal Elimination of Drugs

Extensive protein binding can affect the action of a drug by restricting distribution, by decreasing penetration into tissues and parts of the body, and by delaying renal excretion. The potential effects of plasma protein binding on the apparent volume of drug distribution and the dynamics of drug elimination are particularly

Table 4.4 Changes in Half-Lives (Hours) of Aminoglycosides with Age

Drug	Age				
	Premature infant		Full-term infant		Adult
	< 1 week	> 1 week	< 1 week	> 1 week	
Kanamycin	18.0[a]	6.0[a]	4.0[b]	3.5[b]	2.0
Streptomycin	7.0[a]	ND	ND	ND	2.7
Gentamicin[b]	6.25	3.25	4.5	3.15	3.15

With permission from Springer Verlag.

[a]Axline and Simon.[44]

[b]McCracken and Jones.[45]

important because binding to plasma proteins results in a reduction in the free (unbound) drug concentration in plasma, and, consequently, the apparent volume of distribution increases in direct proportion to the extent of binding. Since the half-life of drug elimination increases with the volume of distribution, the time of elimination is also lengthened.

The combined effects of variation in protein binding and in renal elimination for drugs eliminated solely by glomerular filtration and exhibiting various degrees of binding can be computed by the mathematical model described by Keen.[48] The computed estimates for newborn infants and adults are compared in Table 4.5. These estimates show the multiple, F, by which plasma protein binding would increase the elimination half-life, assuming the initial free drug concentration is the same for newborns and adults.

Table 4.5 shows the greatest potential effect of protein binding on elimination half-life in both newborns and adults occurs for a drug confined to plasma water. For a highly bound drug (90% or more), there is at least a 10-fold increase in elimination half-life. The increase is the same in both age groups because the plasma water space, about 4–5% of the body weight, is the same in both groups. In contrast, when the drug is distributed in extracellular water, or total body water, plasma binding has smaller effects on the rate of drug elimination. In newborns,

Table 4.5 The Potential Effect of Plasma Protein Binding on Time of Drug Elimination in Newborns versus Adults after a Single Dose of Drugs Excreted by Glomerular Filtration[a]

Plasma protein binding (% bound)	Drug distributed in								
	Plasma water			Extracellular water			Total body water		
	V_D	$t\frac{1}{2}$	F	V_D	$t\frac{1}{2}$	F	V_D	$t\frac{1}{2}$	F
Newborn infant (3,400 g)	ml (140 ml)	Minute		ml (1,530 ml)	Minute		ml (2,630 ml)	Minute	
0	140	32	—	1,530	354	—	2,650	612	—
50	280	64	2	1,670	387	1.10	2,790	645	1.05
80	700	160	5	2,090	484	1.37	3,210	740	1.21
90	1,400	320	10	2,790	646	1.84	3,910	900	1.47
95	2,800	640	20	4,190	970	2.74	5,310	1220	2.00
Adult (70,000 g)	(3,000 ml)			(12,000 ml)			(41,000 ml)		
0	3,000	16	—	12,000	64	—	41,000	218	—
50	6,000	32	2	15,000	80	1.25	44,000	234	1.07
80	15,000	80	5	24,000	128	2.00	53,000	281	1.29
90	30,000	160	10	39,000	208	3.25	68,000	362	1.66
95	60,000	320	20	69,000	368	5.75	98,000	521	2.38

With permission from Springer Verlag.

[a]Calculated from Equations 5 and 12 of Keen.[48] F is the factor by which plasma protein binding increases the time for which the free drug concentration exceeds any given value assuming the initial free drug concentration is the same in each case.

the half-life is lengthened 2.74 times and in adults 5.75 times for a highly bound drug. The increase is dampened more effectively in newborns because the extracellular water accounts for a larger proportion of the body weight in newborns compared to adults (45% vs. 17%). The smaller difference in half-lives between newborn infants and adults for a drug distributed in total body water (1.47 vs. 1.66) is explained by similar reasoning.

For a 1-year-old child, the potential effect of protein binding on drug elimination by glomerular filtration and distributed in total body water, or in plasma water, should be approximately the same as for an adult because of the similarity of these compartments in these two age groups. On the other hand, extracellular water space does not reach the adult level by 1 year of age, so there is still a difference in elimination half-life as protein binding increases between a 1-year-old child and an adult. These relationships are graphically illustrated in Figure 4.2.

The effects described in Table 4.5 apply to a *single* dose of drug, but Keen's model[48] also applies to the potential effects of protein binding on plasma drug concentration and elimination in response after *repeated* drug dosing (Table 4.6). The effects on single dosing (Table 4.5) and on repeated dosing (Table 4.6) follow a similar pattern. Notice that for a highly bound drug, there is a 50% decrease in the maximum blood level of the drug, and the minimum level of the free drug can decrease to zero between doses. As with single dosing, the greatest potential effects occur when the drug is confined to plasma water in both newborn and adult, but when it is distributed in extracellular water, or in total body water,

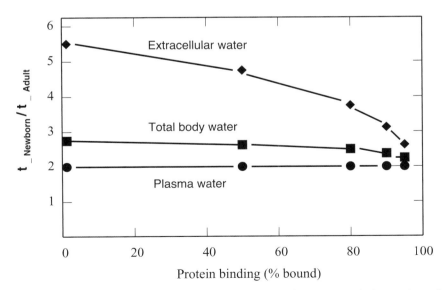

Figure 4.2 Effect of plasma protein binding on the relative rate of elimination of drugs excreted by glomerular filtration by newborn infants and adults.

Table 4.6 The Potential Effect of Plasma Protein Binding on Drug Plasma Levels and Time of Drug Elimination in Newborns versus Adults after Repeated Dosing of Drugs Excreted by Glomerular Filtration[a]

Plasma protein binding (% bound)	$t_{1/2}$	Drug distributed in												
		Plasma water			Extracellular water				Total body water				
		Max blood level	F'	Variation	$t_{1/2}$	Max blood level	F'	Variation	$t_{1/2}$	Max blood level	F'	Variation		
					Newborn infant (3,400 g)									
0	32	200	1	200→100	304	200	1	200→100	612	200	1	200→100		
50	64	133	0.67	133→33	387	187	0.94	187→87	645	193	0.97	193→93		
80	160	103	0.52	100→3	484	163	0.82	163→63	740	176	0.88	176→76		
90	320	100	0.50	100→0	646	130	0.70	139→39	900	156	0.78	156→56		
95	640	100	0.50	100→0	970	117	0.59	117→17	1220	133	0.67	133→33		
					Adult (70,000 g)									
0	16	200	1	200→100	64	200	1	200→100	218	200	1	200→100		
50	32	133	0.67	133→33	80	172	0.86	172→72	234	191	0.96	191→91		
80	80	103	0.52	100→3	128	133	0.67	133→33	281	169	0.85	169→69		
90	160	100	0.50	100→0	208	112	0.56	112→12	362	146	0.73	146→46		
95	320	100	0.50	100→0	368	102	0.51	102→2	521	124	0.62	124→24		

[a]Values tabulated were calculated assuming a single dose of drug gives a blood level of 100 units and is eliminated by a first-order process. For a first-order process with a rate constant k (time^{-1})

$$kt = 2.303 \log a/(a - x)$$

where $a =$ amount of drug present at time zero, $x =$ amount gone after time t, and $a - x =$ amount remaining after time t. It can be shown that

$$t_{1/2} = 2.303 \log 2/k$$

If we set $a = 1$, then

$$t_{1/2} = - \log (1 - x)/0.301$$

where $(1 - x)$ is the fraction of drug remaining. Also, since dose (here 100) $=$ (fraction drug gone at t), then the

maximum drug level$= 100/x$

and the variation in blood level is

$$100/x - 100$$

when the drug is given at intervals of time t. F' is the factor by which plasma binding decreases the maximum blood level assuming the initial free drug concentration is the same in each case, as described in Table 4.5.

plasma protein binding exerts smaller effects on maximum and minimum drug levels.

In healthy, elderly persons, age-dependent changes in plasma protein binding are generally not clinically relevant because drug elimination increases when the free (unbound) drug concentration is enhanced.[22] A decrease in plasma protein binding may thus obscure an age-related decrease in drug clearance.[8] Acidic drugs, such as diazepam, phenytoin, warfarin, and salicylic acid, bind principally to albumin, whereas basic drugs such as lignocaine and propanolol bind to α_1-acid glycoprotein. However, neither of these proteins has been observed to exhibit substantial changes in their concentrations in elderly persons.[18]

PHARMACODYNAMIC VARIATION

Pharmacology holds that a drug must be present at receptor sites to produce its characteristic response. The magnitude of the response depends on the concentration of the drug at the receptor sites (pharmacokinetics) as well as the number of receptors and the ability of the cells to respond to receptor occupation (pharmacodynamics). Pharmacodynamics contributes, independent of pharmacokinetics, to the total individual variability in drug response. Studies that combine measures of pharmacokinetic and pharmacodynamic variation are most illuminating, but technically they are more difficult to carry out. Since pharmacodynamic variation depends on the drug under consideration, broad generalizations are difficult. Hence, less information of a more limited character is available from which to determine the pharmacodynamics of drug responses in developing and aging persons.

Physicians often attempt to optimize the dose administered from the concentration of the drug in plasma. Because it is commonplace to have a 5-fold range of concentrations for the same dose, the drug concentration is usually a better predictor of drug effect than the dose administered. Nevertheless, there are drugs for which the opposite is true. The total variation accumulating along the way from drug administration to drug effect can be split into three parts[49]: (1) that due to the distribution of the drug from its site of administration into plasma, (2) that due to its distribution from plasma to target tissue, and (3) that due to the action of the drug in the receptor compartment. They show that part 2 may contribute more to the total variation than part 1. This is not a new idea, but heretofore it has been somewhat neglected because of the technical problems that limit accessibility of the target compartment. In the past few years there has been the development of innovative, noninvasive technologies (such as magnetic resonance spectroscopy, single-photon emission computed tomography) that permit measurements in defined regions and tissues, and for a few classes of drugs, preliminary data suggest that they permit measurement of the drug concentration in target tissue. Thus it may be possible in the future to improve on measuring the effect of development and aging on pharmacodynamics by paying less attention to plasma concentration measurements and focusing more on a target concentration strategy.

Prenatal Studies and Studies in Infants and Children

Pharmacotherapy based on studies in adults can lead to inappropriate handling of pediatric disorders because the actions of drugs on infants and children may differ sharply from those in mature individuals. Considerable evidence from rodent and other animal models indicates that receptor ontogeny is important during development and maturation, and that distinct patterns of change of opioids, adenosine A1, and serotonergic, dopaminergic, and adrenergic receptors have been observed prenatally and postnatally. The extent to which these findings are applicable to humans, though, is uncertain because few correlative human data are available.

The pediatric literature contains many clinical observations in which infants and children were found to be more susceptible than older children and adults to increased risk of toxicity from treatment with an assortment of drugs. A lengthy list includes impaired growth due to chronic treatment with adrenocorticosteroids, enamel dysplasia of developing teeth due to tetracycline antibiotics, dystonic reactions and seizures due to antiemetics such as metoclopramide and prochlorperazine, respiratory depression due to opioid antitussive agents, supratachyarrhythmias due to verapamil, and hepatoencephalopathy due to the anticonvulsant valproic acid. Infants and children may also be less susceptible to toxicity than adults from certain drugs. Examples include oto toxicity and renal toxicity from aminoglycoside antibiotics such as streptomycin, mild liver toxicity from acetaminophen, liver toxicity due to the general anesthetic, halothane, and isoniazid-induced hepatotoxicity. Most of these observations represent anecdotal observations from the older literature and, for the most part, the mechanisms by which they occurred were not investigated.

A recent survey of receptor pharmacogenetics based on the PubMed database turned up an abundance of information on a number of nuclear and cell surface receptors.[50] Among the most prevalent of the nuclear receptors for the most recent 5-year period for which data were available (1999–2003) were polymorphic receptors for glucocorticoids, mineralocorticoids, androgens, estrogens, retinoic acid, vitamin D, and arylhydrocarbon hydroylases, and among cell surface receptors were polymorphic receptors for ion channels, sulfonylurea, chemokines (CCR5, CCR2), angiotensin II Type 1, and receptors implicated in asthma (β_2-adrenergic, the high-affinity receptor for IgE, FcϵRI-β) and the Toll (TLR4) receptor implicated in endotoxic shock. A similar search for developmental changes among these receptors for infants and children failed to yield any citations for years 1996–2006. However, the search did identify citations on the developmental pharmacodynamics of the GABA receptor complex, neurotransmitter receptors in fetal brain, cyclosporine, warfarin, the cystic fibrosis transmembrane conductance regulator (CFTR), and the arachadonic cascade.

Consider first the actions of drugs that act at the GABA$_A$ receptor complex such as benzodiazepines and barbiturates. Children require larger doses than adults of numerous drugs including benzodiazepines and barbiturates. Chugani and associates[51] used positron emission tomography (PET) imaging, with a tracer,

[^{11}C]flumazenil, that binds specifically to α-subunits of the GABA$_A$ receptor to measure changes in flumazenil binding in various brain regions of nonhuman primates and epileptic children 2–17 years of age. Flumazenil PET has been used extensively to measure the GABA$_A$ receptor complex in a number of diseases including epilepsy. The flumazenil volume of distribution due to specific receptor binding was highest in children 2 years of age and declined exponentially to 50% of peak values by 17 years of age. These findings reveal changes in receptor ontogeny in a critical period of human development and help explain the requirement for larger doses of drugs acting at GABA$_A$ receptors in developing individuals.

The ability to manufacture neurotransmitters or their receptors is a common feature of developing cells. During development, receptor stimulation uniquely communicates with the genes that control cell differentiation, changing the ultimate fate of the cell, so that there are permanent alterations in responsiveness. In a series of elegant experiments employing nicotine as a tool to disrupt the natural flow of events in developing tissue, Slotkin and his associates have demonstrated that nicotine targets specific neurotransmitter receptors in the fetal brain, eliciting abnormalities of cell proliferation and differentiation, leading to shortfalls in the number of cells and eventually to altered synaptic activity. Apart from demonstrating the adverse effects of nicotine, Slotkin's studies have revealed the close regulatory association of cholinergic and catecholaminergic systems. They also show that disruption of multiple transmitter pathways may have immediate developmental consequences in the fetal brain, but also the eventual programming of synaptic competence.

Marshall and Kearns[52] investigated why and to what extent infants exhibit a greater immunosuppressive response to cyclosporine than older children and adults. They found that peripheral blood monocytes of infants showed a 2-fold lower mean IC$_{50}$ (peripheral blood monocyte proliferation) and 7-fold lower mean IC$_{90}$ (interleukin-2 expression) than peripheral blood monocytes from older subjects in response to cyclosporine. They believe these findings are related to the immaturity of the T-lymphocyte response in infants and are independent of pharmacokinetic differences in cyclosporine.

The study of warfarin enantiomers in Japanese children by Takahashi and colleagues provides another example of developmental changes in pharmacodynamics.[53] The anticoagulant response to warfarin is greater in prepubertal children than in pubertal children and adults independent of plasma S-warfarin and vitamin K concentrations. A greater inhibition of thrombin generation and lower plasma concentrations of protein C associated with a significantly greater international normalized ratio (INR) were observed in prepubertal persons compared to adults even though the mean vitamin K and S-warfarin concentrations were not different between the age groups. This suggests a greater sensitivity to warfarin in prepubertal children. The fact that vitamin K and S-warfarin concentrations did not differ seems to rule out a pharmacokinetic mechanism, although the exact pharmacodynamic mechanism remains to be determined.

Developmental changes in the CFTR gene and regulation of its developmental expression have been studied in great detail. In their recent assessment of the topic, McCarthy and Harris[54] review the structure and organization of the CFTR gene, a gene that encodes a 1480 amino acid protein that functions as an epithelial chloride channel. This protein is a member of the ATP-binding cassette (ABC) membrane transporter superfamily and is known to regulate other ion channels including the epithelial sodium channel (ENaC) and the volume-activated channel. Studies of mRNA *in situ* hybridization reveal the expression of the CFTR gene is tightly regulated temporally and spatially during development. The gene is expressed in pulmonic and pancreatic epithelia from before the start of the second trimester of human development and expression levels are high in the mid-trimester pancreas. Between the second trimester of gestation and postnatal life, CFTR expression levels in most tissues show little fluctuation. In lung epithelia, the high expression levels of CFTR mRNA that persist throughout fetal life are in contrast with the much lower levels at birth and into adulthood. However, there appears to be a shift in the cellular profile of CFTR expression as gestation advances. During the first trimester, CFTR expression in the trachea was intermediate and diffuse. In the second trimester, expression was reduced and was limited to a subset of tracheal epithelia. And by the third trimester, only individual cells expressed CFTR, but at very high levels. In postnatal human lung epithelium significant CFTR expression is limited to specific cells of the submucosal glands and individual cells in the airway surface epithelium. In the pancreas, small intestine, and colon, high levels of CFTR expression are present from an early gestational age, but in contrast to lung expression patterns, levels in these tissues remain constant throughout gestation.[55] Investigators have suggested that the higher levels of CFTR expression in the airway epithelium during the second trimester may correspond to an important functional change of CFTR at this developmental stage. For example, it might be a consequence of the change in function of the respiratory epithelium for chloride secretion to sodium absorption near term; recent data indicate that ENaC is inhibited by CFTR, and the decline in CFTR expression mRNA and protein would be compatible with enabling ENaC activity. An additional possibility is that CFTR expression in fetal lung epithelium has an as yet undefined role in the normal maturation of lung development. Thus, although lung epithelia pathology in cystic fibrosis is uncommon at birth, there is often evidence of inflammation in the absence of functional CFTR protein.

The arachadonic acid cascade provides an excellent example of how metabolic and receptor-related aspects of development may be so closely entwined as to be virtually inseparable. More than a decade ago, Nebert proposed that oxidative metabolism by the P450-mediated metabolism of xenobiotics and endogenous ligands involved in growth and differentiation were both components of a much broader set of functions implicit in fetal development involving the concerted actions of genes during organogenesis as receptor and signal transduction systems are established and as organ function matures.[56] CYP3A7 is involved in the placental biosynthesis of the endogenous ligand, estriol, but it may have additional functions of potential importance during gestation by protecting the fetus from the inhibitory effects of high concentrations of dehydroepiandrosterone 3-sulfate (DHEA-S) on cell proliferation and progesterone synthesis, and by protecting it from the embryotoxic effects of retinoic acid, particularly from exogenous sources.[29] In a study by Leeder and associates, CYP3A7 was found to be the most abundant CYP3A mRNA in a panel of fetal livers.[57] They observed that the hydroxylation of testosterone and DHEA-S hydroxylation vary by 175- to 250-fold across the entire panel, and mRNA by about 10-fold (634-fold if five outliers with extremely low values were included). Some other features of CYP3A7 relevant to developmental changes in hepatic drug-metabolizing activity of the human fetus were considered above. Given its potential importance on fetal development, Leeder's laboratory investigated the effect of the developmental expression of CYP3A7 on various nuclear receptors[58] such as the pregnane X receptor (PXR) and the constitutive androstane receptor (CAR), receptors whose expression is known to be induced by various xenobiotics including therapeutically important drugs such as phenobarbital and rifampin. They found that RNA of PXR and CAR was expressed at low and highly variable levels in prenatal and neonatal liver compared to those in older children, whereas mRNA expression of RXRα was less variable and did not differ appreciably between the prenatal and postnatal liver. Still further, CYP3A7 mRNA expression was significantly correlated with PXR and CAR mRNA in the fetal liver, but associations were weaker than those for CYP3A4 mRNA in the postnatal liver. These findings support the contention put forward recently by Handschin and Meyer[59] that nuclear receptors can act as sensors of xenobiotics, coordinating the metabolism and elimination of xenobiotics in fetal life.

As a result of studies, CYP2J2, one of the newer members of the CYP2 family involved in the P450-mediated cascade of arachadonic acid metabolism, has emerged as one of the major enzymes in the formation of eicosatetraenoic and eicosatrienoic acids (EETs) in extrahepatic tissues.[60] Because EETs have such a wide tissue distribution, are highly conserved, and play a critical role in the regulation of renal, pulmonary, and cardiovascular function of adults, they may also be functionally crucial in human development. Quantitative studies of CYP2J2 expression performed on fetal liver and various other fetal tissues showed the presence of CYP2J2 in postnatal liver samples.[61] The amounts of immunoreactive protein varied substantially among samples without an apparent relationship to the transcript number or genotype, and Western blot analysis revealed a qualitative change in the protein pattern between prenatal and postnatal liver samples. Whether CYP2J2 has unidentified effects on receptor populations of the fetus similar to that of CYP3A7 remains to be determined, warranting further study of the mechanisms leading to variable amounts of immunoreactive protein and distinct prenatal and postnatal CYP2J2 protein patterns.

Studies in Aging Persons

Aging is associated with a broad range of important changes in the major organ and bodily systems.[1,10,18,62] Modern noninvasive techniques increasingly have provided a means to investigate the time course and extent of morphological and functional changes in aging populations. The cardiovascular system is exemplary for analyses by echocardiographic and plethysmographic methods, and for laser

Doppler measurements of cardiac output and regional blood flow that have greatly facilitated the identification of true age-related changes. Such studies have demonstrated a reduction in the elasticity and compliance of the great arteries, in left ventricular ejection and the rate of cardiac relaxation, in the prolongation of isotonic contraction, and in the decrease in its velocity. Moreover, extensive studies of neurohormonal mechanisms controlling the cardiovascular system have confirmed classically defined changes in vascular control systems[63] and revealed novel peripheral control vascular mechanisms for autonomic nerve transmitters, autocoid mediators, smooth muscle receptors, and ion channel mechanisms linked to age-related alterations of endothelial and vessel wall functions.[64,65] In the neuroendocrine system as another example, age-related changes in response to psychosocial or physical stress have been observed in the hypothalamic–pituitary–adrenal (HPA) axis. For instance, excessive HPA activation and hypersecretion of glucocorticoids can lead to dendritic atrophy in neurons of the hippocampus, resulting in impairment of learning and memory. The potential for further damage to hippocampal neurons caused by elevated glucocorticoid concentrations may result from impaired feedback inhibition of the HPA axis and glucocorticoid secretion.

Table 4.7 Some Clinically Important Pharmacodynamic Changes Associated with Aging[18]

Drug	Pharmacodynamic effect	Age-related change
Adenosine	Heart rate response	No significant change
Diazepam	Sedation, postural sway	Increase
Diltiazem	Acute and chronic antihypertensive effect	Increase
	Acute PR interval prolongation	Decrease
Diphenhydramine	Postural sway	No significant change
Enalpril	Angiotensin-converting enzyme inhibition	No significant change
Furosemide	Peak diuretic response	Decrease
Heparin	Anticoagulant effect	No significant change
Isoproterenol	Chronotropic effect	Decrease
Morphine	Analgesic effect	Increase
	Respiratory depression	No significant change
Phenylephrine	α_1-Adrenergic responsiveness	No significant change
Propranolol	Antagonism of chronotropic effects of isoproterenol	Decrease
Scopolamine	Cognitive function	Decrease
Temazepam	Postural sway	Increase
Verapamil	Acute antihypertensive effect	Increase
Warfarin	Anticoagulant effect	Increase

Some important age-related pharmacodynamic changes, many of which involve cardiac or neuroleptic drugs, are listed in Table 4.7.[18] The exact mechanisms responsible for these changes are unknown, but it seems reasonable to expect that the constitutional changes alluded to above may have a bearing on their occurrence.

SUMMARY

Drug disposition and the dynamics of drug responsiveness change with maturation and aging. Such changes tend to occur in an orderly sequence at predictable stages in life, but their onset and extent can vary widely from one person to another. During infancy and childhood, these changes are usually rapid and are either periodic or cyclic, whereas they tend to occur more gradually but asynchronously with advancing age so that individual variability in disposition and response increases substantially among elderly persons. In general, bodily clearance of therapeutic agents and toxicants is an age-related function of metabolic and renal capacity. During infancy, transitory insufficiency in metabolic pathways explains the reduced metabolism of most drugs, while maturation of existing renal structures accounts for the low level of drug clearance. Consequently, the dose and/or time of administration of most drugs is decreased during the first few weeks after birth to avoid toxicity. In elderly persons, a reduction in hepatic and renal clearance prolongs drug elimination, and pharmacodynamic changes may alter the sensitivity to many drugs that are frequently used in older persons. However, broad generalizations are difficult, and less information of a more limited character is available because pharmacodynamic variation depends on the specific drug under consideration.

REFERENCES

1. Shock NW. Age changes in some physiologic processes. Geriatrics 1957; 12(1):40–48.
2. Nyhan WL. Toxicity of drugs in the neonatal period. J Pediatr 1961; 59:1–20.
3. Done AK. Developmental pharmacology. Clin Pharmacol Ther 1964; 5:432–479.
4. Szorady I. Developmental pharmacology. Trends Pharmacol Sci 1982; 3(Apr):142–144.
5. Yaffe SJ, Arand JV. Neonatal and Pediatric Pharmacology. Therapeutic Principles in Practice, 3rd ed. Philadelphia: Lippincott Williams & Wilkins, 2004.
6. Crooks J, Stevenson IH. Drugs and the Elderly. Baltimore: University Park Press, 1979.
7. Weber WW, Cohen SN. Aging effects and drugs in man. In: Gillette JR, Mitchell JR, editors. Concepts in Biochemical Pharmacology. New York: Springer-Verlag, 1975: 213–233.
8. Turnheim K. Drug therapy in the elderly. Exp Gerontol 2004; 39(11–12):1731–1738.
9. Cusack BJ. Pharmacokinetics in older persons. Am J Geriatr Pharmacother 2004; 2(4):274–302.
10. McLean AJ, Le Couteur DG. Aging biology and geriatric clinical pharmacology. Pharmacol Rev 2004; 56(2):163–184.

11. Schmucker DL. Age-related changes in liver structure and function: Implications for disease? Exp Gerontol 2005; 40(8–9):650–659.

12. Hollingsworth JW, Hashizume A, Jablon S. Correlations between tests of aging in Hiroshima subjects—an attempt to define "physiologic age." Yale J Biol Med 1965; 38(1):11–26.

13. Norris AH, Shock NW. Aging and variability. Ann NY Acad Sci 1966; 134:591–601.

14. McMahon T. Size and shape in biology. Science 1973; 179(79):1201–1204.

15. Stahl WR. Organ weights in primates and other mammals. Science 1965; 150(699): 1039–1042.

16. Butler AM, Richie RH. Simplification and improvement in estimating drug dosage and fluid and dietary allowances for patients of varying sizes. N Engl J Med 1960; 262:903–908.

17. Kearns GL, Abdel-Rahman SM, Alander SW, Blowey DL, Leeder JS, Kauffman RE. Developmental pharmacology—drug disposition, action, and therapy in infants and children. N Engl J Med 2003; 349(12):1157–1167.

18. Mangoni AA, Jackson SH. Age-related changes in pharmacokinetics and pharmacodynamics: Basic principles and practical applications. Br J Clin Pharmacol 2003; 57(1):6–14.

19. Friis-Hansen B. Body water compartments in children: Changes during growth and related changes in body composition. Pediatrics 1961; 28:169–181.

20. Morselli PL, Franco-Morselli R, Bossi L. Clinical pharmacokinetics in newborns and infants. Age-related differences and therapeutic implications. Clin Pharmacokinet 1980; 5(6):485–527.

21. Thummel KE, Shen DD, Isoherranen N, Smith HE. Design and optimization of dosage regimens: Pharmacokinetic data. In: Brunton LL, Lazo JS, Parker KL, editors. Goodman and Gilman's The Pharmacological Basis of Therapeutics. New York: McGraw-Hill, 2006: 1787–1888.

22. Benet LZ, Hoener BA. Changes in plasma protein binding have little clinical relevance. Clin Pharmacol Ther 2002; 71(3):115–121.

23. Asteriadou-Samartzis E, Leikin S. The relation of vitamin K to hyperbilirubinemia. Pediatrics 1958; 21(3):397–402.

24. Silverman WA, Andersen DH, Blanc WA, Crozier DN. A difference in mortality rate and incidence of kernicterus among premature infants allotted to two prophylactic antibacterial regimens. Pediatrics 1956; 18(4):614–625.

25. Weiss CF, Glazko AJ, Weston JK. Chloramphenicol in the newborn infant. A physiologic explanation of its toxicity when given in excessive doses. N Engl J Med 1960; 262:787–794.

26. Nelson DR, Zeldin DC, Hoffman SM, Maltais LJ, Wain HM, Nebert DW. Comparison of cytochrome P450 (CYP) genes from the mouse and human genomes, including nomenclature recommendations for genes, pseudogenes and alternative-splice variants. Pharmacogenetics 2004; 14(1):1–18.

27. Guengerich FP. Human cytochrome P450 enzymes. In: Ortiz de Montellano PR, editor. Cytochrome P450. Structure, Mechanism, and Biochemistry. New York: Kluwer Academic/Plenum, 2005: 377.

28. Hines RN, McCarver DG. The ontogeny of human drug-metabolizing enzymes: Phase I oxidative enzymes. J Pharmacol Exp Ther 2002; 300(2):355–360.

29. Sim SC, Edwards RJ, Boobis AR, Ingelman-Sundberg M. CYP3A7 protein expression is high in a fraction of adult human livers and partially associated with the CYP3A7*1C allele. Pharmacogenet Genomics 2005; 15(9):625–631.

30. Lacroix D, Sonnier M, Moncion A, Cheron G, Cresteil T. Expression of CYP3A in the human liver—evidence that the shift between CYP3A7 and CYP3A4 occurs immediately after birth. Eur J Biochem 1997; 247(2):625–634.

31. Ward RM. Drug disposition in the late preterm ("near-term") newborn. Semin Perinatol 2006; 30(1):48–51.

32. McCarver DG, Hines RN. The ontogeny of human drug-metabolizing enzymes: Phase II conjugation enzymes and regulatory mechanisms. J Pharmacol Exp Ther 2002; 300(2):361–366.

33. Le Couteur DG, McLean AJ. The aging liver. Drug clearance and an oxygen diffusion barrier hypothesis. Clin Pharmacokinet 1998; 34(5):359–373.

34. Muiras ML, Verasdonck P, Cottet F, Schachter F. Lack of association between human longevity and genetic polymorphisms in drug-metabolizing enzymes at the NAT2, GSTM1 and CYP2D6 loci. Hum Genet 1998; 102(5):526–532.

35. Rane A. Drug metabolism and disposition in infants and children. In: Yaffe SJ, Arand JV, editors. Neonatal and Pediatric Pharmacology. Therapeutic Principles and Practice. Philadelphia: Lippincott Williams & Wilkins, 2004: 32–43.

36. Sotaniemi EA, Arranto AJ, Pelkonen O, Pasanen M. Age and cytochrome P450-linked drug metabolism in humans: An analysis of 226 subjects with equal histopathologic conditions. Clin Pharmacol Ther 1997; 61(3):331–339.

37. Wynne HA, Cope LH, Mutch E, Rawlins MD, Woodhouse KW, James OF. The effect of age upon liver volume and apparent liver blood flow in healthy man. Hepatology 1989; 9(2):297–301.

38. Schmucker DL. Liver function and phase I drug metabolism in the elderly: A paradox. Drugs Aging 2001; 18(11):837–851.

39. Cotreau MM, von Moltke LL, Greenblatt DJ. The influence of age and sex on the clearance of cytochrome P450 3A substrates. Clin Pharmacokinet 2005; 44(1):33–60.

40. Pratt WB. The entry, distribution and elimination of drugs. In: Pratt WB, Taylor P, editors. Principles of Drug Action. The Basis of Pharmacology. New York: Churchill Livingstone, 1990: 201–296.

41. Barnett HL, Hare K, McNamara H, Hare R. Measurement of glomerular filtration rate in premature infants. J Clin Invest 1948; 27(6):691–699.

42. West JR, Smith HW, Chasis H. Glomerular filtration rate, effective renal blood flow, and maximal tubular excretory capacity in infancy. J Pediatr 1948; 32:10–18.

43. Davies DF, Shock NW. Age changes in glomerular filtration rate, effective renal plasma flow, and tubular excretory capacity in adult males. J Clin Invest 1950; 29(5):496–507.

44. Axline SG, Simon HJ. Clinical pharmacology of antimicrobials in premature infants. I. Kanamycin, streptomycin, and neomycin. Antimicrobial Agents Chemother (Bethesda) 1964; 10:135–141.

45. McCracken GH Jr, Jones LG. Gentamicin in the neonatal period. Am J Dis Child 1970; 120(6):524–533.

46. Barnett HL, McNamara H, Shultz S, Tompsett R. Renal clearances of sodium penicillin G, procaine penicillin G, and inulin in infants and children. Pediatrics 1949; 1949:418–422.

47. Axline SG, Yaffe SJ, Simon HJ. Clinical pharmacology of antimicrobials in premature infants. II. Ampicillin, methicillin, oxacillin, neomycin, and colistin. Pediatrics 1967; 39(1):97–107.

48. Keen P. Effect of binding to plasma proteins on the distribution, activity and elimination of drugs. In: Brodie BB, Gillette JR, editors. Concepts in Biochemical Pharmacology. Berlin: Springer-Verlag, 1971: 213–233.

49. Fick DM, Cooper JW, Wade WE, Waller JL, Maclean JR, Beers MH. Updating the Beers criteria for potentially inappropriate medication use in older adults: Results of a US consensus panel of experts. Arch Intern Med 2003; 163(22):2716–2724.

50. Weber WW. Receptors. In: Kalow W, editor. Pharmacogenetics. New York: Taylor & Francis, 2005: 71–108.

51. Chugani DC, Muzik O, Juhasz C, Janisse JJ, Ager J, Chugani HT. Postnatal maturation of human GABAA receptors measured with positron emission tomography. Ann Neurol 2001; 49(5):618–626.

52. Marshall JD, Kearns GL. Developmental pharmacodynamics of cyclosporine. Clin Pharmacol Ther 1999; 66(1):66–75.

53. Takahashi H, Ishikawa S, Nomoto S, Nishigaki Y, Ando F, Kashima T, et al. Developmental changes in pharmacokinetics and pharmacodynamics of warfarin enantiomers in Japanese children. Clin Pharmacol Ther 2000; 68(5):541–555.

54. McCarthy VA, Harris A. The CFTR gene and regulation of its expression. Pediatr Pulmonol 2005; 40(1):1–8.

55. Broackes-Carter FC, Mouchel N, Gill D, Hyde S, Bassett J, Harris A. Temporal regulation of CFTR expression during ovine lung development: Implications for CF gene therapy. Hum Mol Genet 2002; 11(2):125–131.

56. Nebert DW. Drug-metabolizing enzymes in ligand-modulated transcription. Biochem Pharmacol 1994; 47(1):25–37.

57. Leeder JS, Gaedigk R, Marcucci KA, Gaedigk A, Vyhlidal CA, Schindel BP, et al. Variability of CYP3A7 expression in human fetal liver. J Pharmacol Exp Ther 2005; 314(2):626–635.

58. Vyhlidal CA, Gaedigk R, Leeder JS. Nuclear receptor expression in fetal and pediatric liver: Correlation with CYP3A expression. Drug Metab Dispos 2006; 34(1):131–137.

59. Handschin C, Meyer UA. Induction of drug metabolism: The role of nuclear receptors. Pharmacol Rev 2003; 55(4):649–673.

60. Roman RJ. P-450 metabolites of arachidonic acid in the control of cardiovascular function. Physiol Rev 2002; 82(1):131–185.

61. Gaedigk A, Baker DW, Totah RA, Gaedigk R, Pearce RE, Vyhlidal CA, et al. Variability of CYP2J2 expression in human fetal tissues. J Pharmacol Exp Ther 2006; 319(2):523–532.

62. Strehler BL. Origin and comparison of the effects of time and high-energy radiations on living systems. Q Rev Biol 1959; 34(2):117–142.

63. Folkow B, Svanborg A. Physiology of cardiovascular aging. Physiol Rev 1993; 73(4):725–764.

64. Andrawis N, Jones DS, Abernethy DR. Aging is associated with endothelial dysfunction in the human forearm vasculature. J Am Geriatr Soc 2000; 48(2):193–198.

65. Lakatta EG, Levy D. Arterial and cardiac aging: Major shareholders in cardiovascular disease enterprises: Part I: Aging arteries: A "set up" for vascular disease. Circulation 2003; 107(1):139–146.

5

Genetics in Pharmacology

By dint of their background and interests, pharmacologists would look for a defect in a drug's pharmacokinetics or pharmacodynamics to explain therapeutic failure or toxicity, but scientists of other biomedical disciplines might interpret the same observations differently. Geneticists, who are more likely to focus on characteristics that differentiate individuals from each other rather than concentrating on their similarities, might view a drug as an exogenous substance on which individuals could exert selective effects. They might consider an unusual drug response as a reflection of a difference in the genetic makeup of normal and unusual responders, and would come up with a different set of testable hypotheses to identify the cause of the difference.

From the 1950s and through the 1970s, investigators combined biochemical and pharmacological approaches with classical genetic methods of analysis to scrutinize unusual drug responses. The person-to-person differences in drug response that they studied in twins and families are excellent models to guide present studies of these phenomena. Technological advances, especially the invention and adoption of recombinant DNA techniques and allied technologies in the 1970s and 1980s, have played a definitive role in pharmacogenetic investigation. Genetic profiling of human drug response was introduced briefly in Chapter 2, and this chapter discusses how this task was combined with pharmacological profiling of drug responses in the era of molecular biology.

THE FINE STRUCTURE OF GENETIC PROFILING HUMAN DRUG RESPONSE

Hereditary differences in human drug responses are broadly characterized by two types of information: the genetics of the inheritance of the trait and the biochemical/molecular basis of the trait. To assess the relative contributions of heredity and environment of pharmacogenetic traits, the principles and tools of classical human and population genetics, biochemistry, and epidemiology are used in concert to analyze pharmacological and toxicological observations of individuals, twins, families, and larger populations. Studies in identical and fraternal twins are used to determine whether the response in question is affected by the presence (or absence) of hereditary elements. Information collected on affected individuals and their families is also used for this purpose, but the patterns of inheritance observed within families can also determine whether a given trait is due to heterogeneity at a single gene locus or at multiple loci. Hereditary peculiarities in human drug response often exhibit genetic heterogeneity (i.e., involve different genes or alleles, in different persons) and many single-gene differences have been found (i.e., only one locus is thought to be responsible in any particular family). Monogenic traits may appear to be more plentiful, but this is probably because they are more easily identified and analyzed, and not because they actually occur more frequently than multifactorial or polygenic traits. Family studies also enable the investigator to discriminate various modes of genetic transmission (sex linkage vs. autosomal linkage), and to determine the dominance–recessivity relationships that characterize the expression of the trait. The sensitivity of a given drug will be due, in certain persons, to new mutations, as is well known for other kinds of human hereditary traits, and just as their genetic and demographic features may vary between different ethnic and geographic populations, the incidence and etiology of pharmacogenetic traits may also vary.

But classical genetic techniques alone do not make it possible to identify the molecular basis of a trait. Their capacity is limited because the existence of allelic variants of genes can be inferred only one gene at a time from information they provide, whereas recombinant DNA techniques and allied technologies enable variant forms of many genes to be described directly. From molecular studies in individuals and in populations, a strong case can be made for large-scale, structural and functional analysis of genetic polymorphisms and genetic diversity aimed at producing a complete catalog of human diversity. By identifying the functions of the natural and variant forms of proteins encoded in the human genome, it is not unreasonable to expect that associations between the genetic makeup of individuals and individual susceptibility to human disease will be discovered. Similarly, by establishing associations with responsiveness to specific therapeutic agents, foods, and other exogenous substances, prospects for better therapies and for predictive biology including individualized medicine will be improved.

Human genetic disorders are due to structural lesions of DNA and based on their size, two groups of genetic disorders are distinguished. There are chromosomal disorders with lesions of several megabases that are large enough to be visualized under light microscopy by cytogenetic techniques, and genic disorders with smaller lesions that can be observed by isolation of the DNA molecules themselves. A few examples of chromosomal pharmacogenetic disorders are known, but the vast majority of known pharmacogenetic traits are genic disorders.

Recombinant DNA technologies have lowered the limit of observation from a few megabases of DNA down to a single base, the smallest unit of heredity. Various methods of specific recognition, such as Southern analysis, Northern analysis, and pulsed field electrophoresis, have extended the range upward through a few kilobases to a few megabases into the cytogenetic range, so that the entire range of lesions has come into view.

SOME ELEMENTARY FEATURES OF THE HUMAN GENOME

The human genome consists of nuclear and mitochondrial DNA sequences. In round numbers, the nuclear sequences of humans consist of approximately three billion base pairs.

The Nuclear Genome

Nuclear DNA is a linear molecule roughly 2 m in length when extended; when folded into the nucleus, it occupies a sphere of about 10 μm in diameter. In human cells, the nuclear DNA sequences are carried on 22 chromosomes plus an X and a Y chromosome in males and two Xs in females. Normally, everyone has two copies of each chromosome (except for the sex chromosomes) and the genes they carry.

Each chromosome has a characteristic length[1] and a distinctive banding pattern. Bands on the long and short arms are numbered from the centromere toward the telomere. Bands on the short arm are designated by "p" and bands on the long arm by "q" followed by the region number, and the band number within that region; subdivisions of bands are designated by a decimal point and a number. Each gene occupies a particular spot on its chromosome. For example, NAT2 is located at 8p21.3–23.1, which means that NAT2 is situated on the short arm of chromosome 8 within band 2, and between region 1, subdivision 3 and region 3, subdivision 1. The glucose-6-phosphate dehydrogenase (G6PD) gene assigned to Xq28 is located in band 2, region 8 on the long arm of the X chromosome.

In eukaryotes and prokaryotes, the genes and the polypeptides they encode are colinear along the DNA molecule, but, unlike prokaryotic genes, almost all eukaryotic genes are divided into exons (*expressed regions*) separated by introns (*intervening regions*). Much of the human genome, as well as those of other higher eukaryotes, consists of sequences whose genetic function is not clearly defined, and for many purposes it is convenient to divide the genome into sequences of three types: the coding sequences along with untranslated regions of exons (UTRs) and their associated promoter regions; the intronic sequences and various repetitive sequences; and the mobile sequences, such as the transposons. Differences in the structure and function between them are relevant to the molecular basis of protein diversity.

Coding sequences encode the messages for synthesis and targeting of proteins. They occupy a small part, 5% or less, of the human genome. Proteins are composed of structural domains that contribute to their three-dimensional architecture and stability, and of functional domains such as binding regions, catalytic sites, and folding elements. Exons are often regarded as units that encode structural or functional domains that remain intact during synthesis and targeting of proteins, and it has been proposed that domain duplication at the protein level corresponds to exon duplication at the DNA level. It has also been suggested that exons can be shuffled independently and that exon shuffling has played a major role in the evolution of higher organisms.[2]

The sequences of eukaryotic nuclear DNA surrounding exons are composed of introns and repetitive sequences. Introns and repetitive sequences may occupy 70% or more of the human genome. Introns may protect exons from mutation, but, except for DNA close to exons, they may not be crucial for their expression as changes in these sequences have no known effect. Repetitive tracts of DNA contribute a variable but significant proportion to the total genomic DNA of eukaryotic chromosomes. The base composition of these sequences is highly heterogeneous. When total genomic DNA is sheared and allowed to reassociate, these elements tend to form "satellite bands" when centrifuged in a density gradient. All such bands have been called satellite DNA from time to time but the term is now usually restricted to tandem repeats of DNA in centromeric and telomeric regions of the chromosome regardless of whether they form bands on a density gradient. Satellite DNAs are often associated with chromatin, although their genetic function has not been clearly defined. Primary sequence analysis of cloned satellite DNA has shown that a great deal of variation occurs within them. In certain instances, a repetitive satellite unit may contain polymorphic sites for restriction endonucleases, and because these polymorphisms are inherited in Mendelian fashion, they are useful in isolation and analysis of hereditary traits as discussed below (see p. 130).

The mobile sequences occupy the remainder of the human genome. They are transposable from one location to a new location and are also referred to as "jumping genes." Transposable elements have been identified as a common feature of prokaryotic and eukaryotic genomes. They are a specific group of genomic elements dispersed throughout the genome, many of which have repetitive sequences present in hundreds or thousands of copies, and they may contain several genes in addition to those essential to their mobility. Transposable elements are responsible for a wide range of mutations and are thought to play a role in shaping evolution, but exactly how they move about and what effects they produce are unknown. Since the mobile sequences may contain other genes with functional regulatory domains, they may also interfere with gene expression. In other instances, insertion of transposons at a new location may interrupt coding sequences, UTRs, or their control regions to inactivate genes.[3]

Evidence for the *de novo* insertion of a transposable element into the blood clotting factor VIII gene on the X chromosome of humans was reported for two hemophilia patients.[4,5] The inserted element was also found to possess reverse transcriptase activity that could represent a potential source of the activity necessary for its relocation. This was one of the first demonstrations that transposable elements can also cause human genetic disease. On the other hand, the scattering of these mobile sequences around the human genome and the effects of mutations in them may, in some instances, benefit the organism by immobilizing them; or they may have been important in the development of whole families of proteins such as the hemoglobins, the cytochrome P450 drug-metabolizing enzymes, and the drug receptors.

Chromosomal translocation is another mechanism by which genes, in this case groups of genes, can move from one location to another in the genome. Reciprocal translocation entails a rupture of the two chromosomes that then fuse their breakpoints to form a chimeric gene. Sometimes a translocation moves a quiescent gene close to an active promoter. Examples of chromosomal translocation of pharmacogenetic importance are glucocorticoid-remediable hypertension[6,7] and resistance to treatment of acute promyelocytic leukemia with all-*trans*-retinoic acid.[8–10]

Additional structural features of DNA that are capable of affecting gene expression are described below (see Chapter 6).

The Mitochondrial Genome

The genetic analysis of the mitochondrial genome (mtDNA), which started as a search for a model system to study gene expression, spanned some 15 years and involved the intimate collaboration of Giuseppe Attardi's laboratory at the California Institute of Technology and Fred Sanger's Laboratory of Molecular Biology at Cambridge University, epitomizes the power of biochemical, electron microscopic, and immunological techniques, and led to the discovery of a genome with unique features of gene organization and expression.[11] Human mtDNA is a compact, circular, double-stranded molecule that contains 16,569 base pairs located within the mitochondrial matrix and anchored at one end to the inner mitochondrial membrane.[12] mtDNA contains 37 genes encoding 22 tRNAs, 12S and 16S ribosomal RNAs, and 13 proteins involved in oxidative phosphorylation. The sequence and organization of human mtDNA differ in several respects from those of the DNA double helix. For example, the genes have none or only a few noncoding bases between them. In many cases, the termination codons are not coded in the DNA but are created posttranscriptionally by polyadenylation of the mRNAs. Additionally, the genetic code differs from the universal code in that UGA codes for tryptophan and not for termination, AUA codes for methionine not isoleucine, and AGA and AGG are termination rather than arginine codons. A 1-kilobase noncoding region contains both promoters and the replication site of origin. The two strands of mtDNA are distinguished as heavy (guanosine rich) and light (cytosine rich). mtDNA does not have DNA repair systems analogous to those of the nucleus, potentially increasing the vulnerability of mtDNA to damage from lipophilic xenobiotics.

At cell division the mitochondria are distributed randomly to daughter cells. If a parental cell contains only normal mitochondria, homoplasmy is said to exist. But if the parental cell contains mutant as well as normal mitochondria, a condition known as heteroplasmy exists, and the proportion of mutant versus normal mitochondria inherited by the heteroplasmic daughter cells will vary. In mammals, less than one mtDNA in a thousand is derived from the father in an average individual, and the transmission of mtDNA occurs almost exclusively through the maternal lineage. A trait that shows maternal inheritance and distributes to sons and daughters could thus be explained by a mutation in a mitochondrial gene.

Mitochondrial genetics is complicated by the unique characteristics of mtDNA inheritance. Mitochondrial disorders are attributed to at least three sources of variation—the particular locus affected, the type of mutation (point mutation, deletion, duplication), and the fraction of mutant mitochondria present in tissues and individuals when heteroplasmy exists; other factors including the nuclear genotype, aging, and the environment, particularly chemical exposure, can also contribute to mitochondrial variation. Typically, a mutation in the mitochondrial genome is sought when clinical findings involve tissues with high energy demands, such as disorders of the brain or skeletal muscle. The same clinical clue would not have suggested mitochondrial mutation in a rare type of maturity-onset diabetes; instead, the pattern of transmission through the maternal line provided that clue. Similarly, the pattern of maternal transmission in aminoglycoside antibiotic-induced deafness provided the clue to the inheritance of this pharmacogenetic trait (see Appendix A).

FRAMEWORK FOR DISSECTING GENETIC VARIATION IN HUMAN DRUG RESPONSE

The basic problem in analyzing the genetics of human variation is to find a means of quantitating the degree of resemblance between related individuals from their overt characteristics. Geneticists have tackled this problem by partitioning the variation in observed characteristics—that is, in the phenotype (from the Greek *phainein* "to show") of individuals in a population—into components attributable to hereditary causes and those attributable to environmental causes. If the relative sizes of the hereditary and environmental components were known (or could be determined), it should be possible, on the further assumption of Mendelian inheritance, to predict the degree of resemblance between related individuals.

These ideas were first put on a quantitative footing in 1918 by Ronald Fisher[13] who proposed the phenotypic variance (V_P) be considered as the sum of the variance of genetic factors (V_G) and the variance embracing all of the environmental factors (V_E). He partitioned the genetic variance into three subcomponents: those due to the additive effects of all allelic genes (V_A), the variance due to dominance effects (V_D), and the variance due to interactions between loci (V_I). The total phenotypic (observed) variance in Fisher's model is thus

$$V_P = V_G + V_E = V_A + V_D + V_I + V_E \qquad (5.1)$$

V_A is a function of the difference between homozygotes—it is usually the most important of the subcomponents that comprise V_G both biologically and numerically. V_D refers to deviations of the heterozygotes from the mean of the two homozygotes. V_I is less well understood, and D.S. Falconer suggested that V_I contributed only a small amount to the total V_G and neglecting it was not likely to introduce a serious error (see Chapters 8 and 9[14]).

Fisher also showed that certain quantitative relationships could be defined from correlations and regressions between relatives of different degrees on the

Table 5.1 Phenotypic Resemblance Between Relatives of Different Degrees[a]

Relatives	Regression (b) or correlation (t)	Covariance
Offspring and one parent	$b = \frac{1}{2}\,[V_A/V_P]$	$\frac{1}{2}V_A$
Offspring and midparent	$b = V_A/V_P$	$\frac{1}{2}V_A$
Half sibs	$t = \frac{1}{4}[V_A/V_P]$	$\frac{1}{4}[V_A/V_P]$
Full sibs	$t = [\frac{1}{2}V_A + \frac{1}{4}V_D + V_E]/V_P$	$\frac{1}{2}V_A + \frac{1}{4}V_D + V_E$

[a]*Source*: Adapted from Falconer,[14] Table 9.4. For a more complete account of the theoretical basis for these relationships, see Falconer, Chapters 8 and 9.[14]

supposition of Mendelian inheritance (Table 5.1). From Table 5.1, the resemblance between relatives of different degrees expressed by the variances composing V_P is apparent. For instance, the regression of offspring on one parent is twice the correlation between half-siblings, and the correlation between full siblings (in the absence of dominance and environmental contributions) is twice the correlation between half-siblings. Intuitively, both of these relationships are reasonable.

TWIN STUDIES

Identical (monozygous) and fraternal (dizygous) twins provide a unique resource for studying the relative importance of heredity and environment. The technique of using twin study, originally devised by Francis Galton during the nineteenth century, has been widely used for the study of human inheritance.

Estimating Heritability from Twin Studies

Many years of research have been devoted to theorizing about ways to assess the importance of heredity in relation to environment, but no completely satisfactory method has been devised as yet. Following Fisher's exposition of a model for quantitating phenotypic variance among related individuals, Karl Holzinger proposed in 1929[15] that differences between the phenotypic variance of fraternal twins (V_{DZ}) and identical twins (V_{MZ}), expressed as a fraction of the variance between fraternal twins, be taken as a decisive index of heritability (H) such that

$$H = [V_{DZ} - V_{MZ}]/V_{DZ} = [r_{MZ} - r_{DZ}]/[1 - r_{DZ}] \qquad (5.2)$$

If the value computed for H derived from concordance rates is 1, the phenotypic variation was assumed to be entirely attributable to heredity; and conversely, if H was 0, the phenotypic variation was assumed to be attributable to environment. This method can yield a deceptively reasonable estimate for heritability, but it has also been shown to give estimates that may be quite different from more soundly based estimates of heritability (see Table 5.2).[16] Although its use has long been used as a measure of heritability in twin studies, the Holzinger index is no longer deemed satisfactory for this purpose and it has been recommended that it be discontinued.[17]

In 1949, Lush defined heritability for quantitative characters in farm animal breeding studies as the fraction of the observed variance (V_P) caused by differences in heredity (V_G),[18] such that

$$\text{heritability} = V_G/V_P$$

Later, two types of heritability were distinguished: (1) "broad sense heritability" ($h_B{}^2$) (Equation 5.3) is the proportion of phenotype difference due to all sources of genetic variance (V_P), regardless of whether the genes operate additively or nonadditively; and (2) "narrow sense heritability" is the proportion of phenotypic variance due solely to additive genetic variance. Thus, if V_G, V_A, and V_D refer to all genetic variance, to additive genetic variance, and to dominance effects, respectively,

$$h_B^2 = V_G/V_P = (V_A + V_D)/V_P \tag{5.3}$$

and

$$h^2 = V_A/V_P \tag{5.4}$$

Table 5.2 Heritability Estimates for Pharmacogenetic Twin Studies[16]

Drug	Measured parameter	$r_{MZ}{}^a$	$r_{DZ}{}^a$	${}^hB^{2\ b}$	H^c (heritability)
Antipyrine	Plasma half-life	0.93	−0.03	>1	0.93
Aspirin	Plasma concentration	0.90	0.33	>1	0.85
	Excretion rate	0.94	0.76	0.36	0.75
Dicumarol	Plasma half-life	0.99	0.80	0.38	0.90
Diphenylhydantoin	Plasma half-life	0.92	0.14	>1	0.91
Ethanol	Plasma half-life	0.64	0.16	0.96	0.57
	Plasma half-life	0.96	−0.38	>1	0.94
	Absorption rate	0.56	0.27	0.58	0.40
Halothane	% of dose	0.71	0.54	0.34	0.37
Isoniazid	% of dose	1.00	0.60	>1	1.00
	Serum concentration	0.95	0.25	0.37	0.93
Lithium	Plasma concentration	0.94	0.61	0.66	0.85
	RBC concentration	0.98	0.71	0.54	0.93
	RBC/plasma concentration	0.84	0.62	0.44	0.58
Phenylbutazone	Plasma half-life	0.98	0.45	0.98	0.96
Salicylate	Steady-state concentration	0.64	0.32	0.64	0.47

[a]Intratwinship correlation.
[b]$2(r_{MZ} - r_{DZ})$.
[c]$(r_{MZ} - r_{DZ})/(1 - r_{DZ})$.

"Narrow sense heritability" (Equation 5.4) is of interest mainly in connection with selective breeding of animals, and is not considered further here. "Broad sense heritability" addresses the relative partitioning of individual differences (say in drug response) into genetic and environmental components, and predicts genotypic values for individuals in a population at a given time.

More recently, Falconer proposed another relationship that approximates broad sense heritability. To give a sense of how Falconer's relationship is derived, some additional statistical concepts, i.e., for "covariance" and "phenotypic correlation," are needed. Since identical (monozygotic, MZ) twins covary completely genetically and also share a familial environment, the covariance for identical twinships is defined as follows:

$$\text{cov}_{MZ} = V_A + V_D + V_{E(MZ)}$$

Fraternal twins have the same genetic components of covariance as full siblings (see Table 5.1), i.e.,

$$\text{cov}_{DZ} = \tfrac{1}{2}V_A + \tfrac{1}{4}V_D + V_{E(DZ)}$$

Thus, the difference between the phenotypic covariances of identical and fraternal twins (assuming equivalent environments) is

$$\text{cov}_{MZ} - \text{cov}_{DZ} = \tfrac{1}{2}V_A + \tfrac{3}{4}V_D$$

Since a phenotypic correlation (r) is defined as a covariance divided by a variance,

$$r_{DZ} = [\tfrac{1}{2}V_A + \tfrac{1}{4}V_D + V_{E(DZ)}]/V_P$$

and

$$r_{MZ} = (V_A + V_D + V_{E(MZ)})/V_P$$

from which the difference between r_{MZ} and r_{DZ} is

$$r_{MZ} - r_{DZ} = (\tfrac{1}{2}V_A + \tfrac{3}{4}V_D)/V_P$$

Doubling this difference gives

$$2(r_{MZ} - r_{DZ}) = (V_A + \tfrac{3}{2}V_D)/V_P \qquad (5.5)$$

This formula (Equation 5.5) is called Falconer's estimate of broad sense heritability. Falconer's formula is an improvement over Holzinger's index for estimating broad sense heritability, but it still appears to be too simple a model for general application to estimate heritability from twin data. The shortcomings of this formula are beyond our present scope (other points may need amplification,[17,19] but one point is easy to see—Falconer's formula overestimates broad sense heritability because it contains 1.5 times the dominance variance).

Table 5.2 represents a fairly complete summary of therapeutic agents that had been investigated by twinship study up to 1978. For several of the agents listed, the values for h_B^2 exceed unity—a result that is disturbing because heritability cannot exceed unity.

Twin Studies in Pharmacogenetics

The acetylation polymorphism (see Appendix A) was one of the first pharmacogenetic traits to be extensively investigated by twin study. In a small series of five identical and five fraternal twinships from a German population, the difference in elimination of isoniazid (as the percentage of dose) was taken as a measure of interindividual variability. Despite the rather small number of twinships studied, it is evident that the intrapair variation observed for identical twinships is consistently much less than for fraternal twinships; this finding suggests heredity is quite influential in isoniazid elimination.

Later, two additional twin studies of the acetylation polymorphism were performed. In the study performed in Japanese twins, a very high intrapair correlation ($r = 0.95$) between the isoniazid blood concentration of identical twinships compared to the correlation ($r = 0.25$) for fraternal twinships was observed—41 of 42 identical twin pairs were concordant, while 7 of 11 fraternal twin pairs were concordant and 4 were discordant. When the results of a third twin study consisting of five identical and four fraternal Caucasian twinships are combined with the German and Japanese studies, the concordance within identical twins is much greater than within fraternal twins (Table 5.3).[20] The difference is highly significant ($\chi^2 = 21.1$, $p < 0.0001$), and this finding provides additional support for the presence of important genetic factors in the control of isoniazid elimination.

Twin studies of antipyrine, dicumarol, and phenylbutazone as well as of several other therapeutic agents (Table 5.2)[16] suggest the major mechanisms controlling variation in the rates of elimination of these drugs are also primarily of genetic origin. The relative importance of heredity and environment to more complicated pharmacological phenomena can also be better appreciated from twin studies (Table 5.4).[21] For example, when two (or more) drugs are coad-

Table 5.3 Twin Studies of Human Acetylation Polymorphism[20]

	Number of twinships		
	Concordant	Discordant	Totals
Identical	51	1	52
Fraternal	12	9	21
Totals	63	10	73

Table 5.4 Plasma Antipyrine Concentrations before and after Administration of Phenobarbital in Identical and Fraternal Twinships[22]

Twin	Age, sex	Plasma antipyrine half-life (hour)		Decrease in half-life (%)	Intratwinship difference (%)	Plasma phenobarbital levels at 156 hours (mg/liter)
		Before	After			
Identical twinships						
Dan E	22,M	13.6	9.6	29.4	0	20.0
Dav E	22,M	13.6	9.6	29.4		20.0
AM	35,F	8.0	6.3	21.2	0	17.5
BZ	35,F	8.0	6.3	21.2		15.0
Bar J	23,F	18.2	8.4	53.8	0	16.8
Bev J	23,F	18.2	8.4	53.8		17.9
BF	26,F	10.8	7.3	32.4	2.6	23.4
BJ	26,F	11.4	7.4	35.0		23.4
Fraternal twinships						
FD	49,M	12.0	10.3	14.2	14.2	19.4
PD	49,M	9.3	9.3	0		18.1
CK	49,M	17.5	5.5	68.6	8.6	
NR	49,M	14.5	5.8	60.0		
HH	47,F	12.3	9.2	25.2	9.8	17.8
PM	47,F	6.5	5.5	15.4		16.0
EW	54,F	15.0	6.9	54.0	30.7	20.0
EE	54,F	9.0	6.9	23.3		20.0

ministered, interactions may occur such as those observed with nortriptyline, an antidepressant drug, and a barbiturate. In part of the study, all subjects were given nortriptyline three times a day for 8 days and all had attained a steady-state concentration of the drug. Identical twins not ingesting other drugs exhibited considerable intertwinship variation but relatively small intratwinship variation. Fraternal twins not ingesting other drugs also exhibited considerable intertwinship variation, and for most twinships (8 out of 12) the intratwinship variability was small, as for identical twins. In 4 out of 12 fraternal twinships, however, there were large intratwinship differences. This finding suggests relatively small numbers of allelic genes are segregating.

Nortriptyline metabolism can be increased by the action of other drugs, especially the barbiturates. In another part of the study referred to above, twinships were encountered in which one or both members were on drug medication, in several instances, barbiturates. Identical twinships in which members were being given other drugs exhibited large twinship variability in nortriptyline steady-state concentrations, and this effect was magnified even more in fraternal twinships in which some members were receiving other drugs. These observations indicate that the nortriptyline steady-state concentration, an index of the individual's capability to metabolize the drug, is the result of genetic constitution and environment (exposure to other drugs), but that heredity exerts a very important influence on the interaction.

To look further into the pharmacogenetics of such interactions, a separate twin study with a barbiturate (phenobarbital) and another drug, antipyrine, was performed. This study revealed that the plasma half-life of antipyrine after phenobarbital was significantly reduced in both identical and fraternal twins, but again the intrapair differences were significantly less in identical than in fraternal twins (Table 5.4).[22]

Identical and fraternal twins are valuable resources for studying the relative importance of heredity and environment. Unfortunately, the genetic interpretation of twin studies may give rise to imprecise estimates of heritability. Furthermore, twin studies do not discriminate between different patterns of inheritance. Because similar drug effects may occur in different persons in similar environments, it is important to study twins who have been reared apart, and who have been exposed to environments as dissimilar as possible.

Epigenetic Influences in Twins

Monozygotic twins share the same DNA and often the same environment, and are considered identical, but sometimes they show striking phenotypic differences. In light of recent epigenetic studies, investigators believe it is time to revisit the problem.[23–25] DNA methylation, which tags cytosine with a methyl group, and chromatin modification, by acetylation, methylation, phosphorylation, etc., are heritable epigenetic mechanisms that together store information and modulate gene expression throughout the genome. Whereas genomic information is uniform among different cells of a complex organism, epigenomic information varies from tissue to tissue, providing a specific identity to each cell type (see Chapter 6).

Recently, Fraga and colleagues, on examining epigenetic differences arising during the lifetime of twins, find that monozygotic twins are epigenetically indistinguishable during the early years of life, but with aging, their epigenetic patterns tend to diverge and exhibit remarkable differences in overall content and genomic distribution of methylated cytosine and modified histones.[26] They found that about a third of monozygotic twins harbored epigenetic differences in DNA methylation and chromatin (histone) modifications. Smoking habits, physical activity, or diet are some environmental factors that might influence epigenetic modifications over the long term. It is also possible that the accumulation of small defects in transmitting through successive cell divisions, or in maintaining it in differentiated cells, might contribute to differences associated with aging. Fraga's comparison of identical twins suggests that environmental and intrinsic factors can affect the phenotype by altering the pattern of epigenetic modification and thereby modulate genetic information. Further studies that address the specific mechanisms responsible for these epigenetic modifications will be of great interest.

INHERITANCE PATTERNS OF MONOGENIC TRAITS

The analysis of inheritance patterns is a key element in the investigation of single-gene pharmacogenetic traits. Despite the addition of important new genomics tools arising from the human genome initiative, many years will pass before we completely understand the role of specific genetic factors and their interactions with environmental factors in health and disease. Until that time, it will be most effective to integrate genotypic data with data gained from the family history to profile individual drug responses and to individualize medical care. The availability of computer-based tools promises to reduce the time needed to obtain, organize, and analyze family history information, and provide a more lasting reminder of the value of this information and a way of keeping it up to date.[27]

This technique involves the collection of data on the family history and transmission patterns of the trait from parents to offspring. Information sought includes the age, sex, health status, and occupations of the parents, siblings, and other close relatives. The exact relationship of the index case (the case that brings the family to the investigator's attention) to the relatives and the occurrence of consanguineous matings, miscarriages, stillbirths, and twinships may provide useful information. Information about the ethnogeographic origin of the parents is important, and a detailed inquiry about the therapeutic agents and environmental exposures that may have occurred in the workplace or elsewhere is also important.

Four inheritance patterns are commonly observed within human families: autosomal dominant inheritance, autosomal recessive inheritance, sex (X)-linked dominant inheritance, and sex (X)-linked recessive inheritance. Another familial pattern attributable to mitochondrial inheritance has been observed, but much less frequently. Pedigrees are charted to show the relationships between the index case and other relatives in the family tree. Symbols commonly used to chart pedigrees are defined in Figure 5.1.

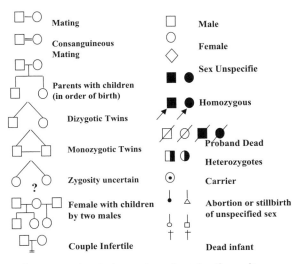

Figure 5.1 Symbols used to chart family pedigrees.

The inheritance patterns of some representative pharmacogenetic traits have been summarized above (see p. 25). The criteria for identifying each of these patterns are reviewed briefly below.

Autosomal Dominant Inheritance

Autosomal dominant inheritance is characterized by transmission of susceptibility from one generation to the next without skipping a generation. Except for new mutants, every susceptible child has a susceptible parent. In matings between a susceptible heterozygote and a normal homozygote, the proportion of susceptible children (the segregation frequency) averages one-half, including father-to-son transmission. The incidence of susceptible persons is the same in males and females. A representative pattern of the autosomal dominant inheritance of malignant hyperthermia is illustrated in Figure 5.2.[28]

Among autosomal dominant traits that cause disease, many are either not very life threatening, or if deleterious, their onset is delayed until later in life, as exemplified by Huntington's disease. In contrast, because of their latency in the absence of exposure to offending environmental agents, several autosomal dominant pharmacogenetic traits may occur predominantly in children and young adults.

Autosomal Recessive Inheritance

Many pharmacogenetic traits are transmitted by autosomal recessive inheritance (also referred to as autosomal codominant inheritance) and a number of those traits are relatively common. Among autosomal recessive traits that cause disease, most are rare and harmful, but the severity of the idiosyncrasy of the susceptible pharmacogenetic phenotype depends on the nature and degree of exposure to environmental agents. Susceptible persons are offspring of phenotypically normal parents who are carriers of the trait. Other susceptible family members occur among siblings of the index case, and not among other relatives. In matings between two phenotypically normal heterozygotes, the probability of having a susceptible child (the segregation frequency) averages 1/4 (Figure 5.3) and that of having a carrier among phenotypically normal children is 2/3. There is an elevated incidence of consanguinity among the parents. The incidence of susceptible persons is the same in males and females.

Sex (X)-Linked Inheritance

Sex-linked inheritance effectively means X-linked inheritance since no male (Y)-linked pharmacogenetic traits have been identified. A sex-(X)-linked dominant trait appears in every generation without skipping and with more affected females than affected males. One or both parents are affected. Affected heterozygous females transmit the trait to half of their children of either sex and affected homozygous females transmit the trait to all of their children. Notice that the pattern of transmission of a sex-linked dominant trait by females is indistinguishable from that of autosomal dominant transmission (Table 5.5).

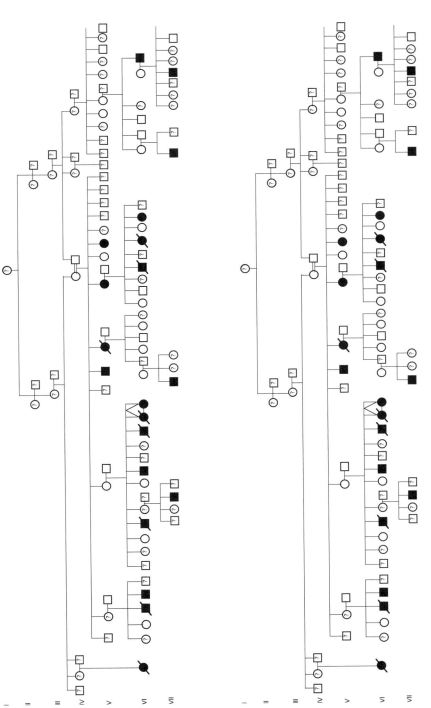

Figure 5.2 Autosomal dominant inheritance of malignant hyperthermia.

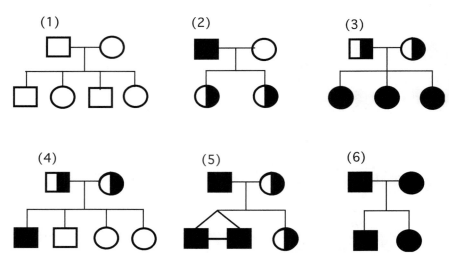

Figure 5.3 Autosomal inheritance of CYP2D6 polymorphism (debrisoquine/spar-sparteine hydroxylation polymorphism).

Most X-linked traits are recessive, or partly recessive. Affected persons are mostly males born of carrier females. They are related to each other through female carrier relatives with a maternal grandfather and grandson being affected, or a maternal uncle and nephew being affected. Among genetic disorders that cause disease, if a recessive trait is harmful, it is usually rare; if it is not very harmful, it may be fairly common. The example chosen to represent a sex-linked pharmacogenetic trait, G6PD deficiency (Figure 5.4),[29] is very common in certain ethnic populations; the severity of the phenotype depends on the nature of the

Table 5.5 Expected Segregation Frequencies among Children with Autosomal and Sex-(X)-Linked Traits

Mode of inheritance	Mating type	Segregation frequency among children		
		Normal	Carrier	Affected
Autosomal dominant	Aa×aa	1/2	—	1/2
	Aa×Aa	1/4	—	3/4
Autosomal recessive	AA×aa	—	1	—
	Aa×aa	—	1/2	1/2
	Aa×Aa	1/4	2/4	1/2

Mode of inheritance	Mating type	Males		Females		
		Normal	Affected	Normal	Carrier	Affected
X-linked dominant	XY×XX	1	—	—	1	—
	XY×XX	1/2	1/2	1/2	—	1/2
X-linked recessive	XY×XX	1	—	1/2	1/2	—
	XY×XX	1/2	1/2	—	1/2	1/2
	XY×XX	—	1	—	1	—

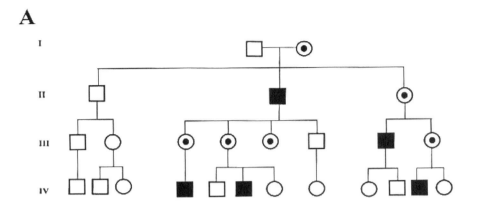

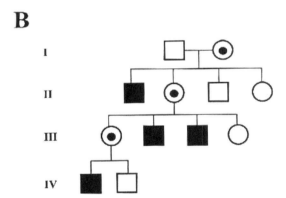

Figure 5.4 Sex (X)-linked inheritance: (*A*) males reproduce; (*B*) males do not reproduce.

enzymatic defect as well as the extent of exposure to therapeutic agents and other environmental agents. The incidence of sex-linked recessive inheritance is very much higher in males than in females. For rare sex-linked traits, parents of affected males are normal, and the only affected relatives are maternal uncles and other male relatives in the maternal ancestry. If an affected male can reproduce, all of his male offspring are unaffected, but all of his daughters are heterozygous carriers. In case the affected male dies before reproducing, or is sterile, transmission is solely by carrier females.

The segregation frequencies expected among offspring of autosomal and sex-(X)- linked traits are summarized in Table 5.5.

Mitochondrial Inheritance

Comparatively few human disorders have been shown to be mitochondrially inherited, and most of these are rare. To date only one mitochondrial (maternally inherited) pharmacogenetic trait has been identified (see Appendix A). The occurrence of this disorder depends on exposure to aminoglycoside antibiotics and its prevalence has not been established.

Mitochondrial DNA (mtDNA) is predominantly inherited from the mother (see p. 103). Male germ cells (spermatozoa) contain very little cytoplasm and are estimated to contribute less than 0.1% of the zygote's mtDNAs. Cells can harbor mixtures of mutant and normal mtDNA (heteroplasmy). Each time a somatic or germ cell line divides, the mutant and normal mtDNAs segregate randomly into daughter cells. The mtDNA genotypes may fluctuate from one cell division to the next, and over many cell divisions the proportion of mutant mtDNAs drifts toward predominantly mutant or normal mtDNA (homoplasmy). The severity of the defect results from the nature of the mtDNA mutation, and the proportion of mutant mtDNAs within the cell; the clinical picture in maternal relatives of heteroplasmic pedigrees varies according to the proportion of mutant mtDNAs that each individual inherits.

While mitochondria are predominantly inherited only from the mother, and some mitochondrial disorders are maternally inherited, recent studies indicate that the great majority—more than 80%—of diseases known to be linked to faulty mitochondria are due to nuclear genes and do not exhibit maternal inheritance. Evidence that mitochondrial proteins are responsible for human disease is growing, but currently, the actual contribution of nuclear genes to mitochondrial disease is unclear because we do not yet know which genes are involved and how they interact with mitochondrial genes.[30]

The possibility of sex (X)-linked inheritance should be considered when maternal transmission is encountered, but can be excluded if both sexes are equally affected, or if males do not transmit the susceptibility to their daughters or to their grandsons through an affected daughter (Figure 5.5).[31]

Certain traits of pharmacogenetic interest do not always follow one of the orthodox patterns of inheritance and may be less straightforward to analyze. For example, responses to exogenous chemicals that involve a combination of monogenic traits usually do not yield such a simple inheritance pattern. Other responses that have been discovered recently and have unorthodox inheritance patterns include traits that are determined by trinucleotide repeats, "jumping genes" or other types of unstable genes, or genes that assume alternate forms and may produce more than one protein.

MATHEMATICAL TREATMENT OF HETEROGENEITY IN HUMAN DRUG RESPONSE

The quantitative treatment of genetic heterogeneity in human drug response is based, in part, on the mathematical concept embodied in the binomial distribution,

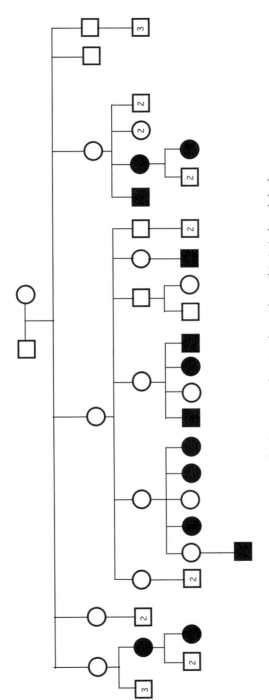

Figure 5.5 Maternal inheritance of aminoglycoside antibiotic-induced deafness.

and a derivative concept, the Hardy–Weinberg law. By applying the principles embodied in these two concepts, a quantitative genetic analysis of the pharmacological characteristics of individuals in families and in populations can be performed.

Binomial Distribution of Discrete Individual Characteristics: The Basic Idea

Important characteristics of interest can be inferred from calculations performed on samples drawn from populations of interest. Suppose we have a population of which a certain proportion p of individuals bears a discrete character, and the fraction $(1-p) = q$ lacks the character. Empirically, we know that if one individual is drawn at random from the population, it has a probability p of bearing the character, and a probability q of lacking the character. In general, whenever there are two alternative characters that an individual may possess, the basic frequency distribution of the characters is usually expected to be binomial, and the mathematical treatment of sampling from such a population makes use of the binomial theorem.

The binomial theorem states that the probabilities of a sample of n individuals having $0, 1, 2, \ldots r, \ldots n$ individuals who bear the character are given by successive terms of the expansion of the binomial $(q+p)^n$. The chance that exactly r individuals bear the character is given by

$$q^n, nq^{n-1}p, \{[n(n-1)]/2\}q^{n-2}p^2, \ldots \{n!/[r!(n-r)!]\}q^{n-r}p^r, \ldots p^n$$

for $r = 0, 1, 2, \ldots r, \ldots n$ individuals, respectively. The probability of r individuals who bear the character in a sample n is given by the general expression

$$P_n^r = n!/[r!(n-r)!]p^r q^{n-r} \tag{5.6}$$

Equation 5.6 is more readily comprehended if it is divided into two parts: the fraction, $n!/[r!(n-r)!]$, equals the number of distinguishable ways of drawing r individuals who have the character [and $(n-r)$ individuals who lack the character] since the joint probability of two independent drawings is the product of their individual probabilities.

Pascal's triangle affords another and a more compact way of presenting the consequences of the binomial concept (Table 5.6). The number of combinations in a given row can be obtained by adding the two numbers on either side of it in the row above. For instance, the probability of drawing two individuals from a set of 5 ($n = 5$) will be given by

$$[5!/2!3!]p^2 q^3 = 10p^2 q^3$$

By reading Pascal's triangle across the row for $n = 5$, we see that 10 is the number of distinguishable ways two individuals who bear the character, and three who do not, can be drawn randomly from a sample of 5: the probability will thus be $10p^2 q^3$.

Table 5.6 Pascal's Triangle of the Binomial Expression

Sample size (n)	Expansion of $(p+q)^n$	Number of combinations $n!/[r!\,(n-r)!]$
1	pq	2
2	$p^2 \quad 2pq \quad q^2$	3
3	$p^3 \quad 3p^2q \quad 3pq^2 \quad q^3$	4
4	$p^4 \quad 4p^3q \quad 6p^2q^2 \quad 4pq^3 \quad q^4$	5
5	$p^5 \quad 5p^4q \quad 10p^3q^2 \quad 10p^2q^3 \quad 5pq^4 \quad q^5$	6
n	$p^n \quad np^nq \ldots \qquad npq^{n-1} \quad q^n$	$n+1$

Some of the general properties of this distribution are used frequently and are worth knowing. It can be seen intuitively, and it can be shown, that the average μ is given by np. It can also be shown that the variance of the mean, $\sigma^2 = npq$, and that r/n has a mean of p and a variance of pq/n.

Familiarity with the basic idea of the binomial distribution, in practice, rests on the performance of numerical calculations for P_n^r. Suppose that the proportion p of a discrete individual character in a given population is known and we wish to examine the distribution of the character on taking repeated samples of a given size from the population. This is given directly by P_n^r (Equation 5.6), which represents the proportion over the long run of p individuals that bear the character in samples of a total of n individuals.

Table 5.7 shows values of P_n^r computed for two values of p with $n = 20$. The frequency distributions for these special cases are shown in Figure 5.6. Readers who are less familiar with the binomial distribution may wish to satisfy themselves of the validity of values tabulated for individual probabilities by computing P_{20}^r for a few specific r values.

The p value has an important effect on the distribution. Consider the case for $p = 0.1$. This means that in repeated samples of 20, it would be expected, on average, that 10%, or 2 of the 20 individuals drawn, would bear the character of interest, and 18 would not. However, the binomial theorem predicts that even though samples with the average number $(r=2)$ have the highest probability, only 29% may be expected to have exactly that number. About 12% of the samples are expected to have no individuals who bear the character, and summing of P_{20}^r from $r = 3$ to $r = 20$ shows that about 32% of the samples will have more than the average number.

For $p = 0.7$ and $n = 20$ (Table 5.8 and Figure 5.6), the long run proportion (average number) of individuals who bear the character is 14 (i.e., $\mu = np$), but as noted above for $p = 0.1$, the expected variation about the mean is substantial. For $p = 0.7$ and $n = 20$, $\sigma^2 = 2.94$. An estimate of r/n is given by $p \pm \sqrt{pq/n} = 0.7 \pm 0.10$.

It is evident that the application of statistical formulas to real situations involves some assumptions. In the cases given above, the most important assumption is that each sample is randomly drawn with respect to the character of interest from the population under investigation.

Table 5.7 Binomial Distribution for Samples of 20 Drawn Randomly from Populations with $p=0.1$ and $p=0.7$

r	P_{20}	$\sum_{r=0}^{r} P_{20}$
	$p=0.1$	
0	0.122	0.122
1	0.270	0.392
2	0.285	0.677
3	0.190	0.867
4	0.090	0.957
5	0.032	0.988
6	0.009	0.997
7	0.002	0.999
	$p=0.7$	
8	0.0038	0.007
9	0.0120	0.019
10	0.0307	0.050
11	0.0655	0.115
12	0.114	0.229
13	0.164	0.393
14	0.192	0.585
15	0.179	0.763
16	0.130	0.893
17	0.071	0.965
18	0.028	0.993
19	0.006	0.999

In summary, whenever two independent alternative characters are randomly chosen from a population, the distribution in a repeated series of trials is expected to be binomial. It follows directly that the variation from the average over the long run is expected to fit a specific well-defined pattern.

The Hardy–Weinberg Law

The basic formula of population genetics is a direct consequence of the binomial theorem. In a randomly interbreeding population segregating for a single gene with two alleles, A and a (i.e., discrete alternative characters), the stable frequency of genotypes is given by $p^2(AA):2pq(Aa):q^2(aa)$. It can be seen that this expression corresponds to the special case given in row 2 of Pascal's triangle (Table 5.6). This concept was gradually derived over the years by longhand arguments involving the origin of evolutionary changes in populations (see Chapter 17 in A.H. Sturtevant's *A History of Genetics*), but it was first expressed in simple algebraic terms independently by Hardy and by Weinberg shortly after the rediscovery of Mendel's laws at the beginning of the 1900s. This idea,

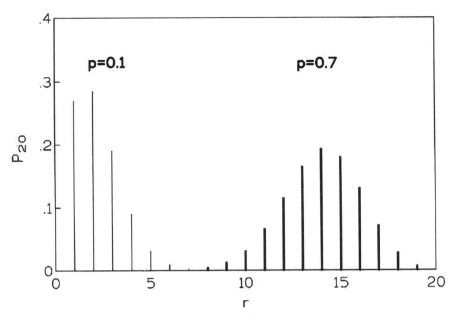

Figure 5.6 Binomial distribution with $n = 20$, $p = 0.1$ and 0.7.

elaborated upon in most textbooks of genetics, is commonly known as the Hardy–Weinberg law or as the Hardy–Weinberg equilibrium.

It is not difficult to see, in retrospect, how the binomial distribution came to be applied to the investigation of variations in Mendelian inheritance if the two primary assumptions implicit in the binomial theorem are fulfilled. The first assumption that two unequivocally distinguishable alternative characters are present in the population of interest is fulfilled by the fact that genes are of a particulate nature and that independent segregation of alleles occurs at meiosis; this mechanism ensures that alternative characters (alleles) are transmitted from parents to offspring. The second assumption that these characters be randomly chosen from the population is in part fulfilled by independent segregation of alleles during the reproductive phase of the cell cycle, but is strictly valid only if mutation, selection, or migration (between populations) is absent, and that mating between interbreeding individuals is random. Many of the further developments in population genetics revolve around the algebraic analysis of the effects of deviations from these stringent requirements. These assumptions are often closely approximated so that the Hardy–Weinberg law is useful in the genetic analysis of human populations.

So far, we have considered the applicability of the Hardy–Weinberg law solely to Mendelian segregation operating in populations that contain different proportions of individuals homozygous and heterozygous for various genes, but the same law is operating within families segregating those genes. It is usually impossible to test for the occurrence of segregation in humans by experimental

Table 5.8 Observed Numbers of Matings Compared with Those Expected by Application of the Hardy–Weinberg Law to Caucasian Subjects[a,b]

Phenotypic matings	Genotypic matings[c]	Expected frequency of matings		Expected occurrence in 53 matings	Observed occurrence
S×S	rr×rr	$p^4 = 0.2728$		14.46	17
R×S	RR×rr	$2p^2q^2 = 0.083$			
	Rr×rr	$4p^3q = 0.4187$	0.4990	26.45	23
R×R	RR×RR	$q^4 = 0.0059$			
	RR×Rr	$4q^3p = 0.0616$			
	Rr×Rr	$4q^2p^2 = 0.1606$	0.2281	12.09	13
Total		0.999		53.00	53

[a]*Source*: From Evans et al.[32]

[b]$\chi^2 = 0.964$, $df = 2$.

[c]R is the allele controlling the dominant character, and r is the allele controlling the recessive character.

crosses, but it is possible to recognize and prove the segregation of a gene by following its effects in several generations of a family tree or family pedigree. In fact, much of our knowledge of heredity in humans has come from pedigree analysis, and the study of sharply alternative pharmacological characters has proven fruitful in testing various pharmacogenetic hypotheses for humans.

Hardy–Weinberg Tests of Pharmacogenetic Hypotheses

Sampling a population whose members differ quantitatively or qualitatively is a situation that arises whenever heterogeneity in individual drug responses is investigated. Studies making use of the Hardy–Weinberg law were performed in the 1930s on phenylthiourea taste testing and in the 1950s on isoniazid acetylation, succinylcholine sensitivity, and G6PD deficiency (see Chapter 1). These are excellent models to illustrate the application of the statistical principles embodied in the Hardy–Weinberg law to the interpretation of pharmacogenetic data. Applications of this principle to an autosomal recessive trait (isoniazid acetylation polymorphism) and a sex-(X)-linked trait (G6PD deficiency) are illustrated below.

Hardy–Weinberg Analysis of Isoniazid Metabolism

A definitive study of isoniazid metabolism was performed on 267 members of 53 complete Caucasian families.[32] The concentration of free isoniazid (measured biochemically) was bimodally distributed because of differences in individual acetylating capacity (see Figure 2.1), Metabolic studies had shown that acetylation was the most important factor in the elimination of isoniazid, and the inheritance patterns in families suggested that individual differences in acetylation measured *in vivo* were controlled by a single gene with two major alleles.

Among 291 unrelated subjects tested, 152 or 52.23% were slow acetylators. The frequency of the slow acetylator allele estimated from the Hardy–Weinberg law is $p = \sqrt{0.5223} = 0.7227$. The frequency of the alternative character, the rapid acetylator allele, is thus $q = 1 - 0.7227 = 0.2773$. The hypothesis that slow acetylation is a recessive character was tested by David Price Evans and colleagues according to the Hardy–Weinberg law (1) by comparing the number of matings observed with those expected in the population sample as shown in Table 5.8, and (2) by comparing the number of children observed with those expected from 53 matings as shown in Table 5.9. Both comparisons show that the data fit the hypothesis (1) that the division into rapid and slow acetylator phenotypes is due to two major alleles and (2) that the slow acetylator phenotype is due to homozygosity of the slow acetylator allele. A test of the alternative hypothesis that rapid acetylation is the homozygous recessive character results in unsatisfactory agreement of observed and expected numbers.

Shortly after the Caucasian study but independent of it, S. Sunahara and co-workers performed a similar analysis of the pharmacogenetics of isoniazid metabolism on Japanese persons and families. It gave results that differed dramatically from those obtained on Caucasians. In the Japanese study, free isoniazid in blood was measured microbiologically instead of biochemically. The more sensitive assay enabled the separation of intermediate rapid (heterozygous) acetylator phenotypes from the homozygous rapid acetylator phenotypes to yield a trimodal frequency distribution (Figure 5.7)[33] instead of the bimodal frequency distribution found for Caucasians (Figure 2.1). Tests of the same hypotheses were performed on the Japanese data by the Hardy–Weinberg law. Comparisons of the observed and expected numbers of matings (Table 5.10) and of the children of each acetylator phenotype for Japanese subjects (Table 5.11) confirmed the conclusions reached for Caucasians even though there are major ethnic differences in the frequencies of the two acetylator phenotypes.

The checkerboard diagram in Figure 5.8 provides an alternative display of the genetic data that complements its presentation in tabular form (Tables 5.8, 5.9, 5.10, and 5.11). The checkerboard helps to explain the Hardy–Weinberg

Table 5.9 Expected Numbers of Children of Each Acetylator Phenotype Compared with Those Observed in 53 Caucasian Matings[a]

Phenotypic matings	Number of matings	Number of children	Number of children of each phenotype				χ^2	df
			Rapid		Slow			
			Exp	Obs	Exp	Obs		
S×S	17	54	Nil	4	54	50	—	—
R×R	23	67	35.88	40	28.10	27	0.075	1
R×R	13	38	31.30	31	6.68	7	0.018	1
Total	53	159		75		84	0.093	2

[a]The hypothesis is made that slow acetylator persons are genetically homozygous recessives.[32]

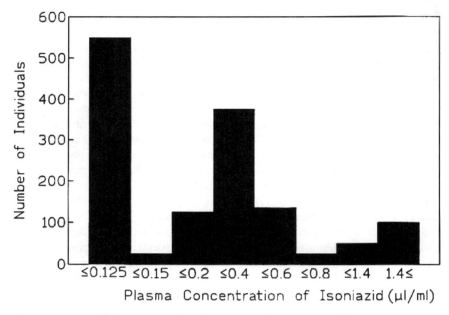

Figure 5.7 Trimodal frequency distribution of plasma isoniazid concentrations in Japanese populations.

calculations because it shows the parental origin of all mating types, as well as the proportion each parental genotype contributes to the genotypes of the offspring. Thus, a proportion p^2q^2 of heterozygote offspring is expected from rr mothers × RR fathers, while an equal proportion p^2q^2 is expected from RR mothers × rr fathers, and another larger proportion $4p^2q^2$ is expected from Rr mothers × Rr fathers. The numbers in Table 5.11 refer to the Japanese study.

Also notice that the information contained in the checkerboard in sum contains information that equals that contained in row 4 of Pascal's triangle (Table 5.6), which represents all possible combinations of the mother's and father's genotypes. The probability of each genotype is given by the product of $(p^2 + 2pq + q^2) \times (p^2 + 2pq + q^2)$.

Since individuals of different racial groups often show significant differences from each other in response to exogenous substances, a comprehensive analysis of any pharmacogenetic trait should include an assessment of the importance of ethnogeographic factors. As illustrated by the studies in Caucasians and Japanese, this requirement poses no analytical problems beyond those already considered for a given population group.

Hardy–Weinberg Analysis of G6PD Deficiency

The first clear indication of the hereditary nature of drug-induced reactions associated with G6PD deficiency came after the development of a bioassay, the

Table 5.10 Observed Numbers of Matings Compared with Those Expected by Application of the Hardy–Weinberg Law to Japanese Subjects[a]

Phenotypic matings	Genotypic matings	Expected frequency of matings[b]	Expected number in 78 matings	Observed number
S×S	rr×rr	$p^4 = 0.01284$	1	1
I×S	Rr×rr	$4p^3q = 0.1012$	7.89	11
R×S	RR×rr	$2p^2q^2 = 0.09973$	7.78	3
I×I	Rr×Rr	$4p^2q^2 = 0.1994$	15.55	15
I×R	Rr×RR	$4pq^3 = 0.3931$	30.66	29
R×R	RR×RR	$q^4 = 0.1937$	15.11	19
Total		1.000	77.99	78

[a]*Source*: Adapted from Sunahara et al.[33]

[b]Calculated assuming a frequency $p = \sqrt{0.115} = 0.3366$ for the slow acetylator allele and $q = 1 - 0.3366 = 0.6634$ for the rapid acetylator allele.

glutathione stability test, which permitted the drug-sensitive red cell to be identified *in vitro*.[34,35] With this test, the distributions of glutathione stability of red cells were determined for 144 male and 184 female black subjects (Figure 5.9) and in black families.[36] These studies revealed two phenotypes among the males (normals and reactors) and three phenotypes among the females (normals, intermediates, and reactors). Family studies showed that transmission of the trait from father to son did not occur.

This pattern of responses suggested a sex-(X)-linked recessive mode of inheritance of the red cell sensitivity. With the aid of the Hardy–Weinberg law, Barton Childs and co-workers tested the hypothesis of sex-linked recessive

Table 5.11 Expected Numbers of Children of Each Acetylator Genotype Compared with Those Observed in 78 Japanese Matings[a,b]

Phenotypic matings[c]	Number of matings	Number of children	Rapid Exp	Rapid Obs	Intermediate Exp	Intermediate Obs	Slow Exp	Slow Obs
S×S	1	2	0	0	0	0	2	2
I×S	11	23	0	1	11.5	11	11.5	11
R×S	3	7	0	0	7	7	0	0
I×I	15	30	7.5	14	15	12	7.5	4
I×R	29	61	30.5	37	30.5	24	0	0
R×R	19	39	39	39	0	0	0	0
Total	78	162						

[a]*Source:* Adapted from Sunahara *et al.*[33]

[b]The hypothesis is made that rapid (R) and slow (S) acetylation is determined by two major alleles without dominance.

[c]I (intermediate) represents the heterozygous phenotype.

Mother

		rr p^2	Rr $2pq$	RR q^2
Father	rr p^2	p^4 0.01284	$2p^3q$ 0.0506	p^2q^2 0.04986
	Rr $2pq$	$2p^3q$ 0.0506	$4p^2q^2$ 0.1994	$2pq^3$ 0.1966
	RR q^2	p^2q^2 0.04986	$2pq^3$ 0.1966	q^4 0.1937

Figure 5.8 Checkerboard diagram showing the segregation of gene-controlling isoniazid acetylation giving genotypes of Japanese parents and offspring.

transmission quantitatively by comparing the numbers of female reactors and male reactors observed in the random populations with the expected numbers; sex-linked recessive inheritance is distinguished from the other modes of inheritance by the fact that the expected frequency of female reactors is given by the square of the expected frequency of male reactors. The data were found to fit this hypothesis (see Table 5.12).

Many years later, the gene that encodes G6PD was shown to be located on the long arm of chromosome Xq28 between the genes for factor VIII and for color

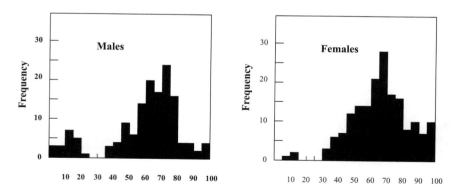

Post-incubation glutathione values

Figure 5.9 Distribution of postincubation glutathione stability values among males and females.

Table 5.12 The Distribution of Glutathione Stability Values among Randomly Selected Negro Males and Females[35]

		Phenotype		
			Observed occurrence	
	Genotype	Expected frequency	Number	Frequency
Females				
Normal	AA	$p^2 = 0.742$	172	0.935
Intermediate	Aa	$2pq = 0.239$	9	0.049
Reactor	aa	$q^2 = 0.019$	3	0.016
Total			184	1.0
Males				
Normal	AY	$p = 0.864$	120	0.833
Intermediate	—	0	3	0.021
Reactor	aY	$q = 0.136$	21	0.146
Total			144	1.0

vision.[37,38] It spans approximately 20 kb and contains a coding sequence of 1548 bp.[39]

Testing for Genetic Association of Human Drug Response

At times, it may be of interest to examine the statistical association between a disorder and genetically determined phenotypes (or genotypes) in a series of studies. The approach of Woolf [40] as modified by Haldane[41] is suitable for this purpose. Evans and colleagues applied this approach to test the association of urinary bladder cancer to slow acetylator phenotype and found about 39% more cancer in slow than rapid acetylators.[42] Bladder cancer is known to occur at a higher rate in subjects exposed to carcinogenic arylamines, in tobacco smoke, and especially among workers in the aniline dye industry.[43] Carcinogenic arylamines are, like isoniazid, substrates for acetylation polymorphism. The data from several human studies of urban and occupationally exposed persons are shown in Table 5.13. Statistical analysis of a series of studies somewhat larger than that of Evans et al. shows the slow acetylator phenotype is significantly associated with about 36% more with bladder cancer than the rapid acetylator phenotype. However, if the persons occupationally exposed to arylamines are analyzed separately, the slow acetylators are associated about 70% more than rapid acetylators, as shown in Table 5.14. Notice that the number of persons with bladder cancer in Ladero's 1985 study exposed to arylamines occupationally (Table 5.14) is smaller than the numbers in Table 5.13 because the latter study combines persons suffering urban and occupational exposure to arylamines. Thus, the association in the larger study is primarily due to the contribution of persons occupationally exposed to arylamines.[44]

Table 5.13 Test of Association between Bladder Cancer and Acetylator Phenotype for Urban Populations and Populations Occupationally Exposed to Arylamines[20a]

Reference	Number of subjects Bladder cancer Slow (h)	Rapid (k)	Controls Slow (H)	Rapid (K)	Approximate relative risk = x^b	$\log_e$ $x = y$	Sampling variance = V^c	Weight I/V^c	Significance of difference from zero = wy^2	wy
Lower et al. (1979) (Danish)	46	25	38	36	1.7288	0.5474	0.2127	8.8968	2.6659	4.8701
Lower et al. (1979) (Swedish)	80	35	79	39	1.1267	0.1193	0.0776	12.8866	0.1834	1.5374
Cartwright et al. (1982) (English)	74	37	118	89	1.5004	0.4057	0.0591	16.8919	2.7803	6.8530
Woodhouse et al. (1982)	21	9	16	11	1.5773	0.4557	0.2876	3.4770	0.7220	1.5945
Miller and Cosgriff (1983)	12	14	18	8	0.3961	−0.9261	0.3073	3.2538	2.7906	−3.0133
Evans et al. (1983)	66	34	510	342	1.2932	0.2571	0.0483	20.6612	1.3657	5.3120
Ladero et al. (1985)	83	47	90	67	1.3111	0.2709	0.05842	17.1174	1.2562	4.6371
Mommsen et al. (1985)	145	83	54	46	1.4867	0.3966	0.05821	17.1791	2.7021	6.8132
Hanssen et al. (1985)	65	40	18	24	2.1418	0.7616	0.1321	7.5660	4.3885	5.7623
Cartwright et al. (1984) (Portuguese)	14	44	10	25	0.7913	−0.2140	0.2183	4.5817	0.2509	−1.0721
Lower (Weber et al., 1983)	13	5	11	8	1.8142	0.5957	0.4380	2.2830	0.8101	1.3600

Weighted mean of $y = \bar{y} = \dfrac{\sum wy}{\sum w} = \dfrac{34.6442}{114.7945} = 0.3018.$

$SE(\bar{Y}) = (\sum w)^{-1/2} = \left(\dfrac{1}{114.7945}\right)^{1/2} = 0.09333.$

95% confidence interval of $\bar{Y} = \bar{Y} \pm t_{10}0.05(\sum w)^{-1/2} = 0.3018 \pm 2.228 \times 0.09333 = 0.5097$ and 0.09386, for 10 df, $t_{10} = 2.228.$

Antilog $\bar{Y} = \bar{X} =$ combined estimates of $x = $ antilog$_e(0.3018) = 1.3623.$

Equivalent $\bar{X}$ values $=$ antilog $(0.5097) = 1.6638$ and antilog $(0.09386) = 1.0984.$

Significance of the difference of $\bar{X}$ from unity $= X_1^2 = \dfrac{(\sum wy)^2}{\sum w} = 10.4554 \ (p<0.01).$

Heterogeneity expression $X_{n-1}^2 = \sum wy^2 - \dfrac{(\sum wy)^2}{\sum w} = 9.4603 \ (p<0.10), = 10 \ df.$

[a] Woolf's method as modified by Haldane.
[b] $x = [(2h+1)(2K+1)] / [(2k+1)(2H+1)].$
[c] $V = [1/(h+1)] + [1/(k+1)] + [1/(H+1)] + [1/(K+1)].$

Table 5.14 Test of Association between Bladder Cancer and Acetylator Phenotype for Populations Occupationally Exposed to Arylamines[20a]

| Reference | Number of subjects | | | | Approximate relative risk $= x^b$ | $\log_e x = y$ | Sampling variance $= V^c$ | Weight $1/V^c$ | Significance of difference from zero $= wy^2$ | wy |
| | Bladder cancer | | Controls | | | | | | | |
	Slow (h)	Rapid (k)	Slow (H)	Rapid (K)						
Cartwright et al. (1982) (English)	74	37	118	89	1.5004	0.4057	0.0591	16.8919	2.7803	6.8530
Lower (Weber et al., 1983)	13	5	11	8	1.8142	0.5957	0.4380	2.2830	0.8101	1.3600
Ladero et al. (1985)	41	14	90	67	1.3111	0.2709	0.05842	17.1174	1.2562	4.6371

Weighted mean of $y = Y = \dfrac{\sum wy}{\sum w} = \dfrac{14.7405}{27.7830} = 0.5306.$

$SE(Y) = \left(\sum w\right)^{-\frac{1}{2}} = \left(\dfrac{1}{27.783}\right)^{\frac{1}{2}} = 0.1897.$

95% confidence interval of $Y = Y \pm t_2 \ 0.05 \left(\sum w\right)^{-\frac{1}{2}} = 0.5306 \pm (4.30)(0.1897) = 1.3463$ and -0.2851 for $2df, t_2 = 4.30.$
Antilog $Y = X =$ combined estimates of $x =$ antilog$_e$ $(0.5306) = 1.7000.$

Equivalent X values $=$ antilog $(1.3463) = 3.8432$ and antilog $(-0.2851) = 0.7519.$

Significance of the difference of X from unity $= X_1^2 = \dfrac{\left(\sum wy\right)^2}{\sum w} = 7.8207 (p < 0.01), 1 df.$

Heterogeneity expression $X_{n-1}^2 = \sum wy^2 - \dfrac{\left(\sum wy\right)^2}{\sum w} = 0.7195 (p > 0.10), 2 \ df.$

[a] Woolf's method as modified by Haldane.
[b] $x = [\backslash lceb 2h + 1)\ (2K + 1)] /[(2k + 1)\ (2H + 1)].$
[c] $V = [1/(h + 1)] + [1/(k + 1)] + [1/(H + 1)] + [1/(K + 1)].$

MOLECULAR PHARMACOGENETICS

Pharmacogeneticists have traditionally relied on phenotypic criteria to analyze individual responsiveness to exogenous chemicals. For genes expressed in accessible tissues, such as peripheral blood cells and skin, the analytical difficulties are not as formidable as for traits whose expression is specific to less accessible tissues such as the liver, skeletal muscle, adrenal, and heart. Investigators have made rapid strides toward the delineation of the structure and organization of human genes and of the pathways by which cells regulate gene expression through the use of recombinant DNA techniques. Since their introduction and widespread adoption about two decades ago, molecular genetic studies have produced a prodigious amount of new information about hereditary susceptibilities to exogenous substances, and profound insights into their underlying mechanisms.

DNA Polymorphism

Every person usually carries two copies of the genes they possess (except for sex-linked genes), but the human genome is highly polymorphic and a given person may possess an alternative DNA sequence at a particular chromosomal site that determines the usefulness of that site for genetic studies. Sites that exhibit alternative sequences are termed DNA polymorphisms, which are useful as genetic markers for the site, or for the chromosome bearing the site. From a pharmacogenetic standpoint, such sites may be useful for identifying individuals who are predisposed to peculiarities in drug response. When these sites are tracked within the context of family studies and in larger populations, inheritance patterns and estimates of their prevalence and significance to humans can be determined. By taking advantage of recombinant DNA techniques, polymorphic sites can be studied at two levels, one employing Southern analysis to survey chromosomal sites for polymorphism and the other employing DNA sequencing to determine the precise location of base changes that define the polymorphism. The latter approach is, in essence, a refinement of the first.

Consider the application of Southern analysis for such a purpose. Restriction enzymes cleave DNA at recognition sites of four to eight bases. An eight-base cutter enzyme, for example, will recognize an appropriate sequence every $4^8 =$ 65,536 base pairs (the probability that a specific base will occur at each of the eight positions); similarly, a six-base cutter will see its sequence every 4096 $(= 4^6)$ base pairs, and a four-base cutter will see its sequence every 256 (4^4) base pairs. If one of the bases at the recognition site of a given restriction enzyme is polymorphic, a panel of six different enzymes of the eight-base cutter type will sample the DNA sites at every $65,536/6 \cong 9400$ base pairs, a six-base cutter will sample the genome at every $4096/6 \cong 680$ base pairs, and a four-base cutter will sample it at every $256/6 \cong 43$ base pairs. Hence, a panel of six of the eight-base cutters would sample a gene of say approximately 30,000 base pairs only about three times $(\cong 30,000/9400)$, the panel of six-base cutters would sample it 44 times $(\cong 30,000/680)$, and the panel of four-base cutters would sample it about 700 times $(=30,000/43)$.

These concepts are illustrated by two studies of the N-acetyltransferase NAT2 gene that is responsible for the isoniazid acetylation polymorphism and is polymorphic in rabbits and humans. In both species the NAT2 gene has a coding region of 870 bases and encodes a protein of approximately 33,000 daltons; additionally, NAT2 is devoid of introns in the coding region and contains 15,000 to 20,000 base pairs. A panel of five six-base cutter restriction enzymes (*Eco*RI, *Hin*dIII, *Xba*I, *Bgl*II, and *Apa*I) was employed to survey the rabbit genome for NAT2 polymorphism,[45] and a panel of three six-base cutter enzymes (*Kpn*I, *Bam*HI, and *Eco*RI) was employed for the human polymorphism.[46] The restriction fragment length polymorphism (RFLP) patterns indicated that the NAT2 of rabbits and humans were both polymorphic; the polymorphism in rabbits was due to a gross deletion of the slow acetylator gene, while the human RFLP patterns suggested that a small genic lesion, possibly a single base substitution, could account for the human polymorphism. Additional studies confirmed this conclusion for human NAT2 polymorphism.[47]

The human genome also contains a variety of short variable DNA repetitive sequences called variable number tandem repeats (VNTR) that contribute to its polymorphic character. Each of these sequences may be repeated 100 times or more in different persons. If a restriction enzyme cuts the DNA on either side of a VNTR, the size of the fragment produced will be proportional to the number of repeats in the VNTR, and the different-sized fragments will migrate differently on an electrophoresis gel.

Gene amplification is another mechanism that generates different-sized DNA fragments that can be observed by Southern analysis. A well-known example of this phenomenon is provided by the study of two families in which amplification of the gene for the debrisoquine hydroxylation polymorphism (CYP2D6) was observed. Restriction analysis with *Eco*RI showed that a single copy of the gene that had undergone amplification was 12.1 kb in length. The RFLP patterns of *Xba*I-cleaved genomic DNA prepared from members of these families revealed restriction fragments of 175 and 42 kb. The 175-kb fragment from the father, daughter, and son of family 1 represented 12 copies of the amplified gene, and the 42-kb fragment from two sons of family 2 represented two copies of the amplified gene.[48]

Unfortunately, RFLP patterns that are generated by VNTR polymorphisms and by other polymorphic fragments that differ by one or only a few bases cannot be resolved by Southern analysis. Also, Southern analysis cannot determine which base is polymorphic. With polymerase chain reaction (PCR), the polymorphic site of DNA can be amplified and its size and boundaries precisely determined.

Many well-characterized polymorphic VNTR DNA sites, now numbering in the thousands, are known. The availability of polymorphic VNTR sites should improve the application of gene mapping techniques to pharmacogenetically important genes. For traits whose identification has been slowed for lack of a sufficient number of markers, these polymorphic sites should remove or reduce this limitation.

Influence of Recombinant DNA Technology on Pharmacogenetics

Prior to the advent of recombinant techniques, knowledge of the biochemical or pharmacological defect for a few traits had led to the discovery of the responsible genes. Certain disorders of hemoglobin and other blood-borne proteins had been attributed to the presence of missense, nonsense, or frameshift mutations that occurred within the coding region of the gene, but recombinant DNA studies revealed that genetic diversity could be created by mutation at various regulatory sites as well as within the coding region of the gene. One entirely unanticipated but particularly notable consequence of these studies was the demonstration that higher organisms had evolved the ability to generate different proteins from a single gene (by alternative splicing mechanisms).

As the pace of mutation detection quickened, it soon became evident that mutations underlying hereditary disorders were most often revealed in one of two ways: (1) by the production of a functionally altered gene product (protein), or (2) by the production of a normal gene product in an altered amount. In the latter case, the amount of the variant protein was most often found to be reduced. There are, however, reports of several traits including serum butyryl cholinesterase sensitivity,[49–51] CYP2D6 polymorphism,[48] and glutathione-S-transferase[52] attributed to increased amounts of the variant protein. To a first approximation, mutations that cause the synthesis of structurally altered polypeptides or proteins usually occur within the coding region of the gene; they include point mutations, frameshift mutations, large deletions or insertions, and chain termination mutations, whereas those that result in altered amounts of protein product include mutations of the transcriptional machinery such as deletions, insertions, mutations of the promoter regions and other regulatory regions, mutations of RNA processing such as those that alter splicing in the 5' untranslated region or 3' adenylation signals, and mutations of the translational machinery that are responsible for the initiation, elongation, and termination of polypeptide chains. The potential for epigenetic modifications that alter gene expression has been recognized more recently as discussed below (see Chapter 6).

These rough guidelines are intended to provide some perspective into the relationship of genetic changes to protein variation that may alter drug responses. It is prudent, however, to keep an open mind about any attempt to classify mutational mechanisms too rigidly from such limited information as it may not be entirely satisfactory. For instance, some traits that appear to be due to a quantitative defect in protein synthesis may on further analysis be found to be due to a structurally abnormal protein that undergoes rapid proteolysis, and others that are genetically heterogeneous could be due to more than a single type of mutational, recombinational, or epigenetic event.

Many pharmacogenetic traits are due to point mutations or other small genic lesions that lead to a functional change in the protein encoded, or to a virtual absence of the protein if the gene that encodes it is deleted entirely or is truncated by the introduction of a premature stop codon. Such alterations occur at specific genetic loci, and hence are useful as genetic markers for diagnosing specific traits. When DNA mutates, recognition sites for restriction enzymes may also change, and such changes can be detected by the difference in the RFLP patterns. The ability to detect minute lesions in DNA, as well as to determine the specific structural change, allows for the diagnosis of the traits in question. Expression and characterization of the mutant and normal proteins may also suggest a plausible explanation of the unusual response.

PCR can provide additional strategies for detecting minute lesions of DNA. Consider, for example, the following experiment. A given gene is amplified in one test tube with "wild-type" primers and cleaved with an appropriate restriction enzyme. In another tube, allele-specific amplification of an aberrant gene is performed with primers made to the mutated site and cleaved with the same restriction enzyme. DNA is needed only for the first amplification because additional amplifications can be performed with PCR-generated template DNA. The resulting fragments are separated on agarose gels (or alternatively on polyacrylamide gels for improved resolution of very faint bands), and the RFLPs are compared for pattern differences. In many applications, allele-specific amplification by PCR is preferable to Southern analysis for comprehensive screening of populations because the latter technique is unable to discriminate many alleles and because PCR analysis is at least an order of magnitude more sensitive than Southern blotting for the detection/amplification of novel sequences, and requires only a small amount of DNA that can be obtained from leukocytes, buccal epithelium, or even dried blood spots.

A number of genes have been found to incorporate microsatellites. Microsatellites are stretches of repetitive DNA sequences, and if mutated, these elements appear to be capable of disrupting cell function. The importance of microsatellite instability has been recognized as a prognostic marker of familial and sporadic colorectal cancer.[53] Microsatellite instability, a striking molecular feature of colorectal cancer seen in more than 90% of cases, refers to somatically acquired variations in the length of repetitive nucleotide sequences in DNA, such as $(CA)^n$ or $(GATA)^n$. Gryfe and colleagues[54] tested the hypothesis that colorectal cancers arising from microsatellite instability have distinctive clinical features that affect outcome. In a population-based series of 607 patients (50 years of age and younger) they found a high frequency of microsatellite instability in 17% of colorectal cancers in these patients. Additionally, they found that these cancers had a decreased likelihood of metastasizing to regional lymph nodes regardless of the depth of tumor invasion. They concluded that high-frequency microsatellite instability reduced the chances of metastases and is an independent predictor of a relatively favorable outcome. In another report, Datta and co-workers[55] describe genetic and phenotypic correlates of colorectal cancer in young patients of age 21 years or younger. Datta's report indicates that there is microsatellite instability in almost half the colorectal cancers in children and young adults.

The genome is well covered by microsatellites, but polymorphisms with these repeats within genes are less abundant. Two methods have been applied successfully to the identification of alleles that cause disease: single-strand conformational polymorphism (SSCP) because of its simplicity, and density gradient gel electrophoresis (DGGE) because of its high, near 100%, sensitivity for allelic differences. Unfortunately, SSCP requires two or three gel conditions for detection and DGGE needs special equipment and more expensive GC-clamped primers. Another method has been described, enzymatic mutation detection (EMD), that promises to be superior to existing techniques in the search for elusive mutations.[56] The technique employs bacteriophage resolvases that are capable of recognizing mismatched bases in double-stranded DNA and cutting the DNA at the mismatch. EMD takes advantage of the mismatch to detect individuals who are heterozygous at the given site—the presence and the estimated position of the mutation are both revealed. In simpler terms, the resolvase can be thought of as a restriction enzyme that recognizes only mutations.

IMPEDIMENTS TO PHARMACOGENETIC INVESTIGATION

Human pharmacogenetic traits encompass an array of responses as broad as the effects evoked by exogenous substances in human subjects, a range that is virtually limitless. Outwardly, there is nothing to distinguish a response of hereditary origin from one that is primarily due to environmental causes. Traditionally, the classic principles of genetics applied to twin studies, family studies, and studies in larger populations are employed to differentiate them.

Assignment of a casual relationship between a clinical event and treatment with a specific drug has been based on the evaluation of individual case reports followed by confirmatory epidemiological studies. If the unusual response involves a long lag between exposure and the outright appearance of clinical manifestations, special epidemiological approaches may be necessary to establish the connection between the response and the influence of heredity. Over the short term, this possibility is exemplified by the predisposition of G6PD-deficient individuals to the hemolytic effect of oxidant drugs and over the long term by the predisposition of glutathione-deficient individuals to cancer of the lung and various other tissues.

Methodological difficulties can arise with a disturbing frequency. The usual recourse to the detection of genetic determinants of drug idiosyncrasy involves a combination of classical and molecular genetic approaches to the study of the disposition of the drug in blood, or urine, its rate of elimination, and so on, as already described. Very few tests for genetic susceptibility to the detection of idiosyncratic drug reactions have been designed that protect sensitive individuals from the risk of injury from further exposure as might occur on repeated testing. Noninvasive tests for traits such as for G6PD deficiency and succinylcholine sensitivity avoid the potential for harm because they are performed on samples of blood or serum removed from the test subject prior to testing. Progress has been made toward the development of such techniques through biochemical studies of leukocytes isolated from peripheral blood, and more recently through the application of recombinant DNA technology to the identification of susceptible phenotypes and genotypes, but this area of investigation needs more emphasis.[57]

An unusual response to a given exogenous agent may be due primarily to the influence of heredity on the one hand, or to the influence of the environment on the other, but the majority of pharmacogenetic traits fall somewhere between these extremes. Changing environmental exposures and the diverse human genetic composition may make the relative contributions of genetic and environmental factors to the idiosyncrasy difficult or impossible to assess from clinical situations or from epidemiological observations alone. Further complications may arise for responses that result from more than one hereditary element. Although the inheritance of monogenic traits is predictable because it obeys Mendelian rules and Hardy–Weinberg expectations, the inheritance of traits caused by the combination of two or more monogenic traits would not follow Mendelian patterns. This point has been addressed for lupus erythematosus induced by hydralazine,[57] and for red blood cell hemolysis induced by sulfones or sulfonamides.[58,59] Other examples of pharmacogenetic importance could arise in connection with responses to therapeutic agents whose actions are mediated by receptor subtypes whose binding specificities overlap, or to carcinogenic chemicals whose metabolism is due to different members of a subfamily of enzymes whose substrate selectivities overlap.

Still further, the extent to which individual responses to certain environmental chemicals or dietary factors[60] is affected even within individuals can be quite variable. The controversy of long-standing surrounding the etiological role of heredity versus environment associated with lung cancer in smokers illustrates this point. Despite the potential for genetic susceptibility of humans to this disorder, and a clear relationship between genetically determined differences in metabolic activation of chemical carcinogens by the cytochrome P450 enzyme CYP1A1[61–63] and susceptibility to cancer in a genetic mouse model, the issue is not completely resolved to everyone's satisfaction.[64–69] Another case in point of the latter possibility has arisen in connection with the contentious association of dopamine D2 receptor gene variants with the abuse of cocaine, alcohol, nicotine (in smoking), as well as other chemical dependency syndromes and addictive–compulsive behavioral disorders.[70]

The determination of the extent and importance of genetically conditioned differences in response to exogenous substances can also be confounded in various ways. For example, Garibaldi's report of an outbreak of isoniazid-induced liver damage with fatal consequences in 1972 drew attention to the extent and severity of this disorder.[71] For more than 15 years after that report, investigators debated the origin of this adverse effect and studied the relevance of the human acetylation polymorphism at clinical, epidemiological, and basic pharmacological levels to this problem in patient populations and animal models. As a consequence, we knew that genetic differences in a single metabolic defect in acetylating capacity acted at an early step in the metabolic pathway of isoniazid, and again later. The polymorphic difference in acetylation that converts isoniazid to the hepatotoxin, monoacetylhydrazine, is almost completely blunted by the acetylation of monoacetylhyrazine to diacetylhydrazine; diacetylhydrazine is a nontoxic metabolite that is excreted harmlessly in urine (Figure 5.10). Both acetylation steps have a bearing on liver damage, but since the second step opposes the first, and other variable metabolic steps intervene, outright prediction of the effect of acetylator status on isoniazid hepatotoxicity is difficult. During the

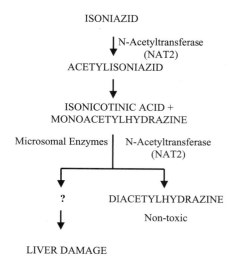

Figure 5.10 Metabolic activation of isoniazid in liver.

decade following Garibaldi's report, epidemiological evidence from retrospective studies could be cited in support of the hypothesis that rapid acetylators were more susceptible, that slow acetylators were more susceptible, or that neither acetylator phenotype was more susceptible.

In 1981, Dickson and co-workers reinvestigated the problem in a prospective study of 111 subjects and on stratifying their data according to age, found three distinct risk levels: rapid acetylators younger than 35 years had very little risk (4%) of developing liver damage, slow acetylators younger than 35 years and rapid acetylators older than 35 years have a moderate risk (13%), or about the population average, and slow acetylators older than 35 years have a very high risk (37%). In 1982, Musch and co-workers observed hepatotoxicity among patients receiving an antituberculosis regimen consisting of isoniazid, rifampacin, and ethambutol in 26 of 56 slow acetylators (46.6%) and only 4 of 30 rapid acetylators. Furthermore, the 12 patients with most severe hepatotoxicity were all slow acetylators. The observations of Dickinson et al.,[72] Musch et al.,[73] and Gurumurthy et al.[74] added another important point: that the significance of the acetylator status as a predictor of susceptibility to liver damage was highly dependent on the index of liver damage chosen. If clinical jaundice was chosen as the index as Gurumurthy did, "liver damage" was unrelated to acetylator status, but if serum transaminase elevations were chosen, as the other investigators did, "liver damage" depended on acetylator status. Clearly, failure to define such terms adequately might lead to loss of valuable information if not invalidation of the conclusions reached.

It may not be possible to identify or anticipate all problems that may arise during the collection of information on human subjects, but in view of the evidence that is required to establish heritability of a given trait, certain criteria can be specified that should be fulfilled in designing and conducting a proper pharmacogenetic study. (1) The distribution of the trait (i.e., of the phenotypes) should be determined in a population of healthy individuals and in an unselected sample of individuals who exhibit the trait; (2) the trait should be demonstrated in healthy individuals including identical and fraternal twins, in families, and in larger populations; (3) the incidence of the trait should be determined in an unselected sample of unrelated individuals; and (4) the presence of the trait should not interfere with the conduct or interpretation of the phenotyping procedure. Additionally, any current disorder being treated at the time of phenotyping should be shown not to interfere with the phenotype determination. Rigorous adherence to these criteria should enhance the reliability of the human data collected and should avoid or minimize the chances of critical gaps in information obtained.

When it is of interest to assess or compare a given trait in different ethnogeographic populations, each of the criteria should be fulfilled for each group or population that is compared. Lastly, because of their importance to the assessment of ethnogeographic factors of human drug response, experienced investigators will want to take account of the potential culturally specific risks that ethnic studies may pose for individual participants or study populations as is considered below (see Chapter 8, p. 249).

SUMMARY

Pharmacogenetic analysis combines the principles and tools of classical and molecular genetics. Adherence to the principles of classical (Mendelian) genetics seeks to partition the pharmacological variation into its hereditary and environmental components. To this end, profiles of information on distinct drug responder phenotypes are collected and analyzed for the variation between individuals, between identical and fraternal twins, within families, and in larger populations. A small degree of variation in response within individuals compared to that observed between individuals, within identical twins compared to that in fraternal twins, clustering of phenotypes within families, and segregation of phenotypes according to Mendelian rules indicates that heritability contributes to phenotypic differences in response. The agreement between the observed numbers of specific drug responder phenotypes and those expected by the Hardy–Weinberg law of population genetics and the association of specific drug responder phenotypes with specific genotypes provides additional support for heritability.

Pharmacogenetic disorders, like genetic diseases, are due to structural lesions of DNA sequences as small as a single base up to an entire chromosome, and DNA technologies are capable of detecting lesions throughout the entire range of interest. These molecular tools enable investigators to produce accurate copies of genes and express the proteins they encode in quantities sufficient for biochemical and pharmacological characterization, permitting an altered response to a therapeutic agent or another exogenous chemical to be associated with its molecular genetic basis.

REFERENCES

1. Daniel A. The size of prometaphase chromosome segments. Tables using percentages of haploid autosome length (750 band stage). Clin Genet 1985; 28(3):216–224.
2. Dorit RL, Schoenbach L, Gilbert W. How big is the universe of exons? Science 1990; 250(4986):1377–1382.
3. Muratani K, Hada T, Yamamoto Y, Kaneko T, Shigeto Y, Ohue T, et al. Inactivation of the cholinesterase gene by Alu insertion: Possible mechanism for human gene transposition. Proc Natl Acad Sci USA 1991; 88(24):11315–11319.
4. Dombroski BA, Mathias SL, Nanthakumar E, Scott AF, Kazazian HH Jr. Isolation of an active human transposable element. Science 1991; 254(5039):1805–1808.
5. Mathias SL, Scott AF, Kazazian HH, Jr., Boeke JD, Gabriel A. Reverse transcriptase encoded by a human transposable element. Science 1991; 254(5039):1808–1810.
6. Lifton RP, Dluhy RG, Powers M, Rich GM, Gutkin M, Fallo F, et al. Hereditary hypertension caused by chimaeric gene duplications and ectopic expression of aldosterone synthase. Nat Genet 1992; 2(1):66–74.
7. Rich GM, Ulick S, Cook S, Wang JZ, Lifton RP, Dluhy RG. Glucocorticoid-remediable aldosteronism in a large kindred: Clinical spectrum and diagnosis using a characteristic biochemical phenotype. Ann Intern Med 1992; 116(10):813–820.
8. Huang ME, Ye YC, Chen SR, Chai JR, Lu JX, Zhoa L, et al. Use of all-trans retinoic acid in the treatment of acute promyelocytic leukemia. Blood 1988; 72(2):567–572.
9. Chen SJ, Zhu YJ, Tong JH, Dong S, Huang W, Chen Y, et al. Rearrangements in the second intron of the RARA gene are present in a large majority of patients with acute promyelocytic leukemia and are used as molecular markers for retinoic acid-induced leukemic cell differentiation. Blood 1991; 78(10):2696–2701.
10. de The H, Vivanco-Ruiz MM, Tiollais P, Stunnenberg H, Dejean A. Identification of a retinoic acid responsive element in the retinoic acid receptor beta gene. Nature 1990; 343(6254):177–180.
11. Attardi G. The elucidation of the human mitochondrial genome: A historical perspective. Bioessays 1986; 5(1):34–39.
12. Anderson S, Bankier AT, Barrell BG, de Bruijn MH, Coulson AR, Drouin J, et al. Sequence and organization of the human mitochondrial genome. Nature 1981; 290(5806):457–465.
13. Fisher RA. The correlation between relatives on the supposition of Mendelian inheritance. Transact R Soc Edinburgh 1918; 52:399–433.
14. Falconer DS. Introduction to Quantitative Genetics. New York: Ronald Press, 1960.
15. Holzinger KJ. The relative effect of nature and nurture influences on twin differences. J Educ Psych 1929; 20:241–248.
16. Propping P. Pharmacogenetics. Rev Physiol Biochem Pharmacol 1978; 83:123–173.
17. Smith C. Concordance in twins: Methods and interpretation. Am J Hum Genet 1974; 26(4):454–466.
18. Plomin R, DeFries JC, McClearn GE. Behavioral Genetics. San Francisco: W.H. Freeman, 1980.
19. Neonatal behaviour and maternal barbiturates. Br Med J 1972; October 14:63–64.
20. Weber WW. The Acetylator Genes and Drug Response. New York: Oxford University Press, 1987.
21. Vesell ES. Recent progress in pharmacogenetics. Adv Pharmacol Chemother 1969; 7:1–52.

22. Vesell ES, Page JG. Genetic control of the phenobarbital-induced shortening of plasma antipyrine half-lives in man. J Clin Invest 1969; 48(12):2202–2209.

23. Jones PA, Laird PW. Cancer epigenetics comes of age. Nat Genet 1999; 21(2):163–167.

24. Beck S. Genome acrobatics: Understanding complex genomes. Drug Discov Today 2001; 6(23):1181–1182.

25. Dennis C. Altered states. Nature 2003; 421(13 Feb):686–688.

26. Fraga MF, Ballestar E, Paz MF, Ropero S, Setien F, Ballestar ML, et al. Epigenetic differences arise during the lifetime of monozygotic twins. Proc Natl Acad Sci USA 2005; 102(30):10604–10609.

27. Guttmacher AE, Collins FS, Carmona RH. The family history—more important than ever. N Engl J Med 2004; 351(22):2333–2336.

28. Britt BA, Locher WG, Kalow W. Hereditary aspects of malignant hyperthermia. Can Anaesth Soc J 1969; 16(2):89–98.

29. Oates NS, Shah RR, Idle JR, Smith RL. Genetic polymorphism of phenformin 4-hydroxylation. Clin Pharmacol Ther 1982; 32(1):81–89.

30. Lane N. Mitochondrial disease: Powerhouse of disease. Nature 2006; 440(7084):600–602.

31. Hu DN, Qui WQ, Wu BT, Fang LZ, Zhou F, Gu YP, et al. Genetic aspects of antibiotic induced deafness: Mitochondrial inheritance. J Med Genet 1991; 28(2):79–83.

32. Evans DA, Manley KA, McKusick VA. Genetic control of isoniazid metabolism in man. Br Med J 1960; 5197:485–491.

33. Sunahara S, Urano M. [Problems of isoniazid metabolism. Hereditary character and variability according to races.]. Med Thorac 1963; 20:289–312.

34. Beutler E, Dern RJ, Alving AS. The hemolytic effect of primaquine. VI. An in vitro test for sensitivity of erythrocytes to primaquine. J Lab Clin Med 1955; 45(1):40–50.

35. Beutler E. The glutathione instability of drug-sensitive red cells: A new method for the in vitro detection of drug sensitivity. J Lab Clin Med 1957; 49(1):84–95.

36. Childs B, Zinkham W, Browne EA, Kimbro EL, Torbert JV. A genetic study of a defect in glutathione metabolism of the erythrocyte. Bull Johns Hopkins Hosp 1958; 102(1):21–37.

37. Beutler E. Glucose-6-phosphate dehydrogenase deficiency. N Engl J Med 1991; 324(3):169–174.

38. Vulliamy TJ, D'Urso M, Battistuzzi G, Estrada M, Foulkes NS, Martini G, et al. Diverse point mutations in the human glucose-6-phosphate dehydrogenase gene cause enzyme deficiency and mild or severe hemolytic anemia. Proc Natl Acad Sci USA 1988; 85(14):5171–5175.

39. Martini G, Toniolo D, Vulliamy T, Luzzatto L, Dono R, Viglietto G, et al. Structural analysis of the X-linked gene encoding human glucose 6-phosphate dehydrogenase. EMBO J 1986; 5(8):1849–1855.

40. Woolf B. On estimating the relation between blood group and disease. Ann Human Gen 1955; 19:251–253.

41. Haldane JBS. The estimation and significance of the logarithm of a ratio of frequencies. Ann Human Gen 1956; 20:309–311.

42. Evans DAP, Eze LC, Whibley EJ. The association of the slow acetylator phenotype with bladder cancer. J Med Genet 1983; 20:330–333.

43. Case RA, Hosker ME, McDonald DB, Pearson JT. Tumours of the urinary bladder in workmen engaged in the manufacture and use of certain dyestuff intermediates in the

British chemical industry. I. The role of aniline, benzidine, alpha-naphthylamine, and beta-naphthylamine. Br J Ind Med 1954; 11(2):75–104.

44. Secko D. A target for Iressa. Scientist 2006; 20(4):67–68.

45. Blum M, Grant DM, Demierre A, Meyer UA. N-Acetylation pharmacogenetics: A gene deletion causes absence of arylamine N-acetyltransferase in liver of slow acetylator rabbits. Proc Natl Acad Sci USA 1989; 86(23):9554–9557.

46. Ohsako S, Deguchi T. Cloning and expression of cDNAs for polymorphic and monomorphic arylamine N-acetyltransferases from human liver. J Biol Chem 1990; 265(8):4630–4634.

47. Vatsis KP, Weber WW. Human N-acetyltransferases. In: Kauffman FC, editor. Conjugation-Deconjugation Reactions in Drug Metabolism and Toxicity. Berlin: Springer-Verlag, 1994: 109–130.

48. Johansson I, Lundqvist E, Bertilsson L, Dahl ML, Sjoqvist F, Ingelman-Sundberg M. Inherited amplification of an active gene in the cytochrome P450 CYP2D locus as a cause of ultrarapid metabolism of debrisoquine. Proc Natl Acad Sci USA 1993; 90(24):11825–11829.

49. Neitlich HW. Increased plasma cholinesterase activity and succinylcholine resistance: A genetic variant. J Clin Invest 1966; 45(3):380–387.

50. Yoshida A, Motulsky AG. A pseudocholinesterase variant (E Cynthiana) associated with elevated plasma enzyme activity. Am J Hum Genet 1969; 21(5):486–498.

51. Soreq H, Zamir R, Zevin-Sonkin D, Zakut H. Human cholinesterase genes localized by hybridization to chromosomes 3 and 16. Hum Genet 1987; 77(4):325–328.

52. McLellan RA, Oscarson M, Alexandrie AK, Seidegard J, Evans DA, Rannug A, et al. Characterization of a human glutathione S-transferase mu cluster containing a duplicated GSTM1 gene that causes ultrarapid enzyme activity. Mol Pharmacol 1997; 52(6):958–965.

53. Offit K. Genetic prognostic markers for colorectal cancer. N Engl J Med 2000; 342(2):124–125.

54. Gryfe R, Kim H, Hsieh ET, Aronson MD, Holowaty EJ, Bull SB, et al. Tumor microsatellite instability and clinical outcome in young patients with colorectal cancer. N Engl J Med 2000; 342(2):69–77.

55. Datta RV, LaQuaglia MP, Paty PB. Genetic and phenotypic correlates of colorectal cancer in young patients. N Engl J Med 2000; 342(2):137–138.

56. Del TB, Jr., Poff HE, III, Novotny MA, Cartledge DM, Walker RI, Earl CD, et al. Automated fluorescent analysis procedure for enzymatic mutation detection. Clin Chem 1998; 44(4):731–739.

57. Shear NH, Spielberg SP, Grant DM, Tang BK, Kalow W. Differences in metabolism of sulfonamides predisposing to idiosyncratic toxicity. Ann Intern Med 1986; 105(2):179–184.

58. Magon AM, Leipzig RM, Zannoni VG, Brewer GJ. Interactions of glucose-6-phosphate dehydrogenase deficiency with drug acetylation and hydroxylation reactions. J Lab Clin Med 1981; 97(6):764–770.

59. Woolhouse NM, Atu-Taylor LC. Influence of double genetic polymorphism on response to sulfamethazine. Clin Pharmacol Ther 1982; 31(3):377–383.

60. Hein DW, McQueen CA, Grant DM, Goodfellow GH, Kadlubar FF, Weber WW. Pharmacogenetics of the arylamine N-acetyltransferases: A symposium in honor of Wendell W. Weber. Drug Metab Dispos 2000; 28(12):1425–1432.

61. Kawajiri K, Nakachi K, Imai K, Yoshii A, Shinoda N, Watanabe J. Identification of genetically high risk individuals to lung cancer by DNA polymorphisms of the cytochrome P450IA1 gene. FEBS Lett 1990; 263(1):131–133.

62. Petersen DD, McKinney CE, Ikeya K, Smith HH, Bale AE, McBride OW, et al. Human CYP1A1 gene: Cosegregation of the enzyme inducibility phenotype and an RFLP. Am J Hum Genet 1991; 48(4):720–725.

63. Wedlund PJ, Kimura S, Gonzalez FJ, Nebert DW. 1462V mutation in the human CYP1A1 gene: Lack of correlation with either the Msp I 1.9 kb (M2) allele or CYP1A1 inducibility in a three-generation family of east Mediterranean descent. Pharmacogenetics 1994; 4(1):21–26.

64. Kellermann G, Shaw CR, Luyten-Kellerman M. Aryl hydrocarbon hydroxylase inducibility and bronchogenic carcinoma. N Engl J Med 1973; 289(18):934–937.

65. Kellermann G, Luyten-Kellermann M, Shaw CR. Genetic variation of aryl hydrocarbon hydroxylase in human lymphocytes. Am J Hum Genet 1973; 25(3):327–331.

66. Paigen B, Minowada J, Gurtoo HL, Paigen K, Parker NB, Ward E, et al. Distribution of aryl hydrocarbon hydroxylase inducibility in cultured human lymphocytes. Cancer Res 1977; 37(6):1829–1837.

67. Paigen B, Gurtoo HL, Minowada J, Houten L, Vincent R, Paigen K, et al. Questionable relation of aryl hydrocarbon hydroxylase to lung-cancer risk. N Engl J Med 1977; 297(7):346–350.

68. Paigen B, Ward E, Steenland K, Houten L, Gurtoo HL, Minowada J. Aryl hydrocarbon hydroxylase in cultured lymphocytes of twins. Am J Hum Genet 1978; 30(5):561–571.

69. Kouri RE, McKinney CE, Slomiany DJ, Snodgrass DR, Wray NP, McLemore TL. Positive correlation between high aryl hydrocarbon hydroxylase activity and primary lung cancer as analyzed in cryopreserved lymphocytes. Cancer Res 1982; 42(12): 5030–5037.

70. Blum K, Sheridan PJ, Wood RC, Braverman ER, Chen TJ, Comings DE. Dopamine D2 receptor gene variants: Association and linkage studies in impulsive-addictive-compulsive behaviour. Pharmacogenetics 1995; 5(3):121–141.

71. Garibaldi RA, Drusin RE, Ferebee SH, Gregg MB. Isoniazid-associated hepatitis. Report of an outbreak. Am Rev Respir Dis 1972; 106(3):357–365.

72. Dickinson DS, Bailey WC, Hirschowitz BI, Soong SJ, Eidus L, Hodgkin MM. Risk factors for isoniazid (NIH)-induced liver dysfunction. J Clin Gastroenterol 1981; 33:271–279.

73. Musch E, Eichelbaum M, Wang JK, Von Sassen W, Castro-Parra M, dengler HJ. [Incidence of hepatotoxic side effects during antituberculous therapy (INH, RMP, EMB) in relation to the acetylator phenotype (author's transl)]. Klin Wochenschr 1982; 60(10): 513–519.

74. Gurumurthy P, Krishnamurthy MS, Nazareth O, Parthasarathy R, Sarma GR, Somasundaram PR, et al. Lack of relationship between hepatic toxicity and acetylator phenotype in three thousand South Indian patients during treatment with isoniazid for tuberculosis. Am Rev Respir Dis 1984; 129(1):58–61.

6

Epigenetics

Epigenetics is the study of heritable changes in gene expression that do not require, or do not generally involve, changes in the genomic DNA sequence. Historically, the term referred mainly to developmental phenomena, but recently the term has been applied more broadly to signify a relation to gene action. Currently, the field is primarily concerned with understanding the handling of genetic information by eukaryotic cells.

Genetic inheritance has been regarded until recently as the sole mode of transmission of information from one generation to the next, but a number of challenges remain in understanding the transmission of genetic information and gene expression despite the successes surrounding the unveiling of the human genome.[1,2] Epigenetic inheritance, which implies modification of gene expression without modifying the DNA sequence, has been proposed as a mechanism complementing genetic inheritance to explain these phenomena. Epigenetic information is transmitted by way of direct modification of DNA or of chromatin. In mammals, DNA methylation of cytosines is the only known physiological modification of DNA, whereas numerous modifications of chromatin have been identified that affect its conformation, but they have proven much more difficult to sort out and their significance is as yet only partially understood.

Many aspects of epigenetics have been examined in abundant detail, particularly within the past 5 years. Although PubMed searches (December 6, 2006) under "epigenetics" for the years 2000–2006 turned up only 533 citations of all kinds including 242 reviews with 197 reviews on humans, it seems apparent that many more epigenetics papers are in the literature, particularly in the older literature before many studies were identified with the term epigenetics. In assembling material for inclusion, an attempt was made to highlight conceptual advances and focus on key steps along the pathway to epigenetics. It is obvious from a timeline of epigenetic research constructed from those PubMed searches that the scope and pace of the investigation changed increasingly over time, particularly since the mid-1970s when a number of new techniques for monitoring the biochemical nature of epigenetic change were developed.

This chapter was written with the purpose of summarizing the emergence, foundations, and status of epigenetics by assembling conceptual approaches, analytical tools, and experimental evidence that led to the emergence of epigenetics as a field of biological inquiry primarily concerned with understanding the handling of genetic information by eukaryotic cells. It concludes with some perspectives on prospects for the field in health and disease.

THE EMERGENCE OF EPIGENETICS

As far back as the eighteenth and well into the twentieth century, biologists debated whether acquired (or adaptive) characters were heritable or not. Often they divided into the "naturalists," who believed that acquired characters were heritable, and the geneticists, who believed only in the inheritance of genetic variants through natural selection. Beginning around 1920, the views of naturalists began to decline while those of geneticists were ascendant, largely as a result of the pioneering studies of heredity in fruit flies by Thomas Hunt Morgan and his students. By the 1940s and 1950s, DNA had been demonstrated to be the genetic material by Oswald, Avery, and McCarty, and the double helix of DNA had been proposed as the molecular basis of modern genetics by Watson and Crick (Table 1.1 and Figure 1.1). During this revolutionary period of experimental biology, epigenetics emerged as a series of isolated observations in three disparate areas, developmental biology, chromosomal biology, and molecular biology, advancing along separate pathways before their convergence in the 1980s.

In attempting to understand how genotypes evolve, developmental biology studies in fruit flies in the 1940s by C.H. Waddington showed that a *crossveinless* phenotype induced by heat shock was assimilated and expressed in nearly 100% of progeny after several generations, even in the absence of heat shock. Waddington hypothesized that a genetic factor was responsible for the assimilation and transmission of this adaptive response.[3] As Waddington's findings were confirmed in other studies (reviewed by Ruden et al.[4]), we next learned how a series of inquiries into chromosomal biology initiated during the 1940s and 1950s began to shed light on X chromosome inactivation and much later how X inactivation was related to the peculiar phenomenon of genomic imprinting. In 1949, Murray Barr demonstrated that a cellular organelle easily visible in male and female animal cells under an ordinary microscope, the so-called "sex chromatin body," could be used to sort tissues and individuals into two groups according to gender.[5] In 1959, Ohno explained that one of the X chromosome pair in female cells remained extended in mitosis while the other assumed a condensed state to form the sex chromatin (Barr) body.[6] Within 2–3 years, Lyon[7] and Beutler and colleagues[8] independently documented the mosaicism of X chromosome expression in female cells, concluding that only one X chromosome was active in each cell of females. While these studies were ongoing, Crouse, in her studies of the mealy bug *Sciara,* discovered another phenomenon having a bearing on X chromosome mosaicism, which she called "parental imprinting" (later also called "genomic imprinting").[9] She used "imprinting" to describe the change in behavior acquired by the chromosome on passing through the male germ line as exactly opposite the imprint conferred on the same chromosome by the female germline.

In 1961, in the course of molecular studies probing the mechanisms of enzymatic replication of DNA in Arthur Kornberg's laboratory, Josse and co-workers made a seminal contribution to the emergence of epigenetics.[10] They found that cytosine in vertebrate genomes occurred at a much lower frequency, about a quarter of that expected from the overall base composition. But several years elapsed before Grippo in Scarano's laboratory clarified this finding. In 1968, Grippo observed the presence of methylases in sea urchin embryos and pointed out that 5-methylcytosine (5mC) was unique among DNA bases in that it was the only methylated base, and that 90% of the methylcytosine is nonrandomly distributed in CpG doublets in this model.[11] Actually, Rollin Hotchkiss had reported the likely presence of methylcytosine in calf thymus DNA in 1948,[12] although he called it "epicytosine." In 1971, Scarano[13] suggested that 5mC was unstable, and would deaminate spontaneously to form thymine (Figure 6.1). Following this suggestion in 1977, Salser[14] showed that the dinucleotide mCpG was indeed unstable, tending to deaminate to TpG. In 1980, Adrian Bird drew attention to the curious species difference in DNA methylation that ranged from very high to intermediate to low in vertebrates, nonarthropod invertebrates, and arthropods, respectively. Bird's analysis of nearest-neighbor dinucleotide frequencies also supported the suggestion that 5mC tended to mutate spontaneously to thymine, and that this tendency caused a CpG deficiency in heavily methylated genomes.[15,16]

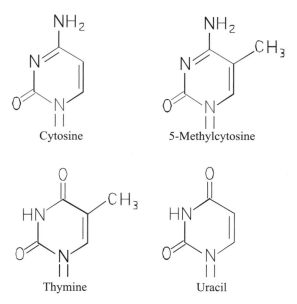

Figure 6.1 The chemical structures of cytosine, methylcytosine, thymine, and uracil.

THE FOUNDATIONS OF EPIGENETICS

DNA Methylation

In 1975, Riggs[17] reviewed the role of DNA methylation on X inactivation, and Holliday and Pugh[18] reviewed the role of DNA modification and gene activity on development. Both reviews proposed that DNA methylation acted as a regulator of gene expression in eukaryotic cells. Riggs pointed out that DNA methylation in eukaryotes had not been examined in the light of accumulating data on changes in the regulation in *Escherichia coli* involving bacterial DNA methylases and their potential for bringing about permanent changes in regulation. Arthur Riggs proposed that DNA methylation of cytosine might have a regulatory role in eukaryotes from the known effect of methylation of adenine on DNA-binding proteins in *E. coli*. Holliday and Pugh noted that the methylation of adenine in DNA in bacterium might present a very different phenotype from one without methylation. They suggested that the same ordered control of gene transcription could be achieved without changes in the DNA sequence by methylation of cytosine followed by its deamination to thymine as discussed by Scarano.[13] Riggs and Holliday and Pugh presented convincing arguments that the methylation of cytosine in CpG doublets merited a more thorough biochemical and genetic study in a higher (eukaryotic) organism.

By 1980, a general consensus had been reached: that methylation of cytosines of CpG doublets was characteristic of genomic DNA, that a deficiency of CpG doublets in genomic DNA was probably due to instability of 5mC through its mutation to thymine, and that the distribution of CpG doublets in genomic DNA was not random. Additional studies then began to reveal connections between DNA methylation and gene expression. In one early study, treatment of a variety of cell lines with the methylation inhibitor 5-azacytidine revealed that a large number of genes were reactivated.[19] However, the chemical mechanism by which cytidine analogs altered at the 5 position perturbed established methylation patterns was not clear. Subsequently, cytidine analogs that had been altered at the 5 position, such as 5-azacytidine and 5-aza-2'-deoxycytidine, became important tools for studying the role of demethylation in gene expression, but it was not realized until investigators in Jaenisch's laboratory showed that incorporation of 5-aza-2'-deoxycytidine into DNA led to covalent trapping of the DNA methyltransferase enzyme. As a result, the cells were depleted of methyltransferase activity and underwent DNA demethylation that led to reactivation of the associated gene.[20]

In an attempt to explain the nonrandom distribution of CpGs, genomic DNAs across various nonvertebrates and vertebrates were compared. They showed that DNA methylation in nonvertebrate genomes was confined to a small fraction of nuclear DNA. This compartmentalization, termed "low-density methylation," was also found in eukaryotes. In fact, most DNA, some 98%, in both nonvertebrate and vertebrate genomic DNA was methylated at low density. But in the remaining 2% of genomic DNA, regions of high-density DNA methylation existed, and their existence was particularly evident in vertebrate DNA. The regions rich in CpG nucleotides were designated as "CpG islands."[21] More recent studies have shown the CpG islands are commonly found at the promoters of genes, in exons, and the 3'-regions of genes.[22] But why the patterns of methylated DNA cytosines in vertebrates and nonvertebrates differed so strikingly remained an enigma.

Questions regarding the significance of DNA methylation engaged the attention of many investigators throughout much of the 1980s. Suppression of transposed elements and other "parasitic" elements had been demonstrated in various model systems, and investigators believed this was the ancestral function of DNA methylation. Studies outside the animal kingdom, as in slime molds and filamentous fungi, provided the strongest evidence in favor of this hypothesis. For example, Rothnie and colleagues[23] had shown that DNA methylation of a single transposable element prevented damaging transposition events, and they inferred that DNA methylation of the foreign element repressed its function and prevented damaging transposition events. Other investigators demonstrated in different model systems that fully infectious proviruses were rendered harmless by methylation,[24] or that demethylation of DNA by 5-azacytidine reactivated quiescent proviral genomes.[25] Based on this information, Bird proposed that DNA methylation in invertebrates was more concerned with suppression of "selfish" elements that could disrupt gene structure and function, whereas vertebrates had retained the so-called ancestral function of DNA methylation, but had also adapted this process as a repressor of endogenous promoters of genes.

DNA Methylation, X Inactivation, and Genomic Imprinting

The effect of parenteral origin on gene expression arises through a mechanism known as genomic imprinting.[9] Experimental evidence for such an effect in mammals was first reported by McGrath and Solter,[26] who demonstrated the failure of mouse embryos derived from purely maternal or paternal genomes to develop beyond implantation. There followed a growing realization that memories of the maternal and paternal genes were permanent, persisting throughout the development and life of the individual, residing in some form of imprinting imposed on the genome during gametogenesis. The incentive to explore molecular mechanisms of genomic imprinting increased following the appearance of a report by Spence et al.[27] consistent with the observations of McGrath and Solter of clinical disorders associated with uniparental disomy. Though little was actually known about the molecular basis of parental imprinting, DNA methylation was considered the best candidate to explain this epigenetic modification.[28,29]

To examine this possibility, Stöger's group investigated the insulin-like growth factor (*Igfr2*), which they had shown earlier by classical mouse genetics to be the only known gene imprinted and expressed exclusively from the maternally inherited chromosome.[29] Stöger and colleagues searched the mouse *Igf2r* locus for the presence of methylation modifications in a parental-specific manner, i.e., for modifications that could act as the imprinting signal permitting the cell's transcription machinery to distinguish genetically identical loci, and they found that different levels of DNA methylation occurred between the maternal and paternal alleles. The *Igf2r* locus was modified by methylation on both paternal and maternal chromosomes. Two regions of the gene were identified, and both were CpG islands as judged by their high GC content and high CpG:GpC ratio. Region 1 contained the CpG island that included the start of transcription and was methylated only on the repressed paternal chromosome, while the expressed maternal locus was methylated at region 2, which was a CpG sequence located in a downstream intron. Methylation of region 1 was acquired after fertilization, whereas methylation of region 2 was inherited from the female gamete. Region 2 differed from region 1 in that it was not associated with the start of transcription of a gene. Stöger proposed that methylation was implicated in the expression of the *Igf2r*, and that methylation of region 2 marked the maternal *Igf2r* locus as an imprinting signal. This was the first clear example of a primary gametic imprint shown to be methylated.[30]

The Chemical Nature of Chromatin

Modern insight into the function of chromatin began with the studies of the cytologist E. Heitz who proposed in 1928 that chromatin has certain genetic attributes. From an earlier time, cytologists had seen an odd assortment of densely stained agglomerations in the cell nuclei of various species of plants and animals. By following chromosomes through cell division cycles, Heitz could distinguish two classes of chromosomal material: euchromatin, which underwent cyclical condensation and unraveling, and heterochromatin, which maintained its compactness in the nucleus. The repressive action of chromatin on gene action had already been recognized at that time and the two chromatin states were viewed as a visible guide to gene action. Nearly 40 years later, Spencer Brown saw the investigation of chromatin as one of the most challenging and diffuse in modern biology in his first-rate review of the subject.[31] Brown believed that resolution of the properties of euchromatin and heterochromatin would eventually improve our understanding of the systems controlling gene action in higher organisms.

More recent research has greatly enhanced our knowledge of the chemical nature of epigenetic modifications and gene expression.[32-34] We now know in affirmation of Brown's prediction that the genomes of many animals including humans are compartmentalized into either transcriptionally competent *euchromatin* or transcriptionally silent *heterochromatin*. Chromatin is a polymeric complex that consists of histone and nonhistone proteins. Genomic DNA in all eukaryotic cells is packaged in a folded, constrained, and compacted manner by a several thousand-fold reduction in association with this polymer. The basic building block of chromatin is the nucleosome, which consists of approximately 146 base pairs of DNA wrapped around a histone octamer that contains two molecules each of core histones H2A, H2B, H3, and H4. These units are organized in arrays that are connected by histones of the H1 linker class. Repeating nucleosome cores are assembled into higher-order structures that are stabilized by linker DNA and histone H1.[33] One of the functional consequences of chromatin packaging is to prevent access of DNA-binding transcription factors to the gene promoter. The

amino termini of histones of chromatin are subject to a variety of posttranslational modifications such as acetylation, phosphorylation, methylation, ubiquina-
tion, and ATP-ribosylation and as chromatin structure is plastic, the potential
exists that an enormous number of combinations of these modifications could
lead to activation or repression of gene expression. It is clear that chromatin remodeling is closely linked to gene expression, but the mechanism or mechanisms
by which this occurs are not well understood.

THE EFFECT OF MOLECULAR BIOLOGY ON EPIGENETICS

During the 1960s and 1970s, observations regarding 5mC raised many more questions than could be answered with the tools that were widely available at that
time. During this same period, however, the genetic code and the rules whereby
cells read information encoded in DNA were established (Figure 1.1), and biologists were more inclined to think of hereditary transactions in terms of the
flow of information from DNA to RNA to protein. The availability of recombinant DNA technologies for cloning, sequencing, and expression of genes, and
the invention of Southern blots for identifying DNA polymorphisms and Northern
blots for determining levels of gene expression, afforded investigators the tools
they needed to relate allelic variants of genes directly to biochemical and pharmacological variants of enzymes, receptors, and other proteins.

But we should recall that the central dogma of molecular biology as formulated
in the 1950s asserted the cardinal function of gene action to be the synthesis
of proteins according to the program of instructions encoded in the DNA that
was subsequently transcribed into RNA and translated into the primary protein
sequence. The gene was judged to be deterministic of *unidirectional* gene expression and for more than 50 years, the bulk of genomics research was guided
by this model. However, recent discoveries have revealed certain inadequa-
cies in this model of the gene–protein relationship. To begin with, the discovery
of reverse transcriptase by Howard Temin and David Baltimore negated the idea
that gene expression was unidirectional. The posttranslational modification of
protein added another twist. More recently, it became apparent that some genes
encoded just one protein, while other genes encoded more than one protein, and
still others did not encode any protein, confounding the predictive value of the
genotype. The identification of previously unknown pathway components illustrated the complexity of cellular events, and recognition of the fact that gene
expression could be altered at the translational, transcriptional, and posttranslational levels by a host of factors necessitated an expanded view of the basic
principles of gene expression and phenotypic expression as originally formulated
(Figure 6.2).

Additional advances in molecular biology in the 1980s are brought into sharper
focus by the cloning and sequencing of a vast number of genes predictive of
disease, the expression of the proteins they encode, and fixing their chromosomal
location in the human genome. The polymerase chain reaction (PCR) combined

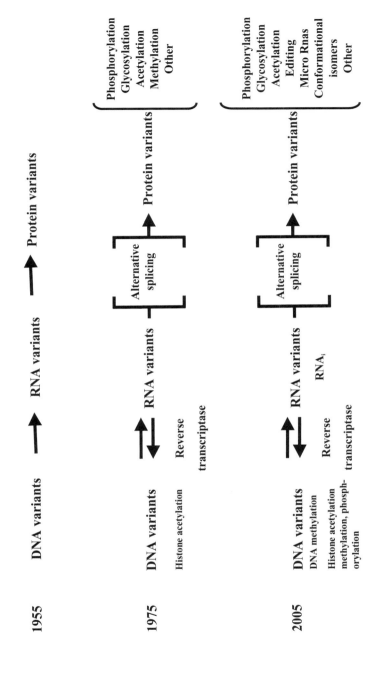

Figure 6.2 Expanding the central dogma of molecular biology. Advances have necessitated revisions of the original proposal formulated in the 1950s that "genes beget RNA, which in turn begets protein." With permission from *The Scientist*.

with gene expression systems afforded the synthesis of well-defined recombinant proteins in quantities sufficient for biochemical and pharmacological characterization. Molecular biological approaches in all forms permeated and dominated biological research setting the stage for the convergence of basic research and clinical medicine. These events not only solidified the foundations of epigenetics and provided novel insights into the multiplicity of factors affecting gene expression, but they also redoubled interest in human epigenetics as a bona fide discipline complementary to human genetics.

Restriction Enzymes Provide the First Clues to Epigenetic Inheritance

Technologies for the identification and quantification of methylated cytosines in DNA that yielded important information about patterns of methylated DNA were developed during the 1950s and 1960s. However, none of these alone could define the distribution of methylated cytosines in eukaryotic DNA or advance our understanding of its function.[35] With the advent of molecular biology, assays capable of sequencing genomic DNA and localizing genotypic differences in genomic targets evolved rapidly in response to demands in research and medicine, and restriction endonucleases were an integral component of many of these assays. Typically restriction endonucleases are bacterial enzymes that recognize palindromic sequences four to eight bases long and make sequence-specific cuts in the phosphate-pentose backbone of DNA to yield "restriction fragments" of the molecule.

Several restriction enzymes include CpG in their recognition sequence such as *Hpa*II (CCGG), *Msp*I (CCGG), *Ava*I (CPyCGPuG), *Sal*I (GTCGAC), and *Sma*I (CCCGGG). Interestingly, some of these enzymes, such as *Hpa*II, do not cut the DNA if the CpG sequence is methylated, while others, such as *Msp*I, cut the DNA regardless of the methylation state.[36] Investigators took advantage of this differential property to determine the pattern of methylation in specific regions of DNA.

In 1975, Edwin Southern combined the specificity of restriction enzymes with slab gel electrophoresis to identify sequence variation in fragments of DNA.[37] He used restriction enzymes to generate predictable fragmentation of genomic DNA, and gel electrophoresis to separate and array the DNA fragments by size. Waalwjik and Flavell[38] used Southern's technique to cut total rabbit genomic DNA with either *Hpa*II or *Msp*I followed by agarose electrophoresis, Southern blotting, and hybridization to a ^{32}P-labeled globin probe. Other investigators applied Southern's technique in experiments similar to that of Waalwjik and Flavell virtually simultaneously. This series of elegant experiments revealed a definitive pattern of methylated cytosines in somatic DNA, that both strands of DNA contained methylated cytosines, and that these patterns were maintained through DNA replication (reviewed in Razin and Riggs[35]). Waalwjik and Flavell were first to demonstrate the pattern and location of methylated cytosines at CpG residues in DNA. Additional studies indicated that unmethylated DNA sequences generally remained unmethylated, and that methylated sequences retained their methyl moieties for at least 50 generations of growth and culture. In this way, the clonal inheritance of the DNA methylation patterns was established; the tissue specificity of these patterns provided further support for this conclusion.

DNA Methylation Involves Two Dynamically Regulated Pathways

Several DNA methylation processes are observed in cells: *de novo* cytosine methylation, maintenance methylation during replication of dsDNA, active demethylation during the absence of replication, and spontaneous demethylation when maintenance methylation is suppressed. CpG sites are the primary sites of cytosine methylation in eukaryotic DNA, but methylation of sites other than CpG occurs.

In vertebrate genomes, approximately 70% of the CpG residues are methylated, the bulk of which occurs in eukaryotes during replication in the S-phase of the cell cycle. However, the regions of the genome termed "CpG islands" were preferentially methylated while other areas were protected from methylation. Reasoning from the properties of DNA methyltransferases in bacteria, a combination of two distinct processes—*de novo* DNA methylation and maintenance DNA methylation—best explained the pattern of genomic methylated sites found in adult eukaryotic tissues (Figure 6.3). *De novo* methylation referred to the enzymatic transfer of a methyl group to CpG dinucleotides that were devoid of methyl moieties and occurred mainly in the early embryo. The embryonic pattern of methylation was maintained by maintenance methylation, which is the process of enzymatic transfer of a methyl group to an unmethylated cytosine paired with a methylated cytosine, i.e., a CpG in which only one strand of DNA was methylated, also referred to as "hemimethylated CpG." Thus, maintenance methylation converted the hemimethylated duplex into a symmetrically methylated form. At the next round of replication when a symmetrically methylated CpG duplex underwent semiconservative replication, hemimethylated sites were formed (Figure 6.3). Hence the pattern of methylation in the parent nucleus was transmitted to the daughter nucleus by only one strand of the DNA double helix. These hemimethylated sites were rapidly converted to symmetrically methylated forms by maintenance methylation, ensuring faithful transmission of the methylation pattern from generation to generation.

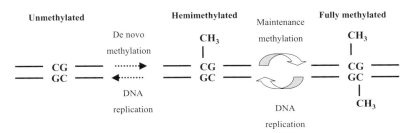

Figure 6.3 *De novo* and maintenance methylation of DNA in eukaryotes.

DNA Methyltransferases

Enzymatic methylation of the C^5-carbon position of cytosine residues in a DNA strand yields 5-methyl-2'-deoxycytidine monophosphate. Enzymes catalyzing this reaction belong to the family methyltransferases (EC 2.1.1, MTs).

Eukaryotic DNA methyltransferase (DNMT) was first cloned and sequenced by Timothy Bestor and Vernon Ingram[39] in 1988. They isolated well-resolved peptides from homogeneous DNA methyltransferase purified from mouse erythroleukemia cells, determined their amino acid sequences by Edman degradation, and used these sequences to design and synthesize a 19-mer oligonucleotide hybridization probe. Screening of λgt11 cDNA libraries prepared from mouse cells with this probe revealed a predicted nucleotide sequence encoding a polypeptide of 1573 amino acid residues that they named Dnmt1. The murine erythroleukemia cells used as a source of Dnmt1 actually contained three very similar species of the enzyme, but their precise relationship was unclear.

The Dnmt1 Family

DNA methyltransferase is a comparatively large molecule of approximately 190 kDa containing 1620 amino acids.[40] Enzymatically catalyzed DNA methylation is a covalent modification of DNA in which a methyl group is transferred from S-adenosylmethionine to the C-5 position of cytosine. Early studies[41] with a prokaryotic methyltransferase (HhaI) showed that the methyl transfer reaction proceeds by an ordered Bi-Bi kinetic mechanism involving the transient formation of a covalent adduct between the enzyme and the methyl donor, S-adenosylmethionine. After transfer of the methyl group to cytosine of DNA the demethylated donor molecule dissociates followed by release of methylated DNA. All DNA methyltransferases that have been studied appear to follow a similar reaction mechanism.

More recently, expression, purification, and characterization of full length recombinant human DNMT1[42] showed that the enzyme prefers hemimethylated DNA compared to unmethylated DNA as a substrate. Under optimal conditions, the preference for methylation between methylated DNA averaged about 15-fold greater than that of unmethylated DNA. DNMT1 was capable of both de novo and maintenance methylation at CG sites, and could also maintain methylation of some non-CG sites.

The carboxyl-terminus of the enzyme represents its catalytic domain, while the amino-terminus has several functions including a targeting sequence that directs it to replication foci[40] (Figure 6.4). Targeting of the DNA methyltransferase to replication foci is believed to permit copying of methylation patterns from parent to newly synthesized DNA of offspring. Functionally, Dnmt1 was found to exhibit a 5- to 30-fold preference for hemimethylated DNA over completely unmethylated DNA. To determine whether de novo methylation and maintenance methylation were performed by the same or different enzymes, a null mutation of this enzyme was generated in mice.[43,44] The null mutant was viable, but retained some capacity (approximately one-third of the wild type) for de novo methyltransferase activity, suggesting the presence of one or more other DNA

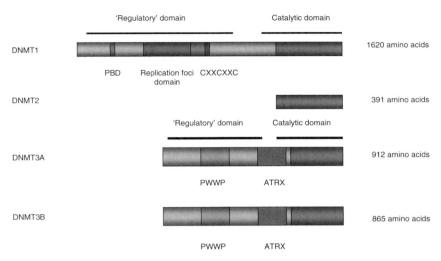

Figure 6.4 Human DNA methyltransferase proteins (DNMTs). All known DNMTs share a highly conserved C-terminal catalytic domain. The regulatory domain located at the N-terminus of DNMT1 differs from the domains of DNMT3A and DNMT3B. Human DNMT3A and DNMT3B are highly homologous and are probably products of gene duplication. DNMT1 shows a strong preference for hemimethylated DNA (maintenance methylation) while DNMT3A and DNMT3B show equal activity for unmethylated and hemimethylated DNA (*de novo* methylation). (*Sources:* Adapted from Bestor,[40] Okano et al.,[51] Bird and Wolffe,[61] and Brueckner and Lyko.[73])

methyltransferase(s) in *Dnmt1* knockout cells.[44] The *Dnmt1* knockout mutation was also found to cause early embryonic lethality indicating that DNA methylation was crucial for normal mammalian development.[43,45] In addition, disruption of *Dnmt1* resulted in abnormal imprinting, and derepression of endogenous retroviruses (summarized in Robertson and Jones[46]). Other targeted mutations in *Dnmt1* produced a number of additional unique phenotypes.[40]

The human homolog, *DNMT1,* mapped to chromosome 19p13.2–13.3.[47]

The Dnmt2 Family

Dnmt1 was the only DNA methyltransferase identified in mammals for about a decade following its cloning and sequencing. Several other groups sought new candidate DNA methyltransferases in mammals by searching expressed sequence tag (EST) databases. Yoder and Bestor[48] reported another potential DNA methyltransferase (*pmt1*$^{+}$) in 1998 in fission yeast, an organism not known to methylate its DNA. Bestor also showed that disruption of *Dnmt2*, the mouse homolog of the yeast enzyme, had no discernible effect on methylation patterns of embryonic stem cells, nor did it affect the ability of such cells to methylate newly integrated retroviral DNA.[40]

About the same time, Van den Wygaert and colleagues reported the identification and characterization of the human *DNMT2* gene.[49] Sequence analysis

indicated that *DNMT2* encoded 391 amino acid residues, but lacked a large part
of the N-terminus that is usually involved in the targeting and regulation of the
MTases. The protein overexpressed in bacteria did not show any DNA methyltransferase activity. Mapping by fluorescent *in situ* hybridization (FISH) showed
the *DNMT2* gene was located on human chromosome 10p13–22. Tissue-specific
expression revealed the human enzyme was relatively high in placenta, thymus,
and testis. However, *DNMT2* was overexpressed in several cancer cell lines consistent with the role of DNA methylation in cancer.

A more recent report has identified and analyzed the human homolog,
DNMT2.[50] The purified enzyme had weak DNA methyltransferase activity at CG
sites. Limited data indicated DNMT2 recognized CG sites in a palindromic
TTCCGGAA sequence context (Figure 6.4).

The Dnmt3 Family

A search by Okano's group[51] for expressed sequence tags using full-length
bacterial methyltransferase sequences as queries identified two methyltransferase
motifs in both mouse and human EST databases. The mouse genes were named
Dnmt3a and *Dnmt3b* because they showed little sequence similarity to either
Dnmt1 or *Dnmt2*. *Dnmt3A* and *Dnmt3B* cDNAs of mice encode proteins of 909
and 859 amino acids; *Dnmt3B* also encoded shorter polypeptides of 840 and 777
amino acid residues through alternative splicing.

Dnmt3a and *Dnmt3b* were both expressed abundantly in undifferentiated cells,
but at low levels in differentiated embryonic stem cells and adult mouse tissues,
and both showed equal activity toward hemimethylated and unmethylated DNA.
The expression pattern plus the substrate selectivity suggested that *Dnmt3a* and
Dnmt3b might encode *de novo* methyltransferases.[51]

The human homologs, *DNMT3A* and *DNMT3B*, were highly homologous to
the mouse genes. *DNMT3A* and *DNMT3B* mapped to human chromosomes 2p
and 20q, and encoded proteins of 912 and 865 amino acids, respectively[40] (Figure
6.4). A human disorder has been attributed to mutations in *DNMT3B* (see p. 164).

DNA Methylation Represses Gene Expression, But How?

As evidence about methylation of DNA accumulated, Arthur Riggs and Abaron
Razin[17,35] recognized that this modification offered a logically attractive explanation for control of gene expression, but experimental support for that idea
remained elusive. They realized from structural studies performed during the
1970s that the conversion of cytosine to 5mC placed a methyl group in an
exposed position in the major groove of the DNA helix. And while methyl groups
in this position would not affect base pairing, and hence would not impede DNA
replication, studies of several proteins such as the lac repressor, histones, and
hormone receptors had demonstrated that changes in the major groove affected
binding of DNA to proteins. Razin and Riggs concluded that 5mC could pro-
foundly affect the binding of proteins to DNA and they suggested that methylated cytosines would modify protein–DNA interactions and could bring about
long-term silencing of gene expression. However, the detailed nature of these

interactions was not clear and further developments were needed to complete the picture.

Methyl-CpG-Binding Proteins

In 1991, Adrian Bird proposed two models[52] to explain how CpG methylation might cause transcriptional repression. Put simply, he postulated in one model— the "*direct*" model, that essential transcription factors saw 5mC as a mutation in their binding site and so were unable to bind, while the other model—the "*indirect*" model, postulated that methylated DNA sites physically blocked the binding of transcriptional factors. Subsequently, two proteins were identified, MeCP1 and MeCP2, that bound specifically to DNA-containing methyl-CpG (MBD1) sites.[52,53] Both proteins were widely expressed in mammalian cells, but MeCP2 was more abundant and more tightly bound in the nucleus than MeCP1, and most importantly was associated with chromatin. Subsequently, MeCP2 was shown to contain both a methyl-CpG-binding domain (MBD) and a transcriptional repression domain (TRD).[54] Bird[55] and colleagues proposed that MeCP2 could bind methylated DNA in the context of chromatin and they suspected this protein contributed to the long-term silencing of gene activity. While this evidence supported inhibition of transcription by the indirect mechanism, it did not clarify the mechanism by which cytosine methylation affected the structure of chromatin.

Searches of the EST database with the MBD sequence as the query enabled Cross et al.[56] to identify the MBD sequence, named MBD1, as a component of MeCP1. Subsequently Hendrich and Bird[54] identified three new human and mouse proteins (MBD2, MBD3, and MBD4) that contain the methyl-CpG-binding domain (Figure 6.5). MBD1, MBD2, and MBD4 were all shown to bind methylated DNA via its MBD region and to repress transcription. The precise significance of MBD3 in mammals was unclear.

Methyl-CpG-Binding Proteins, Histone Deacetylation, and Chromatin Remodeling

In 1998, Nan et al.[57] and Jones et al.[58] reported independently that MeCP2 resided in a complex with several histone deacetylases (HDACs). The complex also contained Sin3A, a corepressor in other deacetylation-dependent silencing processes, plus several additional unidentified proteins. Both laboratories demonstrated that transcriptional silencing could be reversed by trichostatin A, a specific inhibitor of histone deacetylases. Additionally, both obtained evidence that histone deacetylation was guided to specific chromatin domains by genomic methylation patterns, and that transcriptional silencing relied on histone deacetylation. Earlier contributions of Vincent Allfrey and of Vernon Ingram, whose laboratories were both engaged in studying biochemical events relevant to gene regulation, should also be acknowledged in the context of transcriptional regulation. Both of these investigators had proposed several years earlier that acetylation (Allfrey) and methylation (Ingram) of histones were linked to gene regulation[59] and that inhibition of histone deacetylation could alter cellular differentiation.[60]

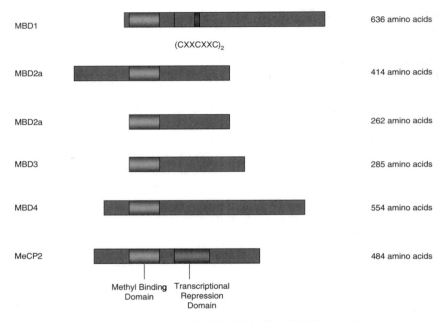

Figure 6.5 Murine methyl-CpG-binding (MBD) proteins.

In commenting on the studies of Nan et al.,[57] Jones et al.,[58] Bestor[60] suggested that deacetylation might exert two structural effects on chromatin that favor gene silencing: First, deacetylation of lysine ε-amino groups might permit greater ionic interactions between the positively charged amino-terminal histone tails and the negatively charged phosphate backbone of DNA, which would interfere with the binding of transcription factors to their specific DNA sequences. Second, deacetylation might favor interactions between adjacent nucleosomes and lead to compaction of the chromatin. The higher affinity of deacetylated histone tails for DNA favored the first explanation while the crystal structure of the nucleosome favored the second. Whether the effects of histone acetylation acted at intra- or internucleosome levels was unclear.[60] Nevertheless, the results of Nan et al.[57] and Jones et al.[58] clearly established a direct causal relationship between DNA methylation-transcriptional silencing and modification of chromatin.

The events of the 1990s can be summed up as follows. At the beginning of this decade, evidence from studies on many model systems had demonstrated that most regions of invertebrate genomes were free of methylation. In contrast, all regions of vertebrate genome were subject to methylation primarily at sites rich in CpG dinucleotides. However, the methylated sites were distributed unevenly throughout the genome in patches of low and high density. At the beginning of this period, Dnmt1 was the only mammalian DNA methyltransferase and no methyl-CpG-binding protein was known. By the close of this decade, the mechanism of the methylation reaction had been worked out; four mammalian Dmnts and five methyl-CpG-binding proteins were known[61] (Figures 6.4 and 6.5).

With these new findings in hand, questions regarding the function of DNA methylation and the relation of histone acetylation and DNA methylation to chromatin remodeling and to repression of gene activity were beginning to yield to experimental scrutiny. Acetylation of conserved lysines on the amino terminals of the core histones was shown to be an important mechanism by which chromatin structure is altered. Histone acetylation was associated with an open chromatin conformation allowing for gene transcription, while histone deacetylation maintained the chromatin in the closed, nontranscribed state. Aided by the tools of molecular biology, investigators had learned how CpG dinucleotides were targeted for methylation, and how the patterns of methylation were read, maintained, and in most cases faithfully transmitted from one generation to the next.

Histone Modifications in Chromatin
Shortly after Nan et al.[57] and Jones et al.[58] reported the role of DNA methylation and modification of chromatin in transcriptional silencing, Ng et al.[62] found that cells deficient in MeCP2 (e.g., HeLa cells) were capable of repressing transcription as determined by reporter constructs. This finding suggested that MeCP2 was probably not the sole connection between the methylation of DNA and transcriptional silencing.

In 2001, Eric Selker and Hisashi Tamaru[63] reported that *dim-5,* a gene that encodes a histone methyltransferase for methylation of lysines of histone tails of chromatin in the fungus, *Neurospora crassa,* was required for DNA methylation. They had accidentally generated a mutation in a previously unknown gene required for DNA methylation. In a series of clever experiments, they mapped the fungal mutant gene to a region homologous to histone methyltransferases and demonstrated through biochemical tests on a recombinant form of the gene that the expressed protein methylated histone H3. In characterizing the mutant gene they found a single nucleotide change (C to G) that generated a stop codon in the middle of a distinctive ~130 amino acid sequence motif called the SET domain,[64] which identified the gene (in *Drosophila*) as required for heterochromatin formation, and possibly was one of the chromatin-associated SET methyltransferases. Substitution of lysine at position 9 with either leucine or arginine in histone H3 caused the loss of DNA methylation *in vivo,* from which they inferred that histone methylation controlled DNA methylation.

The study of Jun-Ichi Nakayama and colleagues[65] provided additional evidence that lysine 9 of histone 3 (H3 Lys[9]) was preferentially methylated at heterochromatin regions of fission yeast (*Schizosaccharomyces pombe*) and that modifications of histone tails were linked to heterochromatin assembly. They proposed that histone deacetylases and histone methyltransferases cooperate to establish a "histone code" that would result in self-propagating heterochromatin assembly. On the basis of conservation of certain transacting proteins that affect silencing (Clr4/SUV39H1 and Swi6/HP1), and the presence of H3 Lys[9]-methyl

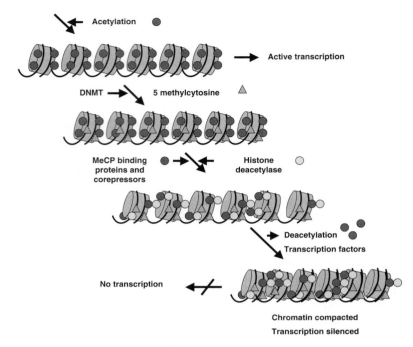

Figure 6.6 DNA methylation and histone modification cooperate to repress transcription. With permission from Elsevier Limited.

modification in higher eukaryotes, they also predicted that a similar mechanism might be responsible for higher order chromatin assembly in humans as well as in yeast (Figure 6.6). However, since the evidence obtained for this "double methylation" system was limited to fungus (*N. crassa*) and fission yeast (*S. pombe*), the extent to which it applies to other eukaryotes, including humans, awaits confirmation.

RNA Interference Regulates Histone Methylation in Eukaryotic Heterochromatin

While the experiments in Selker's laboratory (see p. 157) were in progress, Andrew Fire and Craig Mello and colleagues[66] discovered that double-stranded RNA (dsRNA) was much more potent than sense or antisense single strands of RNA at silencing gene expression in *Caenorhabditis elegans*. They found that only a few molecules of dsRNA were required to cause silencing. They suggested that a catalytic or amplification step might be involved, and named this phenomenon RNA interference (RNAi).

In a study using fission yeast (*S. pombe*) as a model, Shiv Grewal and Robert Martiennssen and colleagues[67] obtained evidence suggesting histone modifications were guided by RNAi by deleting several genes (argonaute, dicer, and RNA-dependent RNA polymerase) that encode part of the molecular machinery of RNAi. Deletion resulted in aberrant accumulation of complementary transcripts from centromeric heterochromatic repeats, as well as transcriptional derepression of transgenes located at the centromere, loss of histone H3 Lys[9] methylation, and loss of centromere function. For intact cells, they explained their findings by the following mechanism: dsRNA derived from repeat sequences in heterochromatin would trigger RNAi that would initiate histone 3 lysine[9] methylation. The covalently modified histone would then signal DNA methylation. This mechanism could guide eukaryotic methyltransferases to specific regions of the genome, such as retroposons and other parasitic elements. They believed this arrangement could be reinforced by maintenance methyltransferase activity as well as by histone deacetylation guided by CpG-methyl-binding proteins.

RNAi is still a comparatively new model in regulatory biology,[68] and the mechanistic complexity of the process and its biological ramifications are only beginning to be appreciated. The technique has been harnessed for the analysis of gene function in several diverse organisms and systems including plants, fungi, and metazoans, but its use in mammalian systems has lagged behind somewhat.[68] The first indication that RNAi could induce gene silencing in mammals came from observations in early mouse embryos and numerous mammalian cell lines, but silencing in these systems was transient. By utilizing long, hairpin dsRNAs, Paddison and colleagues[69] have recently succeeded in creating stable gene silencing in mouse cell lines substantially increasing the power of RNAi as a genetic tool. The ability to create permanent cell lines with stable "knockdown" phenotypes extends the utility of RNAi in several ways, one of which will be its application to epigenetics research.

EPIGENETICS IN HEALTH AND DISEASE

Nearly three decades have elapsed since Salser attached the mutability of CpG dinucleotides to instability of 5mC.[14] This event was closely linked in time with the invention of recombinant DNA techniques. The simplicity and elegance of those technologies rapidly facilitated their adoption in many laboratories, but more recently, they have been applied to the identification of the natural patterns of genomic methylation in DNA sequences, and unraveling of the mechanisms that initiate and maintain epigenetic silencing.

In the course of screening for restriction fragment length polymorphisms (RFLPs) in human DNA sequences, David Barker and his co-workers were among the first to recognize the importance of polymorphisms at CpG islands.[70] They identified nine polymorphic loci at CpG sites among 31 arbitrarily selected loci and estimated that the likelihood of polymorphisms in CpG sequences might be some 10-fold higher than for other bases. In 1983, Andrew Feinberg and Bert Vogelstein discovered global hypomethylation of various human cancers as a feature common to many cancers of different types. Aberrant hypermethylation of CpG islands in promoter regions reported subsequently by Manel Esteller, Steve Baylin, and colleagues was another feature common to breast cancer, lymphomas, and lung cancers.[71] In 1988, David Cooper and Hagop Yousoufian found that CpG mutations within the coding regions of genes associated with human disease were some 42-fold higher than random mutation predicted and they proposed that methylation of DNA contributed to human disease.[72]

The study of epigenetics and its health consequences holds an attraction for clinical investigators of human disease, particularly those with specialized interests in developmental abnormalities and cancer. They are learning whether or not the natural patterns of DNA methylation are disturbed in human neoplasia and other human disorders, and why. During the last 5–10 years, innovative approaches and technical refinements have advanced the identification and characterization of epigenetic markers for human disease, improved the diagnosis of various human disorders, and enhanced our knowledge of the contribution of epigenetic silencing to human illness.[73–75]

Tools for Dissecting Epigenetic Pathways

Detailed studies have identified many of the components and basic principles of epigenetic mechanisms of gene expression. So far, the evidence indicates that stable but reversible alteration of gene expression is mediated by patterns of cytosine methylation and histone modification, the binding of nuclear proteins to chromatin, and interactions between these networks. The positioning and occupancy of nucleosomes are likely to be important factors in gene expression because these structures may modulate the binding of transcription factors as well as the movements of transcribing RNA polymerases, and there may be other, yet unknown factors that contribute to epigenetic mechanisms of gene regulation. The availability of specific, sensitive, and quantitative analytical tools has played a crucial role in dissecting epigenetic patterns and networks. Some of the important methods that have advanced our understanding of their architecture and function are described in this section.

Analytical techniques for monitoring the methylation state of DNA may be divided into two groups: those designed to determine the *level of global methylation* of studied genomes, and those designed to determine *regional patterns of methylation,* mostly CpG islands, of studied genomes. Established methods for measuring the methylation status include routine chromatographic methods, electromigration methods, and immunoassays,[76] and modifications of these older techniques continue to evolve.[76] Semiautomatic detection of methylation at CpG islands,[77] oligonucleotide-based microarrays, and tissue microarrays[78–80] are some of the newer methods that have been reported. In addition, immunodetection offers the possibility of obtaining spatially resolved information on the distribution of 5mC on metaphase chromosomes.[81]

The choice of a proper method for a particular investigation rests with the aims and the specific requirements of the investigation. The important features of several widely used methods that employ 5mC as a marker for DNA methylation are summarized below and in Table 6.1. For details of protocols, the reader is referred to the recent review of Havlis and Trbusek[76] as well as additional references cited in Table 6.1.

Table 6.1 Tools for Monitoring DNA Methylation in Epigenetic Disease

Method	Detection	DNA amount needed	Sensitivity	Comments	Selected references
High-performance thin layer chromatography	Scintillation	5 μg	20 fmol	Simple, low cost, rapid, good for large-scale screening	82
High-performance liquid chromatography	Optical—UV scintillation fluorescence MS	<1 μg	400 fmol	Quantitative, reproducible, sensitive	83
Capillary electrophoresis	MS	<1 μg	100 fmol	Automation possible, high sample throughput	84
Immunoassay	Fluorescence	NA	1.5 fmol	Spatial resolution on metaphase chromosomes previously stained by the Giemsa method	81
Modification-sensitive restriction enzymes (MSRE)	Gel electrophoresis, Southern blot	>5 μg	NA	Methylation site specific	85, 86
Bisulfite sequencing	Gel electrophoresis	10 ng	2.5 fmol	Sensitive, easy, best for analysis of different sequences in a small number of samples	87, 88
Bisulfite sequenceing + chloroaldehyde	Fluorescence	10 ng	175 fmol	Slow and chloroaldehyde is toxic, does not require extensive purification of DNA	89
Combined bisulfite restriction analysis (COBRA)	Gel electrophoresis	1 μg	125 fmol	Rapid, sensitive, quantitative and can be used with paraffin sections	90
Methylation-sensitive single nucleotide primer extension (MS-SNuPE)	Gel electrophoresis	5 ng	500 fmol	Avoids MSRE and is automatable; target sequence should contain only A, C, and T, while primer should contain only A, G, and T	91

Chromatographic Methods

Chromatographic methods include thin-layer chromatography (TLC), high-performance liquid chromatography (HPLC), and affinity chromatography. Large-scale screening is the primary advantage of TLC; other advantages of TLC are its simple instrumentation, low cost, and speed. HPLC is the most commonly used chromatographic technique for global methylation analysis. It is sensitive, quantitative, and highly reproducible and it can use fluorescent detection, but separations are slow. Affinity chromatography is an important component of ICEAMP,[82] a method that allows identification of methylation changes without the necessity of knowing the target sequence region and has no need for modification-sensitive restriction enzymes.

Slab Gel Electrophoresis

From the very beginning of recombinant DNA technology, slab gel analysis has been a favorite technique to separate DNA fragments. In epigenetic analysis, it is used in combination with restriction enzymes (MSREs) sensitive to 5mC for RFLP/Southern blot analyses, or with specific sequencing protocols such as bisulfite and hydrazine/permangante sequencing. More recently, slab gel analysis has often been replaced by separation techniques that are more sensitive, less labor intensive, and automatable. In recent years, bisulfite sequencing has been used as the standard method to detect DNA methylation at CpG islands. Genomic DNA first reacted with bisulfite converts unmethylated cytosine to uracil while leaving 5mC unchanged (Figure 6.1). The conversion to uracil is detected with specifically designed PCR primers. Methylation-specific restriction enzymes employed in combination with PCR provide a very sensitive, commonly used technique that requires much less DNA than traditional Southern blot analysis. A widely used combination of MSREs for detection of methylated cytosines is MspI/HpaII isoschizomers, although other restriction enzymes afford alternatives to one or both of these. For instance, detection of the methylation state of the FMR1 gene promoter used analysis of EcoRI and EagI digests of DNA from fragile X patients to distinguish the normal genotype, the premutation, and the full mutation.[83] Bisulfite sequencing is straightforward and efficient and in the event that a site is only partially methylated, it has the added advantage of enabling the determination of the proportion of cells that is methylated. Bisulfite sequencing has been combined with other methodologies such as "combined bisulfite restriction analysis and amplification," abbreviated COBRA.[84] COBRA is relatively easy to use, quantitatively accurate, and compatible with paraffin sections. Another method that uses bisulfite sequencing is "methylation-sensitive single nucleotide primer extension," abbreviated MS-SNuPE. This approach uses very small amounts of DNA, can be used with microdissected material, and avoids the use of restriction enzymes.

The MS-SNuPE technique has also been adapted to semiautomatic detection of DNA methylation at CpG islands.[77]

Immunological Methods

Pfarr and co-workers have recently described a technique that renders possible immunodetection of 5mC on human chromosome metaphase spreads.[81] A monoclonal antibody tagged with fluorescent dye is used to image the chromosomes after they have been previously stained by the Giemsa method. The technique can be used to obtain a fast and global overview of changes in genomic methylation patterns during the development of various types of cancer. Potential applications of the technique include characterization of disease-related methylation patterns on a genomic scale for diagnostic purposes and monitoring of patient responsiveness to therapy.

Microarrays

Many genes and signaling pathways controlling cell proliferation, death, and differentiation, as well as genomic integrity are implicated in the development of cancer and other diseases. New techniques that can measure the expression of thousands of genes simultaneously are needed to establish the diagnostic, prognostic, and therapeutic importance of each emergent cancer gene candidate. The development of microarrays for DNA methylation analysis may afford a potential solution to this problem.

Several microarray methods have been developed to map methylcytosine patterns in genomes of interest.[85] One set of methods uses methylation-sensitive restriction enzymes. For example, Huidong Shi and colleagues have devised an oligonucleotide-based microarray technique that measures hypermethylation in defined regions of the genome.[78] DNA samples from various tumor types are first treated with bisulfite and specific genomic regions are then PCR amplified converting the modified UG to TG and conserving the originally methylated dinucleotide as CG. Primers were designed so that they contained no CpG dinucleotides and were complementary to the flanking sequences of a 200- to 300-bp DNA target. This permitted unbiased amplification of both methylated and unmethylated alleles by PCR. PCR-amplified target DNAs were subsequently purified and labeled with fluorescent dyes (Cy5 or Cy3) for hybridization to the microarray. The fluorescently labeled PCR products are hybridized to arrayed oligonucleotides (affixed to solid supports, e.g., microscope slides) that can discriminate between methylated and unmethylated alleles in regions of interest. Shi et al. employed their technique to distinguish two clinical subtypes of non-Hodgkin's lymphomas, mantle cell lymphoma and grades I/II follicular lymphoma, based on the differential methylation profiles of several gene promoters.

Shi's technique for profiling methylation patterns[78] could also afford an alternative approach to predict and discover new classes of cancer in a manner similar to that pioneered by Todd Golub,[86,87] and by other investigators.[88–91] Additionally, this technology might be used to monitor the effects of new pharmacological agents in patients under treatment and provide valuable information regarding the outcome of epigenetic therapies.

Chuan-Mu Chen and associates have developed another, somewhat different, microarray technique, called methylation target array (MTA), for analysis of hypermethylation.[79] The technique is similar to that developed for tissue microarrays by Juha Kononen et al.[80] Methylation targets are affixed to a solid support and different CpG island probes are hybridized to the array one at a time. The technique can interrogate hypermethylation of CpG islands in hundreds of clinical samples simultaneously. Its applicability to cancer-related problems was demonstrated by determining hypermethylation profiles of 10 promoter CpG islands in 93 breast tumors, 4 breast cancer cell lines, and 20 normal breast tissues. A panel of 468 MTA amplicons, which represented the whole repertoire of methylated CpG islands in these tissues and cell lines, was arrayed on nylon membrane for probe hybridization. Positive hybridization signals, indicative of DNA methylation, were detected in tumor amplicons, but not in normal amplicons, indicating aberrant hypermethylation in tumor samples. The frequencies of hypermethylation were found to correlate significantly with the patient's hormone receptor status, clinical stage, and age at diagnosis. Because a single nylon membrane can be used repeatedly for probing with many CpG island loci, this technique may be advantageous clinically for rapid assessment of potential methylation markers for predicting treatment outcome.

Transcription factors, nucleosomes, chromatin-modifying proteins, and epigenetic markers together form extremely complex regulatory networks. Recently, Bas van Steensel described two microarray approaches that have been developed for genome-wide mapping of the binding sites of regulatory proteins and the distributions of methylation patterns and histone modifications.[85] In one of these, chromatin immunoprecipitation (ChIP) is combined with microarray detection. Cells are treated with a cross-linking reagent such as formaldehyde, the chromatin is isolated and fragmented, and immunoprecipitation is used to identify the protein of interest along with the attached DNA fragments. To identify the DNA fragments, the cross-links are reversed and the DNA fragments are labeled with a fluorescent dye and hybridized to microarrays with probes corresponding to regions of interest. The other method, called DamID, utilizes a different principle. In this case, a transcription factor or chromatin-binding protein of interest is fused to DNA adenine methyltransferase (Dam). When this fusion protein is expressed, Dam will be targeted to binding sites of its fusion partner resulting in methylation of adenines in DNA near the binding sites. To identify these sites, the methylated regions are either purified or selectively amplified from genomic DNA, fluorescently labeled, and hybridized to a microarray. Because adenine methylation does not occur endogenously in mammals, the binding sites of targeted methylation can be derived from the microarray signals. So far, only limited comparisons with ChIP are available, but studies of one regulatory protein, the GAGA factor, indicate the two methods can yield similar results. However, ChIP-chip requires a highly specific antibody against the protein of interest, while DamID does not. On the other hand, DamID is suited for the detection of histone or other posttranslational modifications. Additional merits and drawbacks of the two methods are considered by van Steensel.[85]

Faulty Epigenetics

Germline Mutations

Germline mutations in genes that encode parts of the methylation machinery have been associated with two human diseases, the immunodeficiency centromeric instability facial anomalies (ICF) syndrome and Rett syndrome (Table 6.2). The salient features of ICF syndrome are immunodeficiency, centromere instability, and facial anomalies. This recessive disorder of childhood is associated with mutations in the DNA methyltransferase gene, *DNMT3B*. The mutations are largely confined to satellite DNA at the centromeric regions of chromosomes 1, 9,

Table 6.2 Epigenetics in Human Disease

Human disorder	Salient clinical features	Molecular pathology	Reference
ICF syndrome	Recessive disorder of children with immunodeficiency, centromere instability and mild facial anomalies causing most ICF patients to succumb to infectious disease before adulthood	Almost completely unmethylated satellite DNA in centromeric regions of chromosomes 1, 9, and 16 attributed to mutations in DMNT3B	92, 93
Rett syndrome[94]	Postnatal neurodevelopmental disorder of infant girls with a variable clinical phenotype characterized by loss of motor and language skills, microcephaly, autistic features, and stereotypic hand movements	Various germline MECP2 mutations may affect the role of MECP2 in higher order chromatin organization and imprinting	95–99
Fragile X syndrome	Mental retardation affecting males primarily; other diagnostic criteria: long face, large everted ears, autism, hand biting, hyperactivity and macroorchidism (large testicles)	Silencing of *FMR1* gene at Xq27.3 containing highly polymorphic, abnormally lengthy CCG repeats in the 5′ region; plus aberrant *de novo* methylation and histone deacetylation of the CpG island upstream of *FMR1*	74, 100
Benign dermoid ovarian teratomas	Tumors contain many tissue types but no placental trophoblast	LOI results in tumors with two maternal chromosomes and no paternal contribution	101
Hydatidform moles	Placental-derived extraembryonic tumors	LOI causes tumors with two paternal chromosomes with no maternal contribution	102
Wilms' tumors	Nephroblastoma of childhood	LOI causes preferential loss of maternal alleles on chromosome 11p15	103, 104

(*continued*)

Table 6.2 (*continued*)

Human disorder	Salient clinical features	Molecular pathology	Reference
Embryonal rhabdomyosarcoma	Tumors of striated muscle		105
Prader–Willi syndrome (PWS)	Deficiencies in sexual development and growth, behavioral and mental retardation; major diagnostic criteria: hypotonia, hyperphagia and obesity, hypogonadism and developmental delay	Prader–Willi and Angelman syndromes (AS) neurogenetic disorders caused by loss of function of imprinted genes at chromosome 15q11–q13; approximately 70% of PWS and AS individuals have a 3–4 megabase deletion in their maternal or paternal chromosome 15q11–q13	106, 107
Angelman syndrome (AS)	Deficiencies in sexual development and growth, behavioral and mental retardation; major diagnostic criteria: ataxia, tremulousness, sleep disorders, seizures, and hyperactivity		106, 107
Beckwith–Wiedemann syndrome	Pre- and postnatal overgrowth, macroglossia and other organomegaly, childhood tumors such as Wilms' tumor of the kidney, hypoglycemia, hemihypertrophy, and other minor complications	LOI results in biallelic expression of *IGF2* (80%), silencing or mutation of *H19* (35%), and silencing of *CDKN1C* (12%)[108]	109

and 16. Normally these satellites are heavily methylated, but in ICF syndrome they are almost completely unmethylated in all tissues.[92] Most affected patients succumb to infectious disease before adulthood.

Rett syndrome is a postnatal neurodevelopmental disorder that occurs almost exclusively in girls.[92–94] It is one of the commonest forms of intellectual disability in young girls and it is characterized by a period of early normal growth and development followed by regression, loss of speech and acquired motor skills, stereotypical hand movements, and seizures. In sporadic cases, affected girls are normal at birth and achieve expected developmental milestones until

6–18 months of age when brain growth slows and growth failure occurs. This disorder is associated with both nonsense and missense mutations of the X-linked gene encoding the methyl-CpG-binding protein, MECP2.

The identification of the genetic cause of Rett syndrome was a major advance in clinical neurology and epigenetics.[95,96] Up to 96% of classic Rett syndrome cases are accounted for by MECP2 mutations. Nearly 70% of the mutations arise from C-T transitions at eight CpG dinucleotides, whereas carboxy-terminal deletions occur in 10–15% of patients. Female patients with phenotypes distinct from the classic presentation of Rett syndrome have also been identified. Males with MECP2 mutations fall into three groups, those with Rett syndrome, those with severe encephalopathy and infantile death, and those with severe neurological and/or psychiatric symptomatology.

Recently, Terumi Kohwi-Shigematsu and colleagues have shown loss of silent-chromatin looping and impaired imprinting of *DLX5* in mice.[97] Using a modified ChIP-based cloning strategy to search for Mecp2 target genes in mouse brain, they identified *DLX5,* a maternally expressed gene on mouse chromosome 6, as a direct target of Mecp2. The importance of *DLX5* lies in the production of γ-aminobutyric acid (GABA). In the Mecp2 null-mouse model, they showed that repressive histone modification at Lys-9 and the formation of a higher order chromatin loop structure were mediated by Mecp2 and specifically associated with silent chromatin at *Dx15–Dx16*. Because loss of imprinting of *DLX5* may alter GABAergic neuron activity, this finding suggests that dysregulation of *DLX5* by mutation of MeCP2 might contribute to some of the phenotypes of this syndrome.[97] Current data, as described by Moretti and Zoghbi,[95] suggest that several putative genes are targeted by MECP2, and that the elucidation of mechanisms that give rise to the characteristic features of Rett syndrome is a key challenge for the future.

Faulty Genomic Imprinting

From estimates made in 1995, only a small minority of genes in the mammalian genome is thought to be imprinted.[98] In humans, more than 25 imprinted genes have been identified, and estimates based on mouse models indicate that as many as 100–200 may exist over the whole genome.[98,99] Imprinted genes are involved in many aspects of development including fetal and placental growth, cell proliferation, and adult behavior.[99] Several inherited disorders have been attributed to faulty genomic imprinting. Certain aberrations of human pregnancy show that loss of genomic imprinting (LOI) plays an important role in embryogenesis (Table 6.2). For example, ovarian dermoid cysts arise from LOI that result in benign cystic tumors that contain two maternal chromosomes and no paternal chromosome. In contrast, the hydatidiform mole contains a completely androgenic genome that arises from LOI, so that these tumors contain two paternal chromosomes and no maternal chromosome.

More recently, additional human genetic diseases and cancers listed in Table 6.2 have been ascribed to faulty genomic imprinting. In 1991, the molecular basis of fragile X syndrome, a common form of heritable mental retardation, was associated with a massive expansion of CGG triplet repeats located in the

5'-untranslated region upstream of the *FMR1* (fragile X mental retardation) gene.[74,100] This syndrome takes its name from the brittle appearance of the X chromosome under a microscope, part of which appears to be dangling by a thread.[101] The fragile X site is located at Xq27.3. This was one of the first of about a dozen identified human disorders that are caused by unstable trinucleotide repeat expansions. In normal individuals, *FMR1* is a highly conserved gene that contains about 30 (range 7 to ~60) CGG repeats while over 230 repeats occur in most affected persons. In the normal transcript the repeats are unmethylated, but in affected persons they are hypermethylated, which silences the *FMR1* gene and causes the absence of the FMR1 protein. Mental retardation is attributed to lack of proper protein expression in neurons during development. Due to X linkage, affected males have more severe phenotypes than affected females, whose phenotype is modulated by the presence of the normal X chromosome.

Several other diseases that are due to faulty imprinting are also listed in Table 6.2. For example, Pal and co-workers observed preferential loss of the maternal alleles on chromosome 11 in 9 of 11 cases of Wilms' tumors where the parental origin of alleles could be followed.[102] Similar observations on five additional cases of Wilms' tumors were made by Schroeder et al.[103] Scrable and colleagues have found that embryonal rhabdomyosarcomas (malignant pediatric tumors of striated muscle origin) could arise from cells that were clonally isodisomic for paternal loci on chromosome 11.[104]

Glenn and associates demonstrated that the *SNRPN* gene, which encodes a small nuclear ribonucleoprotein subunit *SmN* thought to be involved in splicing of pre-mRNA, is expressed only from the paternally derived chromosome 15q11–q13 in humans with Prader–Willi syndrome.[105] More recently, Horsthemke and colleagues performed a molecular analysis at the *SNURF-SNRPN* locus in 51 patients with Prader–Willi syndrome and 85 patients with Angelman syndrome that revealed that the majority of these defects were epigenetic mutations. Seven patients with Prader–Willi syndrome (14%) and eight patients with Angelman syndrome (9%) had an imprinting center deletion. Sequence analysis of 32 Prader–Willi syndrome patients and no imprinting center deletion and 66 AS patients and no imprinting center deletion did not reveal any point mutation in imprinting center elements. In patients with Angelman syndrome, they found the imprinting defect occurred on the chromosome that was of maternal grandparental origin, whereas in the patients with Prader–Willi syndrome and no imprinting center deletion, the imprinting defect occurred on the chromosome inherited from the paternal grandmother.[106] The fact that epimutations on the maternal chromosome were often present in a mosaic form suggested that in patients with Angelman syndrome and no imprinting center deletion that aberrant DNA methylation responsible for the imprinting defect occurred after fertilization.

Mannens et al. carried out cytogenetic and DNA analyses on patients with Beckwith–Wiedemann syndrome.[107] They refined the localization of the syndrome at chromosome 11p15.3-pter to two regions, BWSCR1 and BWSCR2. They found that LOI was involved in the etiology of the Beckwith–Wiedemann syndrome with BWSCR2 since all balanced chromosomal abnormalities observed at this region were maternally transmitted. Loss of imprinting can cause either biallelic expression (such as *IGF2*) or silencing (such as *CDKN1C*) that is found in most sporadic cases of Beckwith-Wiedemann syndrome (Table 6.2).

Another interesting aspect of imprinting is that imprinted genes tend to be clustered in the genome. In humans, the two major clusters are associated with the two major imprinting disorders (Table 6.2). The cluster at chromosome 15q11–13 is linked to the Prader–Willi and Angelman syndromes, and the one at 11p15.5 is linked to the Beckwith–Wiedemann syndrome.

Cancer

Cancer develops through a combination of genetic instability and selection that results in clonal expansion of cells that have accumulated an advantageous set of genetic aberrations. Genetic instability may occur as a result of point mutations, chromosomal rearrangements, DNA dosage abnormalities, or perturbed microsatellite sequences while epigenetic instability may result from faulty imprinting as previously discussed, or from aberrant patterns of DNA or histone methylation. The abnormalities may act alone or in concert to alter the function or expression of cellular components. Cancers sometime retain a history of their development, but this may be difficult to decipher because some aberrations may be lost or obscured by subsequent events.

Epigenetic Hallmarks of Cancer

Salser's observation in 1977 that 5mC was responsible for the mutation of CpG dinucleotides prompted investigators to determine whether the natural patterns of methylation were disturbed in human neoplasia.[14] The first change to be reported for a number of cancers by Andrew Feinberg and colleagues was loss of methylation at the level of individual genes and globally.[108,109] In four of five patients, representing two different types of cancer, Southern blots revealed substantial hypomethylation in genes of cancer cells compared to their normal counterparts; in one of these patients hypomethylation was progressive in a metastasis.[108] Such a loss appeared to be ubiquitous for human neoplasms, whereas hypomethylation was the only type of change observed in benign neoplasms. A generalized decrease in genomic methylation was also noted as cells age, and this gradual loss could result in aberrant gene activation.

The second notable change observed in many human cancers was hypermethylation, particularly of CpG islands at gene promoters.[110] A very recent study has shown that promoter hypermethylation of genes involving important cellular pathways in tumorigenesis is a prominent feature of many major human tumor types.[71] Hypermethylation, which is often accompanied by global hypomethylation, could act as an alternative to mutations that inactivate tumor-suppressor genes and it also could predispose to genetic alterations through inactivation of DNA repair genes.

The third important change is LOI. In cancer, LOI can lead to activation of growth-promoting genes such as IGF2, and to silencing of tumor suppressor genes,[111–113] as already noted.

The full range of epigenetic change that occurs in human cancers is not known, but hypomethylation, hypermethylation at CpG islands, and LOI occur most frequently.[114] An early study of p53 illustrates what might be learned from a study of 5mC mutations in human tissues.[115] p53 is a well-known tumor suppressor gene that has been studied intensively. Normally in a cell, p53 is kept at very low levels, but DNA damage results in a rapid increase and its activation as a transcription factor. As a transcription factor, p53 either arrests the cells in the G1 phase of the cell cycle or triggers apoptosis.[116] More than 4500 mutations have been identified in the p53 gene, and p53 mutations are found in 50–55% of all human cancers. Three codons in p53 (175, 273, and 248) are of particular interest because they are hotspots for point mutations that impair p53 function in cancer. Sequencing indicates that all three of these codons contain 5mC which is mutated in various tumors. Rideout et al. found that as many as 43% (9 of 21) of the p53 somatic mutations at these sites are due to 5mC. There are 82 CpGs in the 2362 nucleotides of the double-stranded coding sequence of p53. The relevance of methylation to mutations in p53 is brought out more clearly by the fact that no more than ~3.5% (82/2362) of the sequence contributed 33–43% of the point mutations, each of which was a transition from 5mC to thymine (or a corresponding G to A)[115] (Figure 6.1).

Significance of Faulty Imprinting in Cancer

Feinberg and colleagues attached special significance to LOI in cancer and they initiated a search for the mechanism by which this epigenetic change might enhance the risk to neoplasia. In the first of two papers, Cui et al. found that LOI of the insulin-like growth factor II (*IGF2*) gene, a feature common to many human cancers, occurred in about 10% of the normal human population.[117] LOI in this segment of the population increased the risk of colorectal cancer about 3.5- to 5-fold, suggesting that faulty imprinting was related to the risk of cancer.

In the second paper, Sakatani et al. created a mouse model to investigate the mechanism by which LOI of *Igf2* contributed to intestinal cancer.[118] They knew from the work of others that imprinting of *Igf2* was regulated by a differentially methylated region (DMR) upstream of the nearby untranslated *H19* gene, and that deletion of the DMR would lead to biallelic expression (LOI) of *Igf2* in the offspring. To model intestinal neoplasia, they used *Min* mice with an *Apc* mutation with or without a maternally inherited deletion, i.e., with or without LOI, and they designed the model to mimic closely the human situation where LOI caused only a modest increase in *IGF2* expression. They created their model of *Igf2* LOI by crossing female heterozygous carriers of deletion ($H19^{+/-}$) with male heterozygous carriers of the $Apc^{+/Min}$. Their results showed that LOI mice developed twice as many intestinal tumors as control littermates, and they also showed a shift toward a less differentiated normal intestinal epithelium. In a comparative study of human tissues, a similar shift in differentiation was seen in the normal colonic mucosa of humans with LOI. These observations suggested that impairment of normal parental imprinting might interfere with cellular differentiation and thereby increase the risk of cancer. In more general terms, the results suggested that mutation of a cancer gene (*APC*) and an epigenetically imposed delay in cell maturation may act synergistically to initiate tumor development.[114]

CpG Island Methylator Phenotype

The causes and global patterns of aberrant methylation, in spite of its frequent occurrence in human cancers, remain poorly defined. In 1999, Toyota and colleagues reported that methylation of CpG islands of normal colonic mucosa was gradually lost as age advanced, and that aberrant methylation was linked to microsatellite instability. To understand these patterns better, these investigators examined the methylation status of CpG islands in 30 differentially methylated loci (including genes known to occur in colorectal cancers such as *p16* and *THBS1*) derived from a panel of 50 primary colorectal cancers and 15 adenomas.[119] Characterization of 26 clones in this study revealed that the majority of CpG island methylation events in 19/26 (73%) clones of colorectal cancers were frequently methylated (averaging 75%, range 30–100%) and related to incremental hypermethylation in normal colon as an age-related phenomenon. Most other methylation events, 7/26 (27%), occurred in a distinct subset of clones from colorectal cancers and adenomas with a significantly lower frequency of methylation (range 10–50%) that appeared to have a new phenotype, designated the CpG island methylation phenotype (CIMP). Age-related hypermethylation was very frequent, affected a large number of cells, occurred in all persons, not just in cancer patients, was gene and tissue specific, and was believed to result from physiological processes. In contrast, cancer-specific hypermethylation was relatively infrequent, and was not found in normal colon mucosa. Next, in a study of 50 colorectal tumors and adenomas, the panel could be divided into two groups according to their hypermethylator status. One group displayed a high level of cancer-specific methylation in which all tumors had methylation of three or more loci (averaging 5.1 loci/tumor), including a high incidence of *p16* and *THBS1*, and the other group in which methylation was extremely rare (an average of 0.3 loci/tumor). In sharp contrast, the frequency of age-related hypermethylation was not significantly different between the two groups of tumors. The CIMP+ tumors included the majority of sporadic colorectal cancers with microsatellite instability related to methylation of the mismatch repair gene hMLH1. The data suggested the existence of a pathway in colorectal cancer that was responsible for the risk of mismatch repair-positive sporadic tumors.[119]

Histone Modifications of Cancer Cells

Considerable effort has been devoted to understanding the relevance of aberrant DNA methylation patterns to human cancer, but much less attention has been focused on histone modifications of cancer cells among many other layers of epigenetic control. Recently, Mario Fraga and colleagues[120] characterized the profile of posttranslational modifications of one of the nucleosomal core histones of chromatin, histone H4, in a comprehensive panel of normal tissues, cancer cell lines, and primary tumors. Using immunodetection, high-performance capillary chromatography, and mass spectrometry, Fraga found that cancer cells overall lost monoacetylation at H4-Lys-16 and trimethylation of histone H4-Lys-20.

These are widely regarded as epigenetic markers of malignant transformation, like global hypomethylation and CpG island hypermethylation. In a mouse model of multistage carcinogenesis, these changes appeared early and accumulated during the tumorigenic process. They were also associated with hypomethylation of DNA repetitive sequences, a well-known feature of cancer cells. The data of Fraga et al. suggest that the global loss of monoacetylation and trimethylation of histone 4 might be another common hallmark of human cancer cells.

THERAPEUTIC POTENTIAL FOR EPIGENETIC DISEASE

Silencing of key nonmutated genes such as tumor suppressor genes and mismatch repair genes is a common event in cancer progression[119,121–128] including cancers of hematological origin.[129–131] Methylation of CpG islands located in promoter regions of cancer cell genes and conformational changes in chromatin involving histone acetylation are two processes that are associated with transcriptional silencing (Figure 6.6). Reversal of these processes and upregulation of genes important in preventing or reversing the malignant phenotype have thus become therapeutic targets in cancer treatment.[132]

Methyltransferase Inhibitors and Demethylating Agents

One possible approach to promote the expression of genes abnormally silenced by methylation is through inhibition of DNA methyltransferases, or alternatively, by agents capable of demethylating DNA.[132] This approach has been studied in hematological and myeloid disorders, although the data are limited. For example, in 1982 Ley et al. reported that the treatment of a patient with severe β-thalassemia with 5-azacytidine as a demethylating agent resulted in selective increases in γ-globin synthesis and in hemoglobin F. Measurement of pretreatment methylation levels compared to posttreatment levels revealed hypomethylation of bone marrow DNA in regions near the γ-globin and the ε-globin genes.[133] Subsequently, several studies examined the use of demethylating agents such as 5-aza-2′-deoxycytidine (decitabine) in the treatment of another heritable hemoglobinopathy, sickle cell anemia. Treatment of this disorder with 2-deoxy-5-azacytidine led to significant increases in hemoglobin F and γ-globin that attained a maximum after 4 weeks of treatment and persisted for 2 weeks before falling below 90% of the maximum.[134] The mechanism of the therapeutic effect was not entirely clear but may have been caused by low pretreatment levels of methylation of the γ-globin gene and altered differentiation of stem cells induced by 2-deoxy-5-azacytidine.

Evidence also points to hypermethylation in the pathogenesis of the myelodysplastic syndromes. Patients with these disorders usually die from bone marrow failure or transformation to acute leukemia. Standard care for this disorder is supportive. In one reported instance, the cyclin-dependent kinase inhibitor, $p15^{INK4b}$, was progressively hypermethylated and silenced in high-grade myelodysplasias, and treatment with 2-deoxy-5-azacytidine resulted in a decrease in *p15* promoter methylation and a positive clinical response in 9 of 12 myelodysplastic patients.[135] Another reported instance involved 191 patients with high-risk myelodysplastic syndromes treated with 5-azacytidine (dose 75 mg/m^2/day) for 7 days every 4 weeks. Statistically significant differences seen in the azacytidine group favored improved response rates, improved quality of life, reduced risk of leukemic transformation, and improved survival compared to supportive care.[136]

The potential reversal of epigenetic silencing by altering methylation levels with methyltransferase inhibitors or DNA demethylating agents has shown promise as a mode of therapy. In 2004, azacytidine was the first agent to receive FDA approval for treatment of several myelodysplastic syndrome subtypes. Cytidine analogs, such as 5-azacytidine and 5-aza-2'-deoxycytidine, achieve their therapeutic effects after a series of biochemical transformations. First, these agents are phosphorylated by a series of kinases to azacytidine triphosphate, which is incorporated into RNA, disrupting RNA metabolism and protein synthesis. Azacytidine diphosphate is reduced by ribonucleotide reductase to 5-aza-2'-deoxycytidine diphosphate, which is phosphorylated to triphosphate and incorporated into DNA. There it binds stoichiometrically DNA methyltransferases and causes hypomethylation of replicating DNA.[136] Most methyltransferase inhibitors are, however, not specific for a particular methyltransferase, and several of them have unfavorable toxicity profiles including severe nausea and vomiting. There are newer agents under development that may improve the targeting of methylation. Among these is MG98, a second-generation antisense oligonucleotide methyltransferase inhibitor that is specific for DNMT1.[132] MG98 produced a dose-dependent reduction of DNMT1 and demethylation of the *p16* gene promoter and reexpression of p16 protein in tumor cell lines. A two-stage Phase 2 trial was performed to assess antitumor activity of MG98 in patients with metastatic renal carcinoma, a solid tumor that has been shown to have hypermethylation of promoter regions of tumor suppressor genes. The study was stopped after the first stage because neither the response nor the progression-free criteria for continuing to the second stage were met. Despite the negative results, the investigators believe the rationale for further study of agents targeting DNA methylation in cancer should not diminish, and that future studies should attempt to assess target effects at the molecular level in cancers thought to be susceptible to this approach.

Histone Deacetylase Inhibitors

Acetylation of DNA-associated histones is linked to activation of gene transcription, whereas histone deacetylation is associated with transcriptional repression. Acute promyelocytic leukemia (APL) provides an excellent model to illustrate the modulation of gene transcription by acetylation and the therapeutic potential of histone deacetylase inhibitors. APL is a hematopoietic cancer that involves the retinoic acid receptor α (*RARα*) gene that maps to the long arm of chromosome 17q21. Ninety-five percent of APL cases arise from a translocation between chromosomes 15 and 17 (t15:17.q21), which leads to the formation of the fusion protein PML-RARα. PML-RARα results in a transcriptional block of the normal granulocytic differentiation pathway. RARα is a member of the nuclear hormone receptor family that acts as a ligand-inducible transcriptional activation factor by binding to retinoic acid response elements (RAREs) in a heterodimer with RXR, a related family of nuclear receptors. In the presence of a ligand (all-*trans*-retinoic acid), the complex promotes transcription of retinoic acid-responsive genes. In the absence of ligand, transcription is silenced by a multistep process involving recruitment of transcriptional regulators, corepressors, and nuclear receptor core repressors such as Sin3 to form a complex. Sin3, in turn, recruits a histone deacetylase that causes condensation of chromatin and prevents accessibility of transcriptional machinery to target genes. The presence of a ligand (all-*trans*-retinoic acid) induces a conformational change in RAR enabling the dissociation of the repressor complex and recruitment of coactivators (such as the *p160* family members). The coactivator molecules possess intrinsic histone acetylase activity that causes unwinding of DNA thereby facilitating transcription and promoting granulocyte differentiation. In an APL patient with a transcriptional block and refractoriness to all-*trans*-retinoic acid resulting in a highly resistant form of APL, Warrell and colleagues showed that treatment with sodium butyrate, a histone deacetylase inhibitor, restored sensitivity to the antileukemic effects of all-*trans*-retinoic acid.[129]

Evaluation of sodium phenyl butyrate (buphenyl) has demonstrated its beneficial effect in the treatment of other disorders including the hemoglobinopathy, β-thalessemia, in acute myelogenous leukemia and in prostate cancer. Phenyl butyrate is one of the older generation of histone deacetylase inhibitors and presently additional inhibitors are being tested in clinical trials.[132] Among these, the inhibitory agent suberoylanilide hydroxamic acid has shown differentiating effects in a bladder cancer cell line. Depsipeptide isolated from *Chrombacterium violaceum* has been demonstrated to have potent cytotoxic activity through several different mechanisms including histone deacetylase inhibition. This agent demonstrated activity against chronic myelogenous leukemia cells resulting in acetylation of histone H3 and H4 as well as expression of apoptotic proteins involving caspase pathways.[132]

Hypermethylation and Histone Deacetylation

The combined manipulation of histone acetylation and cytosine methylation in chromatin presents another strategy for gene-targeted therapy through epigenetic modification. These two epigenetic processes are linked as was shown by Nan et al.[57] and Jones et al.[58] (see p. 155) who showed that the repressive chromatin structure associated with dense methylation was also associated with histone deacetylation. Methylated DNA binds the transcriptional repressor MeCP2 at the MBD, which recruits the Sin 3A/histone deacetylase complex to form transcriptionally repressive chromatin. This process was reversed by trichostatin A, a specific inhibitor of histone deacetylase.

Since little was known about the importance of methylation relative to histone deacetylation in the inhibition of gene transcription, Cameron et al. examined this question.[137] They found that trichostatin alone did not reactivate several hypermethylated genes [*MLH1, TIMP3, CDKN2B (INK4B, p15)*, and *CDKN2A (INK4, p16)*] under conditions that allowed reactivation of nonmethylated genes. These findings suggested that dense CpG island methylation in gene promoter regions was dominant over histone deacetylation in maintaining gene repression. They then induced partial CpG island demethylation by treatment with the demethylating agent 5-aza-2'-deoxycytidine in the presence or absence of histone deacetylase inhibition. They observed robust expression (4-fold increase) of the genes tested by combined drug treatment (trichostatin plus 5-aza-2'-deoxycytidine) in an experiment in which low-level reactivation was seen with 5-aza-2'-deoxycytidine treatment alone. These results indicated that histone deacetylation may not be needed to maintain a silenced transcriptional state, but histone deacetylase has a role in silencing when levels of DNA methylation are reduced. Bisulfite sequencing showed that the increase in gene expression brought about by the combination of the two drugs occurred with retention of extensive methylation in the genes tested. They also found that inhibition of deacetylase activity can induce gene expression without a large-scale change from repressive to accessible chromatin in agreement with the work of others. Taken together the data suggested that decreased methylation is a prerequisite for transcription following histone deacetylase inhibition.

In experiments similar to those of Cameron et al., Chiurazzi and colleagues examined the relative roles of methylation and histone deacetylation in silencing the *FMR1* gene in fragile X syndrome.[138,139] Hypermethylation of CGG repeats in this disorder silences the *FMR1* gene to cause the absence of the FMR1 protein that subsequently leads to mental retardation (see p. 154). In their first paper, Chiurazzi et al. found that the demethylating agent 5-aza-2'-deoxycytidine partially restored FMR1 protein expression in B-lymphoblastoid cell lines obtained from fragile X patients confirming the role of *FMR1* promoter hypermethylation in the pathogenesis of fragile X syndrome.[138] In their second paper, they found that combining 5-aza-2'-deoxycytidine with histone deacetylase inhibitors such as 4-phenylbutyrate, sodium butyrate, or trichostatin resulted in a 2- to 5-fold increase in FMR1 mRNA levels over that obtained with 5-aza-2'-deoxycytidine alone. The marked synergistic effect observed revealed that both histone hyperacetylation and DNA demethylation participate in regulating *FMR1* activity. These results may help pave the way for future attempts at pharmacologically restoring mutant *FMR1* activity *in vivo*.[139]

Methylation and histone deacetylation thus appear to act as layers for epigenetic silencing. Cameron et al. believe that one function of DNA methylation may be to firmly "lock" genes into a silenced chromatin state.[137] They suggested that this effect may be involved in transcriptional repression of methylated inactive X chromosomal genes and imprinted alleles. They proposed that to achieve maximal gene reactivation, it might be necessary to block simultaneously both DNA methylation and histone deacetylation, both of which are essential to the formation and maintenance of repressive chromatin.

SUMMARY

Epigenetics constitutes the study of the heritable changes in gene expression that do not require or generally involve changes in the genomic DNA sequence. The field began as a series of isolated observations on developmental phenomena in three disparate areas of biology more than 60 years ago, but following the advent of genomic technologies, epigenetics became primarily concerned with understanding the handling of genetic information by eukaryotic cells. The treatment of cancer and other diseases of epigenetic interest has spawned a new area of clinical investigation. *In vitro* studies and small clinical studies of various chemotherapeutic agents in the treatment of cancer and other diseases of epigenetic interest have demonstrated intriguing results while several second-generation drugs are in development or are undergoing evaluation at various early stages of clinical trial, resulting in a new area of clinical investigation. Today the field is recognized as a stand-alone discipline complementary to genetics and pharmacogenetics.

REFERENCES

1. Silverman PH. Rethinking genetic determinism. Scientist 2004; 18(10):32–33.
2. Baltimore D. Our genome unveiled. Nature 2001; 409(6822):814–816.
3. Waddington CH. Canalization of development and the inheritance of acquired characters. Nature 1942; 150:563–565.
4. Ruden DM, Garfinkel MD, Sollars VE, Lu X. Waddington's widget: Hsp90 and the inheritance of acquired characters. Semin Cell Dev Biol 2003; 14(5):301–310.
5. Barr ML, Bertram EG. A morphological distinction between neurones of the male and female, and the behaviour of the nucleolar staellite during accelerated nucleoprotein synthesis. Nature 1949; 163(Apr 30):676–677.
6. Ohno S, Kaplan WD, Kinosita R. Formation of the sex chromatin by a single X-chromosome in liver cells of Rattus norvegicus. Exp Cell Res 1959; 18:415–418.
7. Lyon MF. X-chromosome inactivation: A repeat hypothesis. Cytogenet Cell Genet 1998; 80(1–4):133–137.
8. Beutler E, Yeh M, Fairbanks VF. The normal human female as a mosaic of X-chromosome activity: Studies using the gene for C-6-PD-deficiency as a marker. Proc Natl Acad Sci USA 1962; 48:9–16.
9. Crouse H. The controlling element in sex chromosome behavior in Sciara. Genetics 1960; 45:1429–1443.
10. Josse J, Kaiser AD, Kornberg A. Enzymatic synthesis of deoxyribonucleic acid. VIII. Frequencies of nearest neighbor base sequences in deoxyribonucleic acid. J Biol Chem 1961; 236:864–875.
11. Grippo P, Iaccarino M, Parisi E, Scarano E. Methylation of DNA in developing sea urchin embryos. J Mol Biol 1968; 36(2):195–208.
12. Hotchkiss RD. The quantitative separation of purines, pyrimidines, and nucleosides by paper chromatography. J Biol Chem 1948; 175:315–332.
13. Scarano E. The control of gene function in cell differentiation and in embryogenesis. Adv Cytopharmacol 1971; 1:13–24.

14. Salser W. Globin mRNA sequences: Analysis of base pairing and evolutionary implications. CSHL 1977; XLVII:985–1003.
15. Bird AP. DNA methylation and the frequency of CpG in animal DNA. Nucleic Acids Res 1980; 8(7):1499–1504.
16. Bird AP, Taggart MH. Variable patterns of total DNA and rDNA methylation in animals. Nucleic Acids Res 1980; 8(7):1485–1497.
17. Riggs AD. X inactivation, differentiation, and DNA methylation. Cytogenet Cell Genet 1975; 14(1):9–25.
18. Holliday R, Pugh JE. DNA modification mechanisms and gene activity during development. Science 1975; 187(4173):226–232.
19. Jones PA, Taylor SM. Cellular differentiation, cytidine analogs and DNA methylation. Cell 1980; 20(1):85–93.
20. Juttermann R, Li E, Jaenisch R. Toxicity of 5-aza-2′-deoxycytidine to mammalian cells is mediated primarily by covalent trapping of DNA methyltransferase rather than DNA demethylation. Proc Natl Acad Sci USA 1994; 91(25):11797–11801.
21. Gardiner-Garden M, Frommer M. CpG islands in vertebrate genomes. J Mol Biol 1987; 196(2):261–282.
22. Takai D, Jones PA. Comprehensive analysis of CpG islands in human chromosomes 21 and 22. Proc Natl Acad Sci USA 2002; 99(6):3740–3745.
23. Rothnie HM, McCurrach KJ, Glover LA, Hardman N. Retrotransposon-like nature of the Tp1 elements: Implications for the organisation of highly repetitive, hypermethylated DNA in the genome of *Physarum polycephalum*. Nucleic Acids Res 1990; 19(2):279–287.
24. Vardimon L, Kressmann A, Cedar H, Maechler M, Doerfler W. Expression of a cloned adenovirus gene is inhibited by in vitro methylation. Proc Natl Acad Sci USA 1982; 79(4):1073–1077.
25. Groudine M, Eisenman R, Weintraub H. Chromatin structure of endogenous retroviral genes and activation by an inhibitor of DNA methylation. Nature 1981; 292(5821):311–317.
26. McGrath J, Solter D. Completion of mouse embryogenesis requires both the maternal and paternal genomes. Cell 1984; 37(1):179–183.
27. Spence JE, Perciaccante RG, Greig GM, Willard HF, Ledbetter DH, Hejtmancik JF, et al. Uniparental disomy as a mechanism for human genetic disease. Am J Hum Genet 1988; 42(2):217–226.
28. Monk M. Genomic imprinting. Memories of mother and father. Nature 1987; 328 (6127):203–204.
29. Stoger R, Kubicka P, Liu CG, Kafri T, Razin A, Cedar H, et al. Maternal-specific methylation of the imprinted mouse Igf2r locus identifies the expressed locus as carrying the imprinting signal. Cell 1993; 73(1):61–71.
30. Barlow DP. Imprinting: A gamete's point of view. Trends Genet 1994; 10(6):194–199.
31. Brown SW. Heterochromatin. Science 1966; 151(709):417–425.
32. Kimmins S, Sassone-Corsi P. Chromatin remodelling and epigenetic features of germ cells. Nature 2005; 434(7033):583–589.
33. Luger K, Mader AW, Richmond RK, Sargent DF, Richmond TJ. Crystal structure of the nucleosome core particle at 2.8 A resolution. Nature 1997; 389(6648):251–260.
34. Luo RX, Dean DC. Chromatin remodeling and transcriptional regulation. J Natl Cancer Inst 1999; 91(15):1288–1294.

35. Razin A, Riggs AD. DNA methylation and gene function. Science 1980; 210(4470): 604–610.

36. Waalwijk C, Flavell RA. MspI, an isoschizomer of hpaII which cleaves both unmethylated and methylated hpaII sites. Nucleic Acids Res 1978; 5(9):3231–3236.

37. Southern EM. Detection of specific sequences among DNA fragments separated by gel electrophoresis. J Mol Biol 1975; 98:503–517.

38. Waalwijk C, Flavell RA. DNA methylation at a CCGG sequence in the large intron of the rabbit beta-globin gene: Tissue-specific variations. Nucleic Acids Res 1978; 5(12):4631–4634.

39. Bestor T, Laudano A., Mattaliano R, Ingram V. Cloning and sequencing of a cDNA encoding DNA methyltransferase of mouse cells. The carboxy-terminal domain of the mammalian enzymes is related to bacterial restriction methyltransferases. J Mol Biol 1988; 203(4):971–983.

40. Bestor TH. The DNA methyltransferases of mammals. Hum Mol Genet 2000; 9(16):2395–2402.

41. Wu JC, Santi DV. Kinetic and catalytic mechanism of HhaI methyltransferase. J Biol Chem 1987; 262(10):4778–4786.

42. Pradhan S, Bacolla A, Wells RD, Roberts RJ. Recombinant human DNA (cytosine-5) methyltransferase. I. Expression, purification, and comparison of de novo and maintenance methylation. J Biol Chem 1999; 274(46):33002–33010.

43. Lei H, Oh SP, Okano M, Juttermann R, Goss KA, Jaenisch R, et al. De novo DNA cytosine methyltransferase activities in mouse embryonic stem cells. Development 1996; 122(10):3195–3205.

44. Li E, Bestor TH, Jaenisch R. Targeted mutation of the DNA methyltransferase gene results in embryonic lethality. Cell 1992; 69(6):915–926.

45. Leonhardt H, Page AW, Weier HU, Bestor TH. A targeting sequence directs DNA methyltransferase to sites of DNA replication in mammalian nuclei. Cell 1992; 71(5):865–873.

46. Robertson KD, Jones PA. DNA methylation: Past, present and future directions. Carcinogenesis 2000; 21(3):461–467.

47. Yen RW, Vertino PM, Nelkin BD, Yu JJ, el Deiry W, Cumaraswamy A, et al. Isolation and characterization of the cDNA encoding human DNA methyltransferase. Nucleic Acids Res 1992; 20(9):2287–2291.

48. Yoder JA, Bestor TH. A candidate mammalian DNA methyltransferase related to pmt1p of fission yeast. Hum Mol Genet 1998; 7(2):279–284.

49. Van den Wygaert, I, Sprengel J, Kass SU, Luyten WH. Cloning and analysis of a novel human putative DNA methyltransferase. FEBS Lett 1998; 426(2):283–289.

50. Hermann A, Schmitt S, Jeltsch A. The human Dnmt2 has residual DNA-(cytosine-C5) methyltransferase activity. J Biol Chem 2003; 278(34):31717–31721.

51. Okano M, Xie S, Li E. Cloning and characterization of a family of novel mammalian DNA (cytosine-5) methyltransferases. Nat Genet 1998; 19(3):219–220.

52. Boyes J, Bird A. DNA methylation inhibits transcription indirectly via a methyl-CpG binding protein. Cell 1991; 64(6):1123–1134.

53. Boyes J, Bird A. Repression of genes by DNA methylation depends on CpG density and promoter strength: Evidence for involvement of a methyl-CpG binding protein. EMBO J 1992; 11(1):327–333.

54. Hendrich B, Bird A. Identification and characterization of a family of mammalian methyl-CpG binding proteins. Mol Cell Biol 1998; 18(11):6538–6547.

55. Meehan RR, Lewis JD, Bird AP. Characterization of MeCP2, a vertebrate DNA binding protein with affinity for methylated DNA. Nucleic Acids Res 1992; 20(19): 5085–5092.

56. Cross SH, Meehan RR, Nan X, Bird A. A component of the transcriptional repressor MeCP1 shares a motif with DNA methyltransferase and HRX proteins. Nat Genet 1997; 16(3):256–259.

57. Nan X, Ng HH, Johnson CA, Laherty CD, Turner BM, Eisenman RN, et al. Transcriptional repression by the methyl-CpG-binding protein MeCP2 involves a histone deacetylase complex. Nature 1998; 393(6683):386–389.

58. Jones PL, Veenstra GJ, Wade PA, Vermaak D, Kass SU, Landsberger N, et al. Methylated DNA and MeCP2 recruit histone deacetylase to repress transcription. Nat Genet 1998; 19(2):187–191.

59. Allfrey VG, Faulkner R, Mirsky AE. Acetylation and methylation of histones and their possible role in the regulation of RNA synthesis. Proc Natl Acad Sci USA 1964; 51:786–794.

60. Bestor TH. Gene silencing. Methylation meets acetylation. Nature 1998; 393(6683): 311–312.

61. Bird AP, Wolffe AP. Methylation-induced repression—belts, braces, and chromatin. Cell 1999; 99(5):451–454.

62. Ng HH, Zhang Y, Hendrich B, Johnson CA, Turner BM, Erdjument-Bromage H, et al. MBD2 is a transcriptional repressor belonging to the MeCP1 histone deacetylase complex. Nat Genet 1999; 23(1):58–61.

63. Tamaru H, Selker EU. A histone H3 methyltransferase controls DNA methylation in Neurospora crassa. Nature 2001; 414(6861):277–283.

64. Rea S, Eisenhaber F, O'Carroll D, Strahl BD, Sun ZW, Schmid M, et al. Regulation of chromatin structure by site-specific histone H3 methyltransferases. Nature 2000; 406(6796):593–599.

65. Nakayama J, Rice JC, Strahl BD, Allis CD, Grewal SI. Role of histone H3 lysine 9 methylation in epigenetic control of heterochromatin assembly. Science 2001; 292 (5514):110–113.

66. Fire A, Xu S, Montgomery MK, Kostas SA, Driver SE, Mello CC. Potent and specific genetic interference by double-stranded RNA in Caenorhabditis elegans. Nature 1998; 391(6669):806–811.

67. Volpe TA, Kidner C, Hall IM, Teng G, Grewal SI, Martienssen RA. Regulation of heterochromatic silencing and histone H3 lysine-9 methylation by RNAi. Science 2002; 297(5588):1833–1837.

68. Hannon GJ. RNA interference. Nature 2002; 418(6894):244–251.

69. Paddison PJ, Caudy AA, Hannon GJ. Stable suppression of gene expression by RNAi in mammalian cells. Proc Natl Acad Sci USA 2002; 99(3):1443–1448.

70. Barker D, Schafer M, White R. Restriction sites containing CpG show a higher frequency of polymorphism in human DNA. Cell 1984; 36(1):131–138.

71. Esteller M, Corn PG, Baylin SB, Herman JG. A gene hypermethylation profile of human cancer. Cancer Res 2001; 61(8):3225–3229.

72. Cooper DN, Youssoufian H. The CpG dinucleotide and human genetic disease. Hum Genet 1988; 78(2):151–155.

73. Brueckner B, Lyko F. DNA methyltransferase inhibitors: Old and new drugs for an epigenetic cancer therapy. Trends Pharmacol Sci 2004; 25(11):551–554.

74. Robertson KD, Wolffe AP. DNA methylation in health and disease. Nat Rev Genet 2000; 1(1):11–19.

75. Egger G, Liang G, Aparicio A, Jones PA. Epigenetics in human disease and prospects for epigenetic therapy. Nature 2004; 429(6990):457–463.
76. Havlis J, Trbusek M. 5-Methylcytosine as a marker for the monitoring of DNA methylation. J Chromatogr B Analyt Technol Biomed Life Sci 2002; 781(1–2):373–392.
77. Hong KM, Yang SH, Guo M, Herman JG, Jen J. Semiautomatic detection of DNA methylation at CpG islands. BioTechniques 2005; 38(3):354, 356, 358.
78. Shi H, Maier S, Nimmrich I, Yan PS, Caldwell CW, Olek A, et al. Oligonucleotide-based microarray for DNA methylation analysis: Principles and applications. J Cell Biochem 2003; 88(1):138–143.
79. Chen CM, Chen HL, Hsiau TH, Hsiau AH, Shi H, Brock GJ, et al. Methylation target array for rapid analysis of CpG island hypermethylation in multiple tissue genomes. Am J Pathol 2003; 163(1):37–45.
80. Kononen J, Bubendorf L, Kallioniemi A, Barlund M, Schraml P, Leighton S, et al. Tissue microarrays for high-throughput molecular profiling of tumor specimens. Nat Med 1998; 4(7):844–847.
81. Pfarr W, Webersinke G, Paar C, Wechselberger C. Immunodetection of 5'-methylcytosine on Giemsa-stained chromosomes. BioTechniques 2005; 38(4):527–528, 530.
82. Brock GJ, Huang TH, Chen CM, Johnson KJ. A novel technique for the identification of CpG islands exhibiting altered methylation patterns (ICEAMP). Nucleic Acids Res 2001; 29(24):E123.
83. Rousseau F, Heitz D, Biancalana V, Blumenfeld S, Kretz C, Boue J, et al. Direct diagnosis by DNA analysis of the fragile X syndrome of mental retardation. N Engl J Med 1991; 325(24):1673–1681.
84. Xiong Z, Laird PW. COBRA: A sensitive and quantitative DNA methylation assay. Nucleic Acids Res 1997; 25(12):2532–2534.
85. van Steensel B. Mapping of genetic and epigenetic regulatory networks using microarrays. Nat Genet 2005; 37(6 Suppl):S18–S24.
86. Golub TR. Genome-wide views of cancer. N Engl J Med 2001; 344(8):601–602.
87. Golub TR, Slonim DK, Tamayo P, Huard C, Gaasenbeek M, Mesirov JP, et al. Molecular classification of cancer: Class discovery and class prediction by gene expression monitoring. Science 1999; 286(5439):531–537.
88. Alizadeh AA, Eisen MB, Davis RE, Ma C, Lossos IS, Rosenwald A, et al. Distinct types of diffuse large B-cell lymphoma identified by gene expression profiling. Nature 2000; 403(6769):503–511.
89. van de Vijver MJ, He YD, van't Veer LJ, Dai H, Hart AA, Voskuil DW, et al. A gene-expression signature as a predictor of survival in breast cancer. N Engl J Med 2002; 347(25):1999–2009.
90. van't Veer LJ, Dai H, van de Vijver MJ, He YD, Hart AA, Mao M, et al. Gene expression profiling predicts clinical outcome of breast cancer. Nature 2002; 415(6871):530–536.
91. Camp RL, Dolled-Filhart M, King BL, Rimm DL. Quantitative analysis of breast cancer tissue microarrays shows that both high and normal levels of HER2 expression are associated with poor outcome. Cancer Res 2003; 63(7):1445–1448.
92. Xu GL, Bestor TH, Bourc'his D, Hsieh CL, Tommerup N, Bugge M, et al. Chromosome instability and immunodeficiency syndrome caused by mutations in a DNA methyltransferase gene. Nature 1999; 402(6758):187–191.
93. Amir RE, Van dV, I, Wan M, Tran CQ, Francke U, Zoghbi HY. Rett syndrome is caused by mutations in X-linked MECP2, encoding methyl-CpG-binding protein 2. Nat Genet 1999; 23(2):185–188.

94. Wan M, Lee SS, Zhang X, Houwink-Manville I, Song HR, Amir RE, et al. Rett syndrome and beyond: Recurrent spontaneous and familial MECP2 mutations at CpG hotspots. Am J Hum Genet 1999; 65(6):1520–1529.

95. Moretti P, Zoghbi HY. MeCP2 dysfunction in Rett syndrome and related disorders. Curr Opin Genet Dev 2006; 16(3):276–281.

96. Miller G. Neuroscience. Getting a read on Rett syndrome. Science 2006; 314(5805): 1536–1537.

97. Horike S, Cai S, Miyano M, Cheng JF, Kohwi-Shigematsu T. Loss of silent-chromatin looping and impaired imprinting of DLX5 in Rett syndrome. Nat Genet 2005; 37(1):31–40.

98. Barlow DP. Gametic imprinting in mammals. Science 1995; 270(5242):1610–1613.

99. Falls JG, Pulford DJ, Wylie AA, Jirtle RL. Genomic imprinting: Implications for human disease. Am J Pathol 1999; 154(3):635–647.

100. Jin P, Warren ST. Understanding the molecular basis of fragile X syndrome. Hum Mol Genet 2000; 9(6):901–908.

101. Miller G. Biomedical research. Fragile X's unwelcome relative. Science 2006; 312(5773):518–521.

102. Pal N, Wadey RB, Buckle B, Yeomans E, Pritchard J, Cowell JK. Preferential loss of maternal alleles in sporadic Wilms' tumour. Oncogene 1990; 5(11):1665–1668.

103. Schroeder WT, Chao LY, Dao DD, Strong LC, Pathak S, Riccardi V, et al. Non-random loss of maternal chromosome 11 alleles in Wilms tumors. Am J Hum Genet 1987; 40(5):413–420.

104. Scrable H, Cavenee W, Ghavimi F, Lovell M, Morgan K, Sapienza C. A model for embryonal rhabdomyosarcoma tumorigenesis that involves genome imprinting. Proc Natl Acad Sci USA 1989; 86(19):7480–7484.

105. Glenn CC, Porter KA, Jong MT, Nicholls RD, Driscoll DJ. Functional imprinting and epigenetic modification of the human SNRPN gene. Hum Mol Genet 1993; 2(12):2001–2005.

106. Buiting K, Gross S, Lich C, Gillessen-Kaesbach G, el Maarri O, Horsthemke B. Epimutations in Prader-Willi and Angelman syndromes: A molecular study of 136 patients with an imprinting defect. Am J Hum Genet 2003; 72(3):571–577.

107. Mannens M, Hoovers JM, Redeker E, Verjaal M, Feinberg AP, Little P, et al. Parental imprinting of human chromosome region 11p15.3-pter involved in the Beckwith-Wiedemann syndrome and various human neoplasia. Eur J Hum Genet 1994; 2(1):3–23.

108. Feinberg AP, Vogelstein B. Hypomethylation distinguishes genes of some human cancers from their normal counterparts. Nature 1983; 301(5895):89–92.

109. Feinberg AP, Gehrke CW, Kuo KC, Ehrlich M. Reduced genomic 5-methylcytosine content in human colonic neoplasia. Cancer Res 1988; 48(5):1159–1161.

110. Baylin SB, Hoppener JW, de Bustros A, Steenbergh PH, Lips CJ, Nelkin BD. DNA methylation patterns of the calcitonin gene in human lung cancers and lymphomas. Cancer Res 1986; 46(6):2917–2922.

111. Feinberg AP. Cancer epigenetics takes center stage. Proc Natl Acad Sci USA 2001; 98(2):392–394.

112. Rainier S, Johnson LA, Dobry CJ, Ping AJ, Grundy PE, Feinberg AP. Relaxation of imprinted genes in human cancer. Nature 1993; 362(6422):747–749.

113. Ogawa O, Eccles MR, Szeto J, McNoe LA, Yun K, Maw MA, et al. Relaxation of insulin-like growth factor II gene imprinting implicated in Wilms' tumour. Nature 1993; 362(6422):749–751.

114. Klein G. Epigenetics: Surveillance team against cancer. Nature 2005; 434(7030): 150.
115. Rideout WM, III, Coetzee GA, Olumi AF, Jones PA. 5-Methylcytosine as an endogenous mutagen in the human LDL receptor and p53 genes. Science 1990; 249(4974):1288–1290.
116. Levine AJ. p53, the cellular gatekeeper for growth and division. Cell 1997; 88(3): 323–331.
117. Cui H, Cruz-Correa M, Giardiello FM, Hutcheon DF, Kafonek DR, Brandenburg S, et al. Loss of IGF2 imprinting: A potential marker of colorectal cancer risk. Science 2003; 299(5613):1753–1755.
118. Sakatani T, Kaneda A, Iacobuzio-Donahue CA, Carter MG, Witzel SD, Okano H, et al. Loss of imprinting of Igf2 alters intestinal maturation and tumorigenesis in mice. Science 2005; 307(25 Mar):1976–1978.
119. Toyota M, Ahuja N, Ohe-Toyota M, Herman JG, Baylin SB, Issa JP. CpG island methylator phenotype in colorectal cancer. Proc Natl Acad Sci USA 1999; 96(15): 8681–8686.
120. Fraga MF, Ballestar E, Villar-Garea A, Boix-Chornet M, Espada J, Schotta G, et al. Loss of acetylation at Lys16 and trimethylation at Lys20 of histone H4 is a common hallmark of human cancer. Nat Genet 2005; 37(4):391–400.
121. Plumb JA, Strathdee G, Sludden J, Kaye SB, Brown R. Reversal of drug resistance in human tumor xenografts by 2′-deoxy-5-azacytidine-induced demethylation of the hMLH1 gene promoter. Cancer Res 2000; 60(21):6039–6044.
122. Ricciardiello L, Goel A, Mantovani V, Fiorini T, Fossi S, Chang DK, et al. Frequent loss of hMLH1 by promoter hypermethylation leads to microsatellite instability in adenomatous polyps of patients with a single first-degree member affected by colon cancer. Cancer Res 2003; 63(4):787–792.
123. Lee WH, Morton RA, Epstein JI, Brooks JD, Campbell PA, Bova GS, et al. Cytidine methylation of regulatory sequences near the pi-class glutathione S-transferase gene accompanies human prostatic carcinogenesis. Proc Natl Acad Sci USA 1994; 91(24):11733–11737.
124. Esteller M, Hamilton SR, Burger PC, Baylin SB, Herman JG. Inactivation of the DNA repair gene O6-methylguanine-DNA methyltransferase by promoter hypermethylation is a common event in primary human neoplasia. Cancer Res 1999; 59(4):793–797.
125. Esteller M, Toyota M, Sanchez-Cespedes M, Capella G, Peinado MA, Watkins DN, et al. Inactivation of the DNA repair gene O6-methylguanine-DNA methyltransferase by promoter hypermethylation is associated with G to A mutations in K-ras in colorectal tumorigenesis. Cancer Res 2000; 60(9):2368–2371.
126. Bastian PJ, Yegnasubramanian S, Palapattu GS, Rogers CG, Lin X, De Marzo AM, et al. Molecular biomarker in prostate cancer: The role of CpG island hypermethylation. Eur Urol 2004; 46(6):698–708.
127. Lynch HT, de la Chapelle A. Hereditary colorectal cancer. N Engl J Med 2003; 348(Mar 6):919–932.
128. Baylin SB, Herman JG. DNA hypermethylation in tumorigenesis: Epigenetics joins genetics. Trends Genet 2000; 16(4):168–174.
129. Warrell RP Jr, He LZ, Richon V, Calleja E, Pandolfi PP. Therapeutic targeting of transcription in acute promyelocytic leukemia by use of an inhibitor of histone deacetylase. J Natl Cancer Inst 1998; 90(21):1621–1625.
130. Stirewalt DL, Radich JP. Malignancy: Tumor suppressor gene aberrations in acute myelogenous leukemia. Hematology 2000; 5(1):15–25.

131. Chim CS, Tam CY, Liang R, Kwong YL. Methylation of p15 and p16 genes in adult acute leukemia: Lack of prognostic significance. Cancer 2001; 91(12):2222–2229.
132. Gilbert J, Gore SD, Herman JG, Carducci MA. The clinical application of targeting cancer through histone acetylation and hypomethylation. Clin Cancer Res 2004; 10(14):4589–4596.
133. Ley TJ, DeSimone J, Anagnou NP, Keller GH, Humphries RK, Turner PH, et al. 5-Azacytidine selectively increases gamma-globin synthesis in a patient with beta+ thalassemia. N Engl J Med 1982; 307(24):1469–1475.
134. Koshy M, Dorn L, Bressler L, Molokie R, Lavelle D, Talischy N, et al. 2-Deoxy 5-azacytidine and fetal hemoglobin induction in sickle cell anemia. Blood 2000; 96(7):2379–2384.
135. Uchida T, Kinoshita T, Nagai H, Nakahara Y, Saito H, Hotta T, et al. Hypermethylation of the p15INK4B gene in myelodysplastic syndromes. Blood 1997; 90(4):1403–1409.
136. Silverman LR, Demakos EP, Peterson BL, Kornblith AB, Holland JC, Odchimar-Reissig R, et al. Randomized controlled trial of azacitidine in patients with the myelodysplastic syndrome: A study of the cancer and leukemia group B. J Clin Oncol 2002; 20(10):2429–2440.
137. Cameron EE, Bachman KE, Myohanen S, Herman JG, Baylin SB. Synergy of demethylation and histone deacetylase inhibition in the re-expression of genes silenced in cancer. Nat Genet 1999; 21(1):103–107.
138. Chiurazzi P, Pomponi MG, Willemsen R, Oostra BA, Neri G. In vitro reactivation of the FMR1 gene involved in fragile X syndrome. Hum Mol Genet 1998; 7(1):109–113.
139. Chiurazzi P, Pomponi MG, Pietrobono R, Bakker CE, Neri G, Oostra BA. Synergistic effect of histone hyperacetylation and DNA demethylation in the reactivation of the FMR1 gene. Hum Mol Genet 1999; 8(12):2317–2323.

7

Genomic Tools

The 1970s marked the beginning of a period of remarkable technical innovation that transformed life science research. Numerous methods were developed for identifying and locating genomic lesions of medical importance while other key technologies were designed that made possible the sequencing of the entire genome of humans and those of many other species. The extensive record of research that defines the field is closely tied to the range of innovative technologies that were developed to explore the composition and function of genomic DNA. As a result, modern genetics experienced a period of rapid growth that has prompted reappraisal and redefinition of the field.

Pharmacogenetic traits are revealed by structural lesions in DNA that can be inferred from family inheritance patterns and demonstrated by direct observation. Finding the genic differences that predispose persons to such traits provides clues that differentiate susceptible persons from those who are not, and on the premise of establishing their molecular basis, we hope to achieve better therapies and improve prospects for predictive biology including new drug discoveries and individualized medicine.

Genic lesions relevant to pharmacogenomics range in size from microscopically visible chromosomal rearrangements to deletions and insertions as large as a single gene and as small as a single DNA base. Single base changes, point mutations, or other small changes in DNA composition that lead to functional changes in a protein are most commonly associated with pharmacogenetic traits. Alternative sequences of DNA that occur at an appreciable frequency, usually set at 1% or greater, are termed DNA polymorphisms. Since these polymorphisms occur at specific loci, technologies for detecting and locating them provide the tools for diagnosing susceptible individuals and for assessing their prevalence, mode of inheritance, and significance in individuals and in populations at large.

CHARTING THE EVOLUTION OF GENOMICS TOOLS

In 1975, Edwin Southern first combined the specificity of restriction endonuclease digestion with gel electrophoresis to identify sequence variations in fragments of genomic DNA (Table 7.1).[1-34] Restriction enzyme digestion generated a collection of controlled, predictable DNA fragments, and gel electrophoresis of DNA fragments immobilized on a membrane provided an efficient, economic means to array the collection of fragments by size. The simplicity and reliability of the method for molecular analysis quickly led to its adoption in many laboratories.[1,2] In 1977 Fred Sanger devised a method for direct sequencing of genomic DNA that used chain termination by dideoxy-nucleotides to specify the genetic change and define its genomic location.[3] In the same year, Alwine developed the "Northern blot" version of Southern's technique,[4] in which a complex RNA sample is size separated and then transferred to an immobilization membrane. This technique established the link between the genomic sequence and messenger RNA (mRNA) expression.

In 1980, Wyman and White showed that probing DNA fragments by restriction enzyme digestion and hybridization yielded altered electrophoretic banding patterns of diagnostic value called restriction fragment length polymorphisms (RFLPs).[5] Wyman and White also reported the accidental discovery of repetitive hypervariable sequences throughout the genome. Because they exhibited variable numbers of repeats within a single locus and between loci, these sequences were termed hypervariable. Encouraged by this report, in 1985 Jeffreys developed the technique of "DNA fingerprinting."[8,35] For this purpose, Jeffreys developed probes that hybridize to these hypervariable loci, which were also dubbed "minisatellites" or "variable number tandem repeats" (VNTRs), and yielded RFLPs arrayed in Southern blots. DNA fingerprinting has been routinely used for genomic mapping and also for individual identification in criminal investigations, paternity disputes, zygosity testing in twins, monitoring transplants, and wildlife forensics.[35]

Subsequently, "dot" blots and "slot" blots were developed.[16,17] "Dot blots" and "slot blots" were also hybridization methodologies that take their name from the circular and slotted wells in templates used to present test samples to a membrane surface. Neither of these methods requires restriction digestion or electrophoresis, and they are faster and easier for hybridization screening than Southern blotting, especially for samples too small or too damaged to undergo purification, digestion, and electrophoresis, or when many samples are to be screened simultaneously using different sets of hybridization probes. They are, however, somewhat less informative because they do not provide RFLP information and are more prone to nonspecific background hybridization. A few years later, after the invention of the polymerase chain reaction (PCR),[12] the "reverse dot blot" was developed. The "reverse dot blot" makes use of probe collections instead of the DNA test samples immobilized on the membrane. DNA to be analyzed is submitted to PCR amplification, labeled with a detectable marker, and hybridized to the array of immobilized probes.[19] With PCR, smaller and smaller amounts of DNA could be analyzed still more rapidly. Reverse dot blot probe sets could be

Table 7.1 Charting the Evolution of Genomics Tools

Year	Genomics Tool	Comment	Reference
1975	Southern blots	DNA sequence variation identified by combining restriction digestion with electrophoresis	1
1977	Direct (Sanger) sequencing	Dideoxy chain termination used for DNA sequencing and for scanning and scoring DNA mutations	3
	Northern blots	The RNA version of Southern blots	4
1980	Restriction fragment length polymorphism (RFLP)	RFLPs are shown to have diagnostic value	5
1982	GenBank established	Part of a larger effort to find new ways of acquiring, storing, and analyzing genomic data	6, 7
1985	DNA fingerprinting	Probes designed to hybridize to minisatellites that yield unique RFLPs for individuals have potential for many biomedical and forensic applications	8
	Microarray analysis of DNA	The first application of microarrays to DNA analysis	9
	Rapid sequence database search tool, FASTA	The method improves the efficiency and sensitivity of amino acid sequence comparisons	10
1986	Automation of DNA sequence analysis	Fluorescent detection, capillary electrophoresis, and computer analysis are combined in the first step to automate DNA sequence analysis	11
1987	Polymerase chain reaction (PCR)	PCR permits DNA from any source to be amplified by a process that starts with a chosen DNA segment and proceeds in successive copying cycles, each of which doubles the number of segments in the reaction	12, 13
	MALDI-TOF mass spectrometry	Mass and composition analysis of proteins embedded in a solid matrix bombarded with laser light of short duration is achieved	14
1988	NCBI established	The National Center for Biotechnology Information (NCBI) was created to house and develop information systems for use in molecular biology	7, 15
1989	Dot blot and slot blot analysis with allele-specific probes	DNA samples placed in circular wells are tested for hybridization with allele-specific probes; dot blots are faster and easier than Southern blotting because restriction digestion and electrophoresis are not required	16, 17

(continued)

Table 7.1 (*continued*)

Year	Genomics Tool	Comment	Reference
	Y2H system	The yeast two-hybrid (Y2H) system made possible identification of interactions between protein pairs without prior purification	18
1990	NCBI scientists publish Basic Local Alignment Search Tool (BLAST)	NCBI-BLAST exists in many different forms (see www.ncbi.nlm.nih.gov/ BLAST/producttable. Html)	
1993	Reverse dot blot analysis	DNA probe collections immobilized on membranes are interrogated by DNA samples	19
1994	Genomic (DNA) profiling by microarrays	The potential utility of arrays of immobilized DNA probe sequences for analysis of cDNA target sequences was tested	20, 21
1995	Gene expression (RNA) profiling by microarrays	Microarrays composed of immbolized *Arabidopsis* cDNAs and expressed sequence tags were used to measure quantitative gene expression of the corresponding genes	22
	Gene expression profiling in cancer	The utility of microarrays to pinpoint gene variants in melanoma cancer cell lines is shown	23
1998	PHRED/PHRAP/CONSED software	Software that emphasizes objective criteria to measure the accuracy of DNA sequences and assemblies	24, 25
	MALDI-TOF DNA sequence analysis	The high resolution needed for the estimation of mass accuracy is substantially improved by (1) increased delay time between ion generation and ion fragmentation, and (2) more efficient salt removal	26
2002	MALDI-TOF analysis for rapid bacterial pathogen identification	Base-specific fragmentation of amplified 16S rRNA gene fragments analyzed by MS offers a tool for rapid identification of bacterial pathogens	27
	MALDI-TOF primer extension analysis in association studies	Primer extension analysis by MALDI-TOF MS provides reliable estimates of allele frequencies in and between pooled DNAs, and of sources of variability in these estimates	28
2003	MALDI-TOF comparative sequence analysis	This high-throughput comparative sequence analysis comprises a homogeneous *in vitro* RNase T1-mediated base-specific cleavage system coupled with MALDI-TOF MS, which enables automated sequence analysis of PCR products up to 1 kb in length to be analyzed	29

(*continued*)

Table 7.1 (*continued*)

Year	Genomics Tool	Comment	Reference
2004	Y2H mapping of the C. elegans interactome	Mapping the protein–protein interactions of *C. elegans* is an instructive step toward determining the human genome interactome	30
	MALDI-TOF discovery of DNA sequence	The first implementation of a comparative sequencing strategy based on analysis of all four base-specific end digests of a targeted nucleic acid sequence	31
2005	Microarray-based genome-wide genotyping	Microarray technology has been adapted to the analysis of the genomic copy number analogous to gene expression profiling, and progress has been made toward genome-wide SNP genotyping	32
	Mass ARRAY MALDI-TOF DNA analysis	An integrated genetic analysis platform based on MALDI-TOF MS to discover SNPs, allele-specific expression, and analyze DNA methylation patterns	33
	MALDI-TOF analysis of DNA methylation patterns	Differential DNA methylation analysis between normal and lung cancer tissue by base-specific cleavage and MALDI-TOF MS aids in detecting disease genes and understanding epigenetic modifications	34

customized by individual investigators for their own applications and commercial suppliers began to develop generic products based on this concept that were widely used throughout the molecular biology community.[36,37]

CONVENTIONAL ANALYTICAL TECHNIQUES

Conventional procedures designed for analysis of molecular variants are of two types: those that scan DNA sequences for unknown or new variants and those that score DNA sequences for known variants. Both types are consequences of the molecular hybridization rules based on Watson–Crick base pairing and recombinant DNA technology. Certain techniques rely primarily on differential hybridization stringency to achieve genotyping specificity, whereas other techniques incorporate enzyme reactions, such as polymerase extension or ligation, to accommodate different molecular processes that specify the genetic change. This distinction is important because procedures that employ an enzymatic reaction, or an enzymatic reaction combined with hybridization to achieve specificity in genotyping, are more robust and exhibit better performance than those that rely solely on hybridization.[38]

Many procedures have been adapted for use with several different platforms, where the term "platform" refers to the specific technology employed to read the genotyping results.[39] Slab gel electrophoresis was the first platform chosen for separating and arraying DNA fragments. This platform gained favor because it was reliable for the analysis of one or a few genes, but difficulties in automation weighed against it, and it has been replaced in many applications by other separation methods[40] such as capillary electrophoresis,[41] high-performance liquid chromatography (HPLC),[42,43] and mass spectrometry.[44–47] Homogeneous assays eliminated the need for the separation of reaction components and increased the popularity of assays based on this platform. The demand for large-scale analysis of sequence variation presented new challenges and led to the development of the platform of solid-phase systems. Solid-phase systems include gene chip/ microarray,[48] bead, and microtiter plate assay formats.[49,50] Adoption of one or another of these platforms has improved the readout of genotyping results, but usually does not alter the fundamental biochemistry that determines the specificity of the approach.[38]

The technique selected for analysis should take account of the expected nature of the variant, its size and the structure of the gene of interest, the availability of mRNA, the degree of sensitivity required, and other resources available. The underlying principle of each procedure, its salient features, and its primary advantages and disadvantages are summarized below. Additional details are available in the references cited.

Procedures used primarily to scan DNA sequences are considered first and separately from those used primarily to score variants.

CONVENTIONAL ANALYSIS OF GENETIC VARIANTS

Scanning for New Variants

Apart from Sanger's direct sequencing methodology, techniques to scan sequences for new mutations take advantage of several unique properties of DNA.[39,51–54] One group of procedures relies on differences in electrophoretic mobilities of wild-type and mutant alleles. Single-strand conformation polymorphism (SSCP), denaturing gradient gel electrophoresis (DGGE or TGGE), and heteroduplex analysis (HET or HA) belong to this group. A second group relies on the ability of proteins or chemicals to recognize a change in double-stranded DNA at the site of a sequence mismatch. Ribonuclease A cleavage (RNase), chemical cleavage of mismatch (CCM), and enzymatic mismatch cleavage (EMC) rely on this principle. A third group is distinguished by reliance on hybridization or hydridization combined with enzyme-based extension.[39] Methods that use scanning and resequencing on microarrays and enzymatic extension from microarrays belong in this group. The protein truncation test (PTT) does not fit into any of the groups as it uses *in vitro* transcription and translation to detect truncation mutations.

Direct Sequencing

Direct sequencing refers to the sequence analysis of PCR products without prior subcloning into sequencing vectors. Direct sequencing is generally accepted as most reliable to scan for new mutations as well as to score for known mutations.

Because of its reliability and low error rate (equal to or less than one in 10,000 bases), the performance of all other analytical methods is traditionally measured against direct (Sanger) sequencing.

Chain termination by dideoxy nucleotides is used to specify the genetic change and precisely defines the location and nature of the alteration.[3,55,56] Initially, Sanger used a polyacrylamide gel platform for fractionation of DNA fragments and autoradiography for detection. Slab gel detection has since been superseded by microcapillary electrophoresis[41] and with the introduction of fluorescent-based sequencing tools, direct sequencing has been automated for high-through-put applications.[57] Since none of the other scanning methods is capable of such precise definition, direct sequencing is the final step to guarantee results obtained by any of the other methods of scanning.

Despite its accuracy and reliability, direct sequencing on a large scale is laborious and expensive. Ideally, the optimal technique for mutation detection would be rapid, could screen large regions of DNA with high sensitivity and specificity, would not require hazardous chemicals or elaborate, expensive equipment, and yet would provide information about the location and nature of the mutation. Numerous procedures have been developed that meet one or more of these conditions, but no procedure is definitive.

Single-Strand Conformational Polymorphism (SSCP) Analysis

Single-stranded nucleic acids differing by a single base form different secondary structures that migrate with different mobilities in a polyacrylamide nondenaturing gel. Orita applied this principle in SSCP analysis to detect sequence differences within the same region of DNA from different individuals.[58] Differences in the electrophoretic patterns obtained are determined visually by nonradioactive means. Under optimal conditions and with the fragment size of the DNA test sample within the range of 150–200 base pairs, 80–90% of base exchanges are detectable.[59]

Recently, high-SSCP analysis has been automated for use with capillary electrophoresis.[60,61] This method has been used to detect point mutations associated with inherited cardiac disorders including the long QT syndrome and hypertrophic cardiomyopathy. The sensitivity was 100% when 34 different point mutations were analyzed on PCR fragments of 166–1223 base pairs in length. Limited experience indicates that the automated technique has advantages of rapidity, robustness, high resolution, and good reproducibility.

Denaturing Gradient Gel Electrophoresis (DGGE or TGGE)

DGGE analysis also relies on differential electrophoretic migration of wild-type and mutant DNA to detect sequence differences.[62,63] Double-stranded DNA molecules differing by a single base substitution exhibit different electrophoretic mobilities compared to homodimers migrating through a gel containing a gradient of increasing concentration of denaturing agent. Detection is by nonradioactive means. When the appropriate primers are used and optimal conditions are attained, DGGE is rapid and highly reliable. This technique is capable of close to 100% accuracy in PCR products up to 1000 base pairs long.[52] Although this method is rapid, it is costly for small numbers of samples because of the require-ment for guanosine–cytosine (GC) clamps.

A refinement of this method (TGGE) replaces the chemical denaturing gradient of DNA in DGGE with temperature as the denaturant.[64]

Heteroduplex Analysis (HET or HA)

In a mixture of wild-type and mutant DNA molecules, heteroduplexes are formed by heat denaturation and reannealing. Heteroduplexes formed between different alleles migrate with different mobilities when subjected to electrophoresis side by side in a nondenaturing polyacrylamide gel.[65] Sequence differences are detected by visually comparing the migration patterns obtained. A level of detection of approximately 80–90%, similar to that obtained in SSCP analysis, is attained with DNA fragments of 200–600 base pairs in length.

In one modification of HET, capillary-based conformation-sensitive gel elec-trophoresis (capillary CSGE), mutation detection is transferred from acrylamide gel to capillary electrophoresis.[66] This modification is capable of detecting every possible single base heteroduplex, all short insertions and deletions (1–4 base pairs), as well as 16 of 22 substitutions of up to approximately 350 base pairs. Multiple PCR products can be resolved by using different fluorescent labels. CSGE can be automated and offers the potential for high-throughput analysis.

Other modifications of HET that enhance heteroduplex resolution have been developed.[67] One modification involves PCR of the region of interest followed by hybridization of the PCR product to a synthetic molecule called a "universal heteroduplex generator" (UHG). This method was used in a study of apolipo-protein E mutations to induce heteroduplex formation. Heteroduplex formation was visualized on a nondenaturing minigel with ethidium bromide. The method was found to be simpler, faster, and more reliable than the current method of choice (RFLP with Hha restriction), and is suitable for high-throughput screening.[67]

Ribonuclease A Cleavage (RNase)

Mismatches between RNA:RNA and RNA:DNA heteroduplexes are cleaved by ribonuclease A.[68] Cleavage of labeled fragments is detected by the presence of shorter fragments on denaturing gels. Fragments as large as 1000 base pairs can be analyzed. Larger fragments are separated under denaturing conditions, but incomplete separation makes interpretation difficult.[69] Only about 70% of muta-tions are detected. The need to prepare RNA as a probe and the inherent insta-bility of RNA as a substrate are additional drawbacks of this technique. For these reasons, this method is less suitable for scanning than other methods.

Chemical Cleavage of Mismatch (CCM)

The principle underlying this method resembles that in ribonuclease A cleavage. The DNA heteroduplex is formed from a mixture of wild-type and mutant DNA heating and annealing. Mismatched T bases of the heteroduplex are modified by osmium tetroxide and mismatched C bases are modified by hydroxylamine. The modified strands of DNA are cleaved at the site of the modification by incubation with piperidine. Fragments are subsequently separated on denaturing polyacrylamide gels and identified by autoradiography. By labeling the antisense strand, adenosine and guanosine mismatches are also detected. This method is capable of detecting at least 95% of mismatches when only the wild type is labeled and 100% when both strands are labeled. PCR products of up to 2 kilobases in length have been studied successfully.[52,70] The precise location and the nature of the mutation can also be determined from the size of the band and the cleaving agent. The primary disadvantage of this method is the use of highly mutagenic and explosive chemicals that are unsuitable for a routine clinical laboratory and limit the potential for automation.

Enzymatic Mismatch Cleavage (EMC)

This strategy exploits the ability of bacteriophage enzymes (resolvases) to recognize and cleave DNA containing unpaired bases. Resolvases can be thought of simply as restriction enzymes that cut DNA only in the presence of mutation. Heteroduplexes created by heat denaturation and renaturation of PCR products are cleaved enzymatically, and subsequently separated by denaturing or nondenaturing polyacrylamide gel electrophoresis. Resolvases that have been used with this technique include T4 endonuclease VII and T7 endonuclease.[71–73] Mutations were detected in DNA fragments between 88 and 940 base pairs[71] and up to 1.5 kilobases in length.[72] An automated version of this technique claims to have improved earlier versions by eliminating the need for sample purification, shortening hybridization time, and increasing the signal-to-noise ratio.[73]

Only a few systematic studies have been conducted with this technique and further evaluation of its reliability is needed. It has been observed that some mutations were poorly recognized by resolvases. Thus, while cleavage of small deletions (1–3 base pairs) is detected, only 13 of 14 point mutations representing all possible nucleotide exchanges were detected.[71] In a second report, only 3 of 4 small deletions and 17 of 18 point mutations were detected.[72] Mutations that are poorly recognized may result in incomplete DNA digestion, and the occurrence of nonspecific bands complicates interpretation of the electrophoretic patterns obtained. Another problem with EMC is that homozygous mutant samples escape detection, but at the same time, non-specific cleavage of homoduplexes is observed where none is expected. As the efficiency and reliability of enzymatic mismatch cleavage remains to be proven, this technique is not yet considered acceptable as a strategy to screen for variants in DNA.

Scanning and Reference-Based Sequence Checking (Resequencing) on Oligonucleotide Microarrays

The DNA microarray is one of more recent promising techniques for mutational analysis. These devices, in their simplest form, exploit direct hybridization. They quickly occupied niches in nearly every area of nucleic acid analysis as several reviews indicate.[74–76] Once hybridization patterns or "signatures" of large numbers of mutant alleles of interest are known, mounting a search for those signatures in many different samples is possible. On the other hand, screening for all possible new mutations with microarrays is more difficult than searching for known mutations.[77]

Several factors may contribute to the potential difficulty in identification: (1) The microarray-based system is more sensitive to detection of homozygous base changes than heterozygous changes. Although it is possible to use microarrays for heterozygous screening,[78] for general use in the detection of heterozygous base changes, accuracy must be improved. It is not yet ready for applications needing >98% heterozygous mutation detection. (2) Variations in target sequence composition, including the presence of repetitive sequence elements, can exert a major influence on the sensitivity of the system, and may lead to unacceptably high false-negative rates. (3) Intramolecular and intermolecular structures, such as hairpins and G-quartets, present in either target or probe can make hybridization less predictable. Variant sequences that disrupt secondary structures may act to increase or decrease the affinity to "perfect match" probes. Deletions and insertions can pose special problems because they may form duplexes containing bulged nucleotides with a wild-type probe that in turn can alter the predictability of the outcome. Unfortunately, few systematic studies have been conducted to determine what steps must be taken to reduce or circumvent the effects of these factors.

The discriminating power that can be achieved by direct hybridization alone can be improved by coupling target hybridization with enzymatic primer extension with DNA polymerase.[77,79] DNA polymerase uses oligonucleotides tethered to the membrane surface, or in a microtiter dish, via the 5'-end linkage to leave exposed the free 3'-OH group. Chain-terminating, labeled dideoxynucleotide triphosphates (ddNTPs) are used in primer extension reactions in which the hybridized target and oligonucleotide probes serve as template and primer, respectively. The enzyme incorporates and extends the primer by only one base, which is complementary to the next base in the target. The enzyme drives the reaction further with greater specificity than is possible with direct hybridization alone under conditions of high stringency. This process is known as "minisequencing"[80] or "genetic bit analysis."[81] Methods similar in principle that use DNA ligase instead of polymerase have been adapted for use with microarrays. A mixture of all four ddNTPs, each labeled with a different fluorescent dye, can be used in the primer extension reactions, and the identity of the extended ddNTP-labeled product is determined by fluorescent microscopy. It should be noted that commercially available Affymetrix™ arrays tethered to the surface through 3'-end linkages are unsuitable for this task.

The Protein Truncation Test (PTT)

The protein truncation test is based on the principle that stop codons generated by point mutations or frameshift mutations lead to a premature stop of translation. The coding region of the gene is amplified by PCR, using a sense primer tailed by a T7 promoter sequence. The amplified PCR product is then used as a template for *in vitro* translation testing. The PTT selectively detects translation-terminating mutations as short peptides. The size of the peptides is determined visually after autoradiography on sodium dodecyl sulfate (SDS)-polyacrylamide gel electrophoresis. It can be anticipated that small differences in the size of the protein fragments created by the truncating mutations may limit applications of the assay. For instance, truncated variants located close to the 5′ binding site that result in very short translation products might be undetectable. Alternatively, for mutations situated close to the 3′ binding site, the truncated and full-length products would be of nearly equal lengths and might not be resolved.

The PTT would be expected to be useful in the diagnosis of disorders to which terminating mutations contribute substantially. It has been used to scan genes related to disease, including familial adenomatous polyposis, hereditary breast and ovarian cancer, Duchenne's muscular dystrophy, and ophthalmic disease.[82] A modification of the standard PTT called digital protein truncation to increase its sensitivity to detect mutations was utilized to detect APC mutations in fecal DNA from patients with colorectal tumors. Mutations were identified in 26 of 46 stool samples tested from patients with neoplastic disease, whereas none was identified in stools from 28 control patients who did not have neoplastic disease.[83]

Scoring for Known Mutations

Gel-Based Methods
Several gel-based methods have been in common use to detect known mutations in DNA sequences. These include RFLP, the allele-specific oligonucleotide assay, allele-specific amplification (ASA), and the oligonucleotide ligation assay (OLA). Some of these methods have been adapted for use with multiple platforms.

Southern Blot Hybridization. Because polymorphic variations in DNA sequences may ablate or create restriction sites, restriction digestion and hybridization probing of DNA samples yield altered banding patterns called RFLPs.[4] RFLP analysis quickly became the standard protocol for the analysis of variants in many molecular biology laboratories. It provides a good first analytical step because no detailed knowledge of the structure and sequence of a gene is required. All types of variants that alter restriction sites are detectable. Polymerase errors may destroy recognition sequences, but when the appropriate restriction enzymes and appropriate controls are used, a specificity of 100% is achieved.

Restriction enzymes are endonucleases that make sequence-specific cuts in the phosphate-pentose backbone of DNA to yield "restriction fragments" of the molecule. Typically, they recognize palindromic sequences four to eight bases long. Restriction enzymes such as *Taq*I, *Msp*I, and *Hae*III are especially useful in scanning for variants by Southern blotting because they are four-base cutter endonucleases (T↓CGA, C↓CGG, and GG↓CC, respectively) and would sample an average size gene (approx 30,000 base pairs) about 700 times. In addition, these endonucleases include CpG dinucleotides in their recognition sequence and they have specificity for mutation-prone CpG dinucleotides.[84]

Genetic polymorphisms in cancer susceptibility genes have been intensely studied for many years. A pharmacogenetic approach to test for polymorphisms would be valuable in cancer studies for routine staging, for tumor marker analysis, and to probe for new prognostic and predictive markers. Several laboratories have applied restriction analysis to DNA recovered from archived paraffin-embedded tumor blocks for these purposes.[85–87] Recently, Rae and associates[87] have demonstrated that fixation and processing did not alter the genotypes of genomic DNA obtained from archived tissues for which peripheral blood was available for comparison. Attempts to extend the method to hematoxylin/eosin or immunohistochemically stained sections were unsuccessful because staining inhibited the PCR reactions. Application of restriction analysis to test for associations between genetic polymorphisms and treatment response may thus have a significant influence on the choice and outcomes of cancer therapy.

Reliability, simplicity, and economy are the primary advantages of restriction enzyme analysis for analyzing one or a few genes, but the original technique is impractical for routine use in the clinical laboratory because it is time consuming, labor intensive, and difficult to automate. Modifications of the method[88,89] have reduced but not eliminated these disadvantages.

Allele-Specific Oligonucleotide (ASO) Hybridization.   ASO hybridization is based on the same principle as RFLP. It has been applied in different formats known as dot blots, slot blots, and reverse dot blots. The characteristics and limitations of ASO hybridization are generally similar to those for restriction enzyme digestion described in the previous section. All mutations are detectable. Hybridization can be performed in solution as well as on solid supports. In modifications of this strategy, hybrids between target DNA and labeled probes are collected onto streptavidin-coated microtitration wells, washed under stringent conditions, and measured by fluorometry. This method has been applied to find point mutations in the Z-allele in α_1-antitrypsin deficiency.[90] ASO hybridization is subject to Taq polymerase error in cloned DNA fragments. The performance and the quality of results depend on adherence to particular technical modifications.

Allele-Specific Amplification (ASA).   ASA relies on hybridization between the primer and target sequence. Assuming amplification occurs only when they match completely, only one allele of either the wild-type or mutant allele is amplified. Two different approaches to ASA have been described. In one, amplification is prevented by a mismatch located at the 3′-terminus of the primer, and in the other, by a mismatch located within the primer. The first is called the "amplification refractory mutation system" (ARMS)[91] and the second is called "competitive oligonucleotide priming" (COP).[92] Either approach detects all base-exchange mutations in homozygous and heterozygous states. However, unless the ratio of variant to wild-type DNA is in the defined range, the specificity and limits of detection may be strongly affected. The possibility of false-positive or false-negative results is the major limitation of this method.

The ARMS technique has been combined with fluorescence polarization in a homogeneous assay format for genotypic analysis. The genotypes determined with the method agree with those obtained by the conventional application of ARMS.[93] Another modification combines ASA with pyrosequencing.[94] The term pyrosequencing is derived from the production of inorganic pyrophosphate (PP_i) formed during primer extension. The incorporation of nucleotides during primer extension produces a long strand of complementary DNA as well as large amounts of PP_i. PP_i is converted to ATP in the presence of adenosine 5'-pyrophosphosulfate, which is detected bioluminetrically with luciferin and luciferase. In the presence of luciferase, ATP initiates the production of visible light proportionate to the number of nucleotides incorporated, while unincorporated nucleotides are degraded by apyrase. Accurate detection of single-nucleotide polymorphisms (SNPs) with frequencies as low as 0.02 is claimed for this technique.

Oligonucleotide Ligation Assay (OLA).   The OLA relies on allele-specific hybridization for mutation analysis. In the original procedure, two probes were used, one that is specific for the wild-type allele and one that is specific for the mutant allele.[95] In a modified strategy, a third fluorescent-labeled common probe is introduced.[96] In the latter case, the 3' terminus of each allele-specific probe is designed to ligate with the 5'-terminus of the common probe. The gene fragment containing the polymorphic site is amplified by PCR and incubated with the probes. In the presence of thermally stable DNA ligase, ligation of the fluorescent-labeled probe occurs only when there is a perfect match between the amplified PCR product and either the mutant probe or the wild-type probe. OLA is capable of detecting all DNA base exchanges. Specificity is dependent on sequences surrounding the polymorphic site, and DNA regions with high GC content complicate optimization and multiplexing.

In an early version of the OLA, ligated and nonligated primers were discriminated by dot blot,[97] but automated versions of the OLA assay have also been developed. One version uses enzyme-linked immunosorbent assay (ELISA)-based oligonucleotides[96] and another uses various combinations of fluorescent dyes and probe lengths[98] to detect multiple mutations in a single reaction. An OLA has also been reported that significantly reduces the time cost of high throughput testing.[99]

Homogeneous Assays

Under homogeneous conditions, mutation analysis is performed in solution and in a single sealed tube.[100,101] These precautions reduce the risk of cross-contamination and enhance speed and simplicity. "Real-time" monitoring and quantitation are possible. Excellent discussions of this topic by Foy and Parkes[100] and by Shi[101] emphasize applications that are emerging in the clinical arena.[100]

Some homogeneous assay platforms incorporate ultrarapid thermocyclers that affect the time for analysis. For example, the thermocycler used in LightCycler™ equipment permits PCR to be performed within 20 minutes in glass capillaries, and that in the ABI Prism 7700 Sequence Detection System™ permits assays to be performed within 2 hours in microtiter plate-based systems. Options for non-PCR-based methods include BDProbeTecET®, which is a platform based on strand displacement and fluorescent detection,[102] and Abbott LCx®, which is a platform that uses a ligase chain reaction for detection.[103]

Both nonspecific and specific homogeneous assay methods are available.[100] Nonspecific methods detect the presence (or absence) of the amplified PCR product but provide no additional information about the product. They are prone to produce false-positive results attributed to undesired products that spuriously increase fluorescence. Specific methods that probe the amplified product are more desirable for molecular genetic diagnostics. Several of the most popular formats for specific methods are non-gel-based, and favor fluorescent signals for detection. Fluorescence resonance energy transfer (FRET)[104] or fluorescence polarization[105] has been utilized for signal generation. The signal appears rapidly and reliably. Examples of FRET-based technologies for specific high throughput detection of mutations include TaqMan® assay, Molecular Beacons®, Scorpion® primers, and the Invader™ assay. The first three techniques use PCR-amplified fragments of DNA while the Invader system enables SNP genotyping without amplification. Fluorescence polarization combined with ARMS as noted above (see p. 195) has also been shown to be a highly sensitive technique for signal generation.[93] The homogeneous assay methods described below are amenable to automation and high-throughput analysis.

Single-Base Primer Extension. The concept of single-base primer extension for mutation analysis, also termed "minisequencing"[80] and "genetic bit analysis,"[81] was developed several years ago. It has attracted a lot of attention and reference to this technique appears under many different names and acronyms. This concept is applicable to several different platforms including gel and capillary electrophoresis, numerous homogeneous assay formats such as ELISA among others, and solid phase assays performed on microarrays and in microtiter plates.[106,107]

The principle of this method in its simplest form involves single-base extension of an oligonucleotide primer annealed to single-stranded DNA at a location adjacent but not overlapping the polymorphic site. This is followed by the addition of DNA polymerase to catalyze extension of the primer in the presence of chain-terminating dideoxynucleotides.[106] Single-base primer extension achieves its specificity through enzyme-based recognition instead of hybridization of the primer. The dideoxynucleotides are labeled by fluorophore or in various other ways to facilitate the identification of the single incorporated nucleotide. The low cost of reagents, robustness, accuracy, and flexibility with respect to platform and scalability from one-gene-at-a time assays to large-scale, high-throughput assays are among the advantages that recommend the method.

A homogeneous assay format using FRET to detect single-base pair exchanges in genomic DNA samples has been applied to detect variants of several genes including the cystic fibrosis gene, the HLA-H human leukocyte gene, and the tyrosine kinase protooncogene.[108] The change in fluorescent intensity during primer extension can be monitored as time passes by a fluorescence spectrophotometer, or at its endpoint by a fluorescence plate reader.

A recent version of this methodology combines the advantages of minisequencing with those of a microarray format that permits highly multiplexed and parallel analysis. The methodology is described in detail by Lovamer and Syvänen.[109]

TaqMan® Assays.   A fluorogenic probe consisting of an oligonucleotide labeled with a fluorophore in close proximity to a quencher dye is included in a typical PCR reaction. When TaqMan DNA polymerase encounters the probe-specific, PCR-amplified product, the 5′-nuclease activity cleaves the probe. Cleavage separates the dye from the quencher and results in an increase in fluorescent intensity.[110] The entire assay is performed using a single thermocycling protocol and a standard method of analysis that enables automated genotyping. By using different reporter dyes, several allele-specific probes can be discriminated in a single analysis.

Allele-specific Taqman probes have been used extensively to detect polymorphisms in drug metabolizing enzymes.[111–113]

Molecular Beacon® Assays.   Molecular Beacons are hairpin-shaped fluorophore-labeled oligonucleotide probes that fluoresce on hybridization.[114] The fluorophore is attached to one end and a quencher is attached to the other end of the hairpin that keeps these two molecules in close proximity, quenching the emitted fluorescence. In the presence of a complementary DNA target, the Molecular Beacon undergoes a conformational change, separating the fluorophore from the quencher, permitting fluorescence to occur. Hairpin probes are advantageous for mutation analysis because they are more specific than linear DNA probes. Molecular Beacons labeled with different fluorophores that emit signals at different wavelengths permit the analysis of more than one allelic combination in the same PCR reaction.

Molecular Beacon probes have been employed to detect the C-to-T point mutation in the methylenetetrahydrofolate reductase gene that is associated with cardiovascular disease.[114]

Scorpion® Primer Assays.   Another method for efficient detection of PCR product uses fluorescent molecules that combine the primer and the probe functions into a single molecule called a "Scorpion" primer.[115] The Scorpion primer is a hairpin-shaped probe element attached via a non-amplifiable segment to the 5′-end primer that carries a fluorophore/quencher pair (similar in principle to the Molecular Beacon). In isolation, the Scorpion primer is fully quenched and does not fluoresce. As the primer extends during PCR, the probe element hybridizes to a target on the newly formed strand from which the hairpin loop opens (but is not cleaved) to separate the fluorophore from the quencher to emit the fluorescent signal.

Application of this system to the analysis of the *BRCA2* gene[115] and the cystic fibrosis gene[116] detected variant forms of these genes in wild-type and variant samples. Comparative fluorescence accumulation patterns showed the sensitivity of Scorpion primers to be approximately equal to that achieved with TaqMan and greater by several-fold under standard conditions than with Molecular Beacons.[115] Another direct comparison between Scorpion, TaqMan, and Molecular Beacons on the Roche-LightCycler™ indicates that Scorpions performed better, particularly under the fast cycling condition.[116] Though experience with the Scorpion primers is limited, it appears that probing of target DNA sequences with unimolecular primers may provide an alternative approach that is beneficial in assay design, reliability, and speed in the analysis of variants.

Invader™ System Assays.   The Invader system relies on naturally occurring and engineered enzymes, referred to as Cleavases® (Third Wave Technologies, Madison, WI), that cleave DNA molecules at particular locations in response to structure rather than sequence.[117] A typical Invader assay includes two downstream allele-specific oligonucleotide signal probes (wild type or variant) plus an upstream Invader probe. The 5′-end of the downstream signal probes contains a "flap" that is not complementary to the DNA target sequence. The Invader system involves sequential primary and secondary reactions. When the 3′-end of the upstream probe overlaps (or invades) the hybridization site of the 5′-end of a downstream probe by at least one base, the "flap" is cleaved by the 5′-exonuclease activity of Cleavase®. The *primary reaction* occurs only when the 3′-end of the upstream probe invades the end of the duplex formed between the downstream probe and the DNA target by at least one base. The "flap" that is cleaved serves as an Invader probe that directs the secondary reaction. The *secondary reaction* uses a synthetic DNA sequence as a target; the second signal probe is hairpin shaped and is labeled with a fluorophore in close proximity to a quencher. Cleavage of the secondary signal probe by the Cleavase® generates the fluorescence signal. Because the sequences of the 5′-flap of the primary signal probe and the secondary signal probes are independent of the target, a universal detector system could be designed.[117,118]

The Invader system thus achieves its specificity by combining hybridization with enzyme recognition but without product amplification. It can use genomic DNA directly to discriminate variant from wild-type genotypes in mixed populations at very low ratios of (1/1000 or lower) of variant to wild type. The technique is rapid and adaptable to large-scale analysis of SNPs that use high-throughput methods of detection such as FRET and matrix-assisted laser desorption/ionization time of flight (MALDI-TOF) mass spectrometry (MS). Applications of the Invader system to Factor V Leiden, factor II (prothrombin), cystic fibrosis, and apolipoprotein E, and to measurement of mRNA levels of ubiquitin demonstrate its versatility and validity for analysis of variants, SNP profiling, and gene expression analysis.[118]

The Invader assay has been combined with multiplex PCR in an automated high-throughput procedure that is capable of genotyping 300,000–400,000 SNPs in 1 day. The amount of DNA needed to assay one SNP is 0.4 ng.[119]

ADVANCES IN GENOMICS TECHNOLOGY

As demands for sequencing, mapping, and identifying human genes moved ahead, so did efforts to find new ways for rapidly acquiring, storing, and analyzing genomic information while maintaining or improving sensitivity and reliability. In numerous instances, scientists whose immediate interests lay outside biology lent their expertise to help achieve these ends.

In 1982, the GenBank database was established to centralize and streamline the storage and accessibility of genomic information and to set in motion the design of tools for computational analysis of genomic information.[120] Then current technology could only read out short lengths of DNA, about 300 bases, and in 1986, investigators first applied fluorescence detection to Sanger's method of analysis to demonstrate the practicality of automated DNA sequence analysis.[11] The concept of immobilizing probe collections on a membrane as in the reverse dot blot methodology led to the idea of DNA microarrays ("gene chips") by generating generic arrays of probe sets and fixing them to solid supports to permit high-throughput screening applications.[121] MALDI-TOF MS, a technology borrowed from chemistry, was adapted to the analysis of proteins and DNA, and the combination of its speed and accuracy gave this technique a role in genome sequencing and diagnosis.[122] The yeast two-hybrid assay system provided a simple and sensitive means of identifying protein–protein interactions that were amenable to large-scale, high-throughput analysis.[18,123] Brief accounts of the origin and development of these revolutionary technologies are presented below.

Computational Biology

During the 1960s, protein chemists began to collect sequences resulting from their own research, from that of their colleagues, and from the literature. Dayhoff and Ledley, who assembled the first major collection of genetic sequence information in the form of atlases of protein sequence and structure, were at the forefront of these efforts. During the 1970s, Berman and colleagues, who assembled a database of X-ray crystallographic protein atomic coordinates, and Kabat and colleagues, who constructed a database on the structure and diversity of immunoglobins, extended these efforts. Additionally, during the 1970s, two computer analysis systems available online, the time-sharing molecular analysis (PROPHET) system, and the Stanford University Medical Experimental Computer Resource (SUMEX), had been developed by government-sponsored groups or in academia.

These databases and computer analysis systems were part of a larger attempt to demonstrate the potential of database facilities for storage and retrieval of molecular data and the importance of computer support for sequence analysis. In 1979, scientists assembled at a workshop sponsored by the National Science Foundation had reached a consensus on the need to establish an international computer database for nucleic acid sequences and recommendations for its establishment had been formally outlined. They knew that computer programs capable of processing large amounts of data would be required to facilitate storage and editing of molecular sequences, to produce copies of a sequence in various forms, to translate into the amino acid sequence that was encoded by a DNA sequence, to search a sequence for particular shorter sequences, to analyze codon usage and base composition, to compare two sequences for homology, to locate regions of sequences that were complementary, and to translate two sequences showing amino acid similarities.[120] Unfortunately, immediate progress toward this goal stumbled because a report of this workshop was not widely distributed, preventing a broad-based discussion of its findings. Subsequent meetings convened in 1980 in rapid succession, notably in Schonau, Germany, on April 24, 1980, and at the National Institutes of Health (NIH) on July 14 and on August 11, 1980, created a sense of urgency about this issue. And submission of proposals on alternative approaches to establish such a resource and further prodding by a number of researchers helped refocus attention on the need to establish a center dedicated to sequence collection and analysis.[6,7] At a final meeting convened at the NIH on December 7, 1980, guidelines were set forth to implement such a project in two phases. Phase I was to establish a centralized nucleic acid sequence database and Phase II was to establish an analysis and software library coupled to the database. In the project implemented, however, only Phase I was supported while Phase II was postponed. Thus, on June 30, 1982, the National Institute of General Medicine announced the award for the establishment of GenBank®, the nucleic acid sequence data bank.

While these attempts to establish GenBank moved ahead in fits and starts, investigators continued to apply rapid DNA sequencing techniques to predict the complete sequence of specific proteins.[124,125] In one notable instance that was concluded in 1978, J.G. Sutcliffe utilized Sanger's "plus-and-minus" method[56] to determine the nucleotide sequence of the ampicillin resistance (penicillinase) gene of *Escherichia coli* that encoded a β-lactamase of approximately 27,000 daltons. Sutcliffe conducted his research in Walter Gilbert's laboratory at Harvard University, and Gilbert knew that investigators in Jeremy Knowles' laboratory at the University of Edinburgh were engaged in direct studies to determine the peptide composition and amino acid sequence of that enzyme.[126] Within 7 months of initiating the project, Sutcliffe had completed the nucleotide sequence[125] and his findings about the hypothetical protein derived from the translation of the DNA sequence were in complete agreement with the amino acid sequence observed in Knowles laboratory.[127] Sutcliffe's study was the first to demonstrate that the derivation of the primary sequence of a protein from its nucleotide sequence was much faster and easier than the sequencing of the protein. His study made a powerful statement about the value of sequencing methodology.[126]

As the number of protein molecules and nucleic acid fragments for which sequences had been determined expanded, the need for efficient, rapid, and economical methods to conduct similarity searches became even more obvious. Early in the 1980s, several different methods were in use for analyzing such similarities, and at that time, all of the software search tools used some measure of similarity between sequences to distinguish biologically significant relationships from chance similarities. Existing methods that had been implemented could be divided into two categories: those for global comparisons where two complete sequences were considered, and those for local searches where the search was limited to similar fragments of two sequences; but these older methods were computationally intensive and expensive when applied to large data banks.[128]

In 1983, Wilbur and Lipman partially resolved this problem by developing a new algorithm that yielded rigorous sequence alignments for global comparisons.

The method substantially reduced search time with minimal loss of sensitivity.[128] Using this algorithm, the entire Protein Data Bank of the National Biomedical Research Foundation (NBRF) could be searched in less than 3 minutes and all eukaryotic sequences in the Los Alamos Nucleic Acid Data base in less than 2 minutes. Waterfield and associates employed this technique to demonstrate that the sequence of platelet-derived growth factor was related to the transforming protein p28sis of simian sarcoma virus.[129] Later, other rapid algorithms such as FASTA and related versions of this program were developed permitting large databases to be searched on commonly available minicomputers.[130]

In 1988, the National Center for Biotechnology Information (NCBI) at the NIH was created to house and develop information systems for use in molecular biology. The NCBI was assigned responsibility for maintaining GenBank® and began to provide data analysis, data retrieval, and resources that operated on the data in GenBank. Since its creation, the purview of the NCBI has greatly expanded and the suite of resources and services currently offered can be grouped into seven categories: (1) database retrieval systems, (2) sequence similarity search programs, and resources (3) for the analysis of gene-level sequences, (4) for chromosomal sequences, (5) for genome-scale analysis, (6) for the analysis of gene expression and phenotypes, and (7) for protein structure and modeling, all of which can be accessed through the NCBI homepage http://www.ncbi.nlm.nih.gov.[15]

In 1990, Altschul and colleagues introduced the basic local alignment search tool (BLAST) as a new approach to rapid sequence comparisons.[131] The basic algorithm was applicable to a variety of contexts including DNA and protein sequence database searches, motif searches, gene identification searches, and the analysis of multiple regions of similarity in long DNA sequences. BLAST had the advantage of being an order of magnitude faster than existing search tools of comparable sensitivity. Since the original version was published, several new versions of BLAST have been developed that improved sensitivity and performance or were customized for high-performance computing.[132,133]

The most frequent type of analysis performed on GenBank data uses BLAST to search for nucleotide or protein sequences similar to a query sequence. To facilitate searches for other purposes or that require other approaches, the NCBI offers specialized versions of the BLAST family and customized implementations of the BLAST family of programs to augment many applications.[15]

For more than 15 years, computational methods for gene finding were based on searches for sequence similarities. These well-established methods proved successful in many cases, but a follow-up study showed that only a fraction of newly discovered sequences had identifiable homologs in current databases.[134] For example, based on sequences in GenBank 2000, when only ~25% of the human genome was available, results of the study suggested that only about half of all new vertebrate genes might be discovered by sequence similarity searches. Recently, another computational approach, the template approach, has been developed. The template approach, more commonly referred to as *ab initio* gene finding, combines coding statistics with signal sensor detection into a single framework. Coding statistics represent measures of protein coding functions, whereas signal sensors are short nucleotide subsequences that are recognized by cell machinery as initiators of certain processes.[135] While many different nucleotide patterns have been examined as signal sensors, those that are usually modeled include promoter elements, start and stop codons, splice sites, and poly(A) sites. Rogic and colleagues have conducted a comparative analysis of several recently developed programs (FGENES, GeneMark.hmm, Genie, Genscan, HMMgene, Morgan, and MZEF) that incorporate coding statistics and signal sensors. The analysis examines the accuracy of predicting gene structure as a function of various structural features such as the $G + C$ content of the sequence, length and type of exons, signal type, and score of exon prediction. The analysis shows that this new generation of programs provides, overall, a substantial improvement over previous programs in predicting some of the complexities of gene structure, and is an important step in deciphering the content of any genome.[134]

The PHRED/PHRAP/CONSED software tools developed by Green and colleagues for DNA sequence analysis should be mentioned as programs that have received recognition and worldwide use in the genomic community.[24,25] A key feature of these programs is their emphasis on objective criteria to measure the accuracy of sequences and assemblies. PHRED reads DNA sequencer trace data obtained from the dideoxy chain-termination method of Sanger,[3] calls bases, and assigns quality values (log transformed error probabilities) to the data. After calling the bases, PHRED writes the sequences in either a FASTA or Standard Chromatogram Format (SCF). PHRAP is a program that assembles shotgun DNA sequence data. It uses a combination of user-supplied and internally computed data to improve accuracy of assembly in the presence of repeats, and constructs a sequence of the highest quality parts of reads. CONSED is a graphic tool for editing PHRAP assemblies into a finished sequence. CONSED implements the finishing strategy. It allows the user to edit the sequence and uses error probabilities from PHRED and PHRAP to guide the editing; the program can also select primers and templates for locations specified by the user, and it automates the process of choosing reads for finishing the sequence.[136]

Thus, comparative analyses of DNA and protein sequences have become an indispensable part of biological research. In 1999, the NIH launched the Mammalian Gene Collection (MGC) program. This program combines and illustrates many of the key features that exemplify computational biology. As originally envisioned, this program was sponsored by 16 NIH institutes and the National Library of Medicine and is led by the National Cancer Institute and the National Institute for Genome Research. It includes components for the production, analysis, and distribution of libraries, clones, and sequences, and technology development, and its major goal was to obtain and identify a full set of human and other mammalian full-length sequences and clones of expressed genes.[137] In the first report of this effort, the MGC program generated and performed initial analysis of more than 15,000 full-length human and mouse cDNA sequences.[137] Among existing gene-identification programs, the prediction of the coding sequence (open reading frame, ORF) of typical genes is an important first step in deciphering the gene content of any genome. In the human portion of the study, a total of 12,419 full ORF human cDNA clones that corresponded to 9530 distinct human genes were sequenced to finished standards. Candidate full ORF clones for an additional 7800 human genes were also identified. This evidence combined with that from the carefully annotated sequence of chromosome 22 indicated that the MGC consists of 52% of all human genes, and that it will grow to 67% in the near future.[138]

Automated DNA Sequence Analysis

In essence, reading the base sequence of any particular segment of DNA using Sanger's dideoxynucleotide chain termination method is achieved through the creation of sequential fragments that match the chain to be sequenced, each fragment being one base longer than the previous one. In four separate reactions, each containing a different terminator dideoxy base (A, G, T, C), one of the four radiolabeled dideoxynucleotides is incorporated into the growing chain of DNA during enzymatic synthesis; its incorporation stops further chain growth resulting in a collection of fragments. The fragments differ in length and they all end in the dideoxynucleotide incorporated during DNA synthesis. The fragment collection that results is then separated according to length by gel electrophoresis. By determining the identity of the final radiolabeled nucleotide in each fragment, the entire sequence could be reconstructed. Manual performance of this process by an experienced investigator permitted the determination of up to about 5000 bases in a week.

In 1985, Hood and colleagues developed a strategy by which the radiolabeled dideoxynucleotides were replaced with fluorescent dyes covalently attached to the oligonucleotide primer used during DNA synthesis; a different colored dye specific for the bases A, G, T, C was used for each synthetic reaction. The reaction mixtures were combined, coelectrophoresed down a single polyacrylamide gel tube, and the fluorescent bands of DNA were separated near the bottom of the tube. The fluorescent bands within the gel were detected by the fluorescence emission spectra excited by an argon laser at four different wavelengths. The sequence was acquired directly by computer. Specialized chemistry that was developed for attaching the dyes to the DNA primer, for fluorescence detection, and for data analysis demonstrated that automated DNA sequence analysis was a practical goal.[11] This first step toward automation eliminated much of the labor associated with DNA analysis and demonstrated that an investigator could read more sequences in a day than could be read manually in an entire week. On the basis of this work, LeRoy Hood in collaboration with colleagues at Applied Biosystems built the first commercial instrument, ABI Model 370, for DNA sequence analysis.

Soon after, a number of innovations and refinements to automatic DNA sequencing were introduced. Simpler chemistry for fluorescent labeling of sequence terminator dyes was devised and with this innovation, the entire sequencing reaction could be performed in a single tube. More powerful computers, increased gel capacity, improvement of the optical systems, and more sensitive fluorescent dyes increased the capacity of the instrument so that the ABI PRISM

Model 377 sequencer introduced in 1995 could sequence more than 19,000 bases per day. Owing to the dependence on slab gel electrophoresis, however, the capacity was limited, time consuming, and cumbersome. Subsequently, this limitation was addressed in the newer machine, the ABI Model 3700 Automated Sequencer, by using capillary electrophoresis for separating DNA fragments. And the technology for DNA sequence analysis has continued to advance. According to Applied Biosystems, the 3730xL sequencer can process 96 capillaries, each with the capacity to call 900 bases, in 3 hours with a 1% error rate.[133]

Two attempts to reduce the time and expense of DNA sequence analysis have recently been reported. The core technology of base-calling from emission wavelength, which had not changed appreciably since Hood's research in 1986,[11] had some disadvantages limiting sensitivity and application to multicomponent systems. Metzker and colleagues presented an approach called pulsed multiline excitation (PME) that uses four different lasers matched to four different dyes to improve sensitivity and broaden application.[139] The higher sensitivity translates into significantly enhanced signal quality that in turn would decrease the cost of fluorescent dye reagents as illustrated in the application to primary DNA sequencing data. In another effort, Margulies and associates searched for alternative methods to reduce the time and cost of DNA sequence analysis. They described a scalable, highly parallel sequencing system with greater throughput than state-of-the-art capillary electrophoresis instruments. They carried out the shotgun sequencing and assembly of the *Mycoplasma genitalium* genome with 96% coverage of 99.96% accuracy in one 4-hour run of the machine. Their apparatus used a new fiberoptic slide of individual wells and could sequence 25 million bases, at 99% or better accuracy, in 4 hours.[140] Shendure and colleagues described a technology that converts an inexpensive epifluorescence microscope to rapid nonelectrophoretic DNA sequencing automation.[6] They used this technology to resequence an evolved strain of *E. coli* at a cost of less than one-ninth that of conventional sequencing and with less than one error per million bases.

DNA Microarrays

Methods for the analysis of DNA have long been recognized as ligand assays, relying on the binding of target molecules to a specific recognition reagent. Techniques for immobilizing DNA on nitrocellulose paper and for detecting the fixed nucleic acid with radioactive probes were widely adopted.[9,141,142] Building on the idea of using immobilized probe collections, as in the "reverse dot blot," Southern developed a method for the parallel, *in situ* synthesis of oligonucleotides using standard nucleotide synthetic reactions as a way to generate oligonucleotide probe arrays on microscope slides for highly parallel hybridization analysis.[20,143,144]

DNA microarrays are assemblies of nucleotide sequences, each of which represents a single gene, splice variant, or another DNA element, attached to a solid surface. Many variations on this central theme have appeared since the origin of the concept. For example, DNA microarrays are distinguished from earlier hybridization methodologies such as reverse dot blots by their relatively high probe density and by their use of miniaturized, solid, nonporous supports. Rigid supports, particularly those that are optically transparent and thermally conductive, are more practical than flexible supports. They are also more practical for interfacing with automatic fluid delivery or printing equipment, and they best accommodate the automatic scanning systems that are used to image arrays. The method of generating probe sets has also been modified in several different ways. In one successful modification, photochemistry and photolithography were incorporated into oligonucleotide synthesis,[21] and in another, piezoelectric nozzles and ink jet heads "printed" DNA synthesis reagents directly onto substrates for *in situ* oligonucleotide synthesis localized by surface chemistry.[145] Thus the idea of generating microarrays, or "gene chips," capable of high-throughput screening took root.

As the amount of available information about the sequence of the entire human genome has emerged, the density of successive generations of DNA microarrays has continued to climb. Recently, several companies have compressed the entire protein-coding portion of the human genome onto a single array—that is, some 30,000 gene sequences are represented on one slide. The result is a dramatic increase in information gathered from each profiling experiment affording the possibility of greater insight into complexities of cellular biology.

Measurements made using DNA microarrays are difficult to optimize to a tightly specified standard because of the high density of information and its parallel nature. It is equally difficult to validate individual probes globally in microarray hybridization assays at every data point, since it is impractical to check every point by a reference assay method. As a result, doubt has persisted about the value of the massive amount of data that microarrays produce. Recently, however, a trio of studies represents a systematic attempt to assess the reliability and reproducibility of microarray data across platforms and between laboratories.[146–148] In each case, by using standard protocols the picture presented is shown to be better than previously thought. They found, first, that both commercial and homemade arrays could deliver good results in experienced hands. They also found that standardized protocols largely solved the problem of poor reproducibility, and finally they found that the majority of microarray data reflects the underlying biology, even when different platforms are used to assess gene expression. On the other hand, the picture was not perfect and these studies called attention to some problem areas or issues. For one, they note that if the investigator is inexperienced, or does not have access to a core facility, use of a commercial chip should be considered. Second, if collaboration with another investigator is possible, the investigator should ensure wherever possible that the same platform and a common set of procedures are used. And third, if comparisons across platforms, say for gene expression, are necessary, a more biologically meaningful and statistically robust approach is to make *relative* rather than *absolute* comparisons.

The first use of microarrays was in immunological assays for diagnostic purposes,[149] but the growth of genome sequencing created a demand for high-throughput, parallel multigene analysis. The uses of DNA microarrays for nucleic acid analysis have come to occupy niches in nearly every area of basic biological research and medical science. Direct sequence analysis of SNPs and entire genomes were made that incorporated both comparative and quantitative measurements. The design and fabrication of microarrays for applications as diverse as genome mapping,[150] genotyping and reference-based sequence checking (resequencing),[77,78] and gene expression profiling[151] were also among some earlier applications. The technology continues to develop and is being transferred into other areas as in the development of proteomic, glycomic, and tissue arrays[152] and G-protein-coupled microarrays,[153] all of which carry the potential as aids for drug discovery. In the biomedical field, potential applications of this technology include the assessment of RNA and protein alterations as diagnostic markers in the clinical arena, particularly in oncology.[154]

In 1999, an appreciation of the different types of microarrays was chronicled in the first of the special series entitled The Chipping Forecast.[74] In 2002, the second in this series focused on new applications of microarrays.[75] A third part in this series published in 2005 dealt with perspectives on the application of microarrays to the assessment of SNP variation, large-scale structural variation, identification of epigenetic markers, bioinformatics of microarray data, and RNA interference.[155] A few current examples of applications of DNA microarrays of particular interest to pharmacogenomics are considered below (pp. 214 and 215).

Mass Spectrometry

The first mass spectrometers were of interest mainly to chemists and physicists, and the design of these instruments was dictated by their use as tools for the structural analysis of hydrocarbons in petroleum chemistry, and for use in specialized tasks of interest to physicists and physical chemists. Structural analysis by MS was accomplished by ionizing a compound of interest with a short burst of energy from an ion beam that caused its fragmentation with the formation of positively charged ions of the compound. The ions so formed were accelerated into a magnetic or an electric field that dispersed them and permitted the measurement of the relative abundance of ions of a given mass-to-charge ratio. But the situation changed in the 1960s when Ryhage invented the "molecular separator" and a combined gas chromatography-mass spectrometry (LKB-9000) was designed for use in biomedical research.[156] Intensive study of fragmentation processes showed that ionization by electron impact or chemical impact was suitable for the analysis of many small molecules of pharmacological and toxicological interest, but these methods or newer means such as fast atom bombardment (FAB) and liquid secondary ion mass spectrometry (SIMS) showed weak signal intensities or poor signal-to-noise ratios and hence were not suitable for the structural analysis of bioorganic compounds in the mass range of 10,000 daltons or larger. These traditional mass spectrometric methods, which were so useful for measuring masses of low-molecular-weight organic molecules, were thus of little use for measuring biopolymers of high molecular masses.

During the 1970s investigators learned that bombardment with short, intense pulses of laser light held the greatest promise for mass spectrometric analysis of large biopolymers within the mass range of a few thousand to a few hundred thousand daltons. After almost two decades of systematic attempts to generate ions of large polymeric molecules, two general principles emerged. First, that lasers emitted at wavelengths at or near the resonant absorption wavelengths were most efficient and controllable for transferring energy to such large molecules, and second, that the energy transfer should be of very short duration to avoid decomposition of the thermally labile biopolymer molecules. The main break-through toward higher masses came when Franz Hillenkamp and Michael Karas realized that embedding a low concentration of the biopolymer in a liquid or solid matrix consisting of small, highly absorbing molecules provided a means of en-ergy transfer that ionized the biopolymer and spared it from decomposition.

In 1988, Hillenkamp and colleagues extended these observations to measure the molecular mass of large peptides (20 kDa) while Tanaka and associates si-multaneously successfully applied them to large proteins (100 kDa).[14] During the same year, Hillenkamp's laboratory introduced MALDI-TOF MS as a rev-olutionary method for the analysis of the mass and composition of large bio-molecules.[157,158] They found that crystals irradiated by a matrix of a protein cocrystallized with a large excess of small aromatic organic molecules, most often organic acids, with a nanosecond laser pulse at a wavelength close to the resonant absorption band of the matrix molecules released ("desorbed") to produce gas-phase matrix ions. When molecules of protein were added to the matrix in solution and dried in the solid matrix crystal, these large molecules were ejected into the gas phase and ionized upon irradiation with the laser, to facilitate mass analysis. The ions are separated by their mass/charge ratio ac-cording to the length of time they require to travel a specific distance in the analyzer of the mass spectrometer. With recent improvements, MALDI-TOF MS is widely recognized to confer speed (the ionization and detection are complete in milliseconds), specificity [the measurement of the mass-to-charge ratio (m/z) was not affected by secondary structure], and high throughput by automation of all steps from sample preparation to acquisition and processing of data. Using MALDI, proteins of up to several hundred thousand daltons were amenable to mass analysis.

In contrast to proteins, DNA molecules were much more difficult to ana-lyze because of their fragile structure, and because of their much lower effi-ciency of detection at high masses. In 1993, Becker and his associates found that modification of the matrix to one composed of 3-hydroxypicolinic acid (3-hydroxypyridine-2-carboxylic acid, 3HPA) reduced some of the deleterious effects and significantly improved the mass range available from 10 to 67 nu-cleotides and the ability to analyze mixed-base oligomers.[159] Still further, by using a mixture of 3HPA and picolinic acid, oligonucleotides that were greater than 500 bases (up to ~200 daltons) in length could be detected. However, the resolution diminished significantly above about 100 bases so that oligomers differing by only one base were poorly separated.

In 1986, Lloyd Smith and colleagues initially proposed MALDI-TOF MS for DNA sequencing as an alternative to the conventional method of detecting fluorescently labeled DNA by gel electrophoresis.[11] Since then, the technology has undergone several key modifications including the matrix used, less expensive, more efficient lasers, and "delayed ion extraction,"[158] and as expected, relying on absolute molecular mass information rather than relative gel electrophoretic mobility has significantly increased sequencing fidelity. Consequently, the range of applications for this platform in basic research, pharmaceutical development, and clinical diagnostics has expanded significantly[33] to include the discovery and identification of SNPs,[29,44,157] the sizing of nucleotide repeats,[160] the estimation of allele frequencies,[28] quantitative analysis of gene expression,[161] and analysis of methylation patterns as a cause of allele-specific expression.[33] The simplicity of the MALDI-TOF MS has increased its popularity among nonexperts in analytical techniques and enhanced its accessibility for rapid detection of bacterial and viral pathogens,[27,29] and for studying the spatial distributions of biomolecules.[162] The latter application has a role in drug discovery to screen for potential drug targets, and for assessing drug distribution in cells, tissues, and organs.[162]

The Yeast Two-Hybrid (Y2H) System

Completion of the yeast genome sequence made possible the systematic analysis of protein–protein interactions for all 6000 yeast proteins by this technique.[163] It was, at the time, the largest genome to be sequenced and was the first genome sequence of a eukaryote to be completed. As a lead organism in the next phase of the campaign to understand how a simple eukaryotic cell works, *S. cervesiae* has several advantageous features: it has a small genome ($\sim$13 Mb) and a small number, 16, of chromosomes, little repetitive DNA, and only a few introns. Additionally, it is unicellular, can grow on chemically defined media permitting complete control of its physiology, and it can grow in either the haploid or diploid state enabling the effect of ploidy on gene action to be determined. And finally, excellent tools exist for its genetic manipulation, permitting the precise deletion of genes under investigation.

As a first step toward understanding how proteins work inside a cell, the yeast two-hybrid system initially described by Stanley Fields and Ok-kyu Song in 1989[18] provides a means of identifying the interactions between pairs of proteins without their prior purification. The basic strategy in a typical two-hybrid assay to determine whether two supposed proteins, say X and Y, interact begins with the creation of two sets of haploid yeast strains. One set contains protein X fused to the DNA-binding region of a transcription factor, while the other set contains protein Y fused to the activator region of the transcription factor (Figure 7.1). The first fusion protein is often referred to as the "bait" while the latter is the "prey." The two strains are then mated to produce diploid cells. If proteins X and Y bind two each other, they will reconstitute the transcription factor and turn on a reporter gene. Under the selective growth conditions of the assay, the product of the reporter permits the yeast to survive. If, on the other hand, the "bait" and "prey" proteins do not interact, the yeast dies.

Several investigators have used the two-hybrid assay to identify interactions between pairs of putative "bait" and "prey" yeast proteins in an effort to produce a comprehensive protein–protein interaction map in yeast. To increase throughput,

Yeast haploid cells

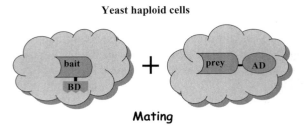

Mating

A diploid cell containing an interacting bait and prey

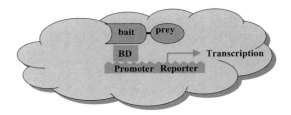

Figure 7.1 A typical yeast two-hybrid assay system.

Ito and colleagues performed a pilot study to examine interaction mating in an array format[164] and subsequently completed this analysis.[165]

These analyses[164,165] and those of others[123] have not only demonstrated the power of the Y2H approach but have also significantly improved the protein interaction map for exploration of genome functions. Recently, applications of this technique have been applied to other more complex, eukaryotic systems. For example, Giot and colleagues present a protein interaction map for the fruit fly based on the Y2H approach.[166] The increased complexity of the fruit fly is shown by the fact that yeast has about 6000 genes and 12 million bases pairs while the fruit fly has approximately 14,000 genes in 165 million bases. Technically, the greatest challenge was moving from cloning from yeast genomic DNA to cloning from *Drosophila* cDNA. A total of 10,623 predicted transcripts were isolated and screened against standard and normalized cDNA libraries to produce a draft of 7048 proteins and 20,405 interactions. This draft was refined to a higher confidence map of 4679 proteins and 4780 interactions with the aid of a computational method to rate the confidence of two-hybrid interactions. The results revealed known pathways, extended pathways, and uncovered previously unknown pathway components.

To better understand protein function in the context of complex molecular networks, Vidal and associates initiated the mapping of protein interactions (or the "interactome") of a large fraction of the genome of the worm metazoan, *Caenorhabditis elegans*.[167] A total of 3024 selected worm proteins were culled to 1873 "baits" that were screened against two different "prey" libraries each with distinct, complementary advantages. They reasoned that interactions detected in two different binding assays were unlikely to be experimental false positives.

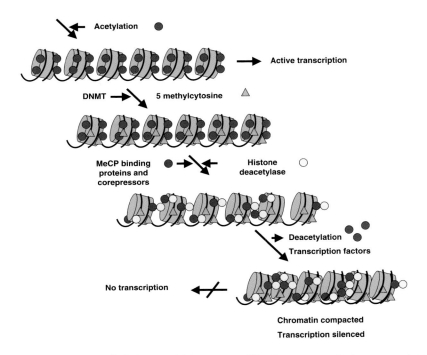

Figure 6.6 DNA methylation and histone modification cooperate to repress transcription. With permission from Elsevier Limited.

B

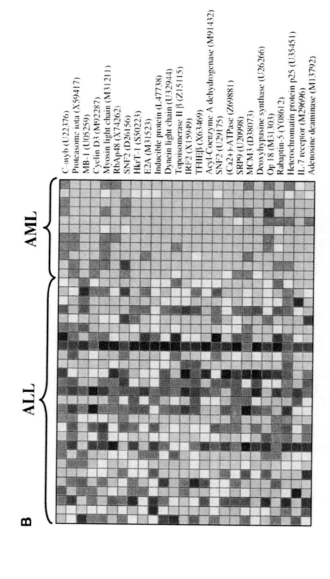

ALL   AML

C-myb (U22376)
Proteasome iota (X59417)
MB-1 (U05259)
Cyclin D3 (M92287)
Myosin light chain (M31211)
RbAp48 (X74262)
SNF2 (D26156)
HkrT-1 (S50223)
E2A (M31523)
Inducible protein (L47738)
Dynein light chain (U32944)
Topoisomerase II β (Z15115)
IRF2 (X15949)
TFIIEβ (X63469)
Acyl-Coenzyme A dehydrogenase (M91432)
SNF2 (U29175)
(Ca2+)-ATPase (Z69881)
SRP9 (U20998)
MCM3 (D38073)
Deoxyhypusine synthase (U26266)
Op 18 (M31303)
Rabaptin-5 (Y08612)
Heterochromatin protein p25 (U35451)
IL-7 receptor (M29696)
Adenosine deaminase (M13792)

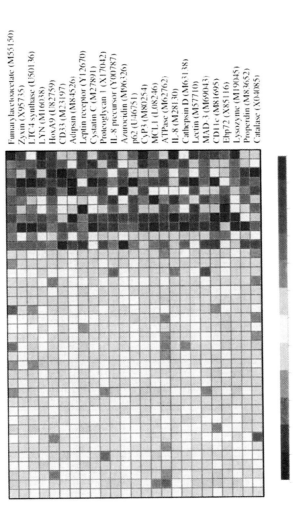

Figure 11.1 Gene expression patterns for acute lymphoblastic leukemia (ALL) and acute myelogenous leukemia (AML). With permission from the *New England Journal of Medicine*.

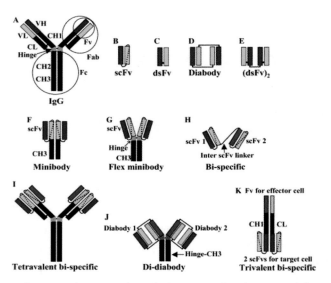

Figure 10.4 Schematic diagram of a whole IgG molecule (*A*) and fragments that have been engineered (*B–K*). With permission from Elsevier Limited.

Additionally, the *C. elegans* interactome network was examined for the presence of highly connected neighborhoods by determining the mutual clustering coefficient between proteins in the network. A total of 4000 interactions were identified by high-throughput Y2H screens. Combining these data with previously described interactions in the literature and of "interologs" (i.e., interactions that are conserved across species) predicted *in silico,* a map containing 5534 interactions was produced. Further analysis of interactions between evolutionarily ancient and new proteins suggested that new cellular functions made use of a combination of ancient and new elements, in line with the idea that evolution modifies and adds to preexisting structures to create new ones.

The *C. elegans* study is an instructive step toward the ultimate goal of determining an interactome map for the human genome.[167] In an attempt to apply similar functional proteomic approaches to large human protein–protein interaction networks, Colland used the two-hybrid system to screen for Smad signaling protein–protein interactions between 11 Smad and related proteins.[168] Smad signaling proteins include members of the tumor growth factor (TGF)-β superfamily, which are involved in many biological processes such as cell growth, differentiation, and morphogenesis, and are associated with several human pathologies including fibrosis, inflammatory disorders, and cancer. Colland's study established a network of 755 interactions, involving 591 proteins, of which 179 were poorly or not annotated. To validate the significance of their findings, the investigators integrated their protein interaction map with various functional assays based on transcriptional responses in mammalian cells. For example, in a set of 14 proteins selected on the basis of favorable interaction scores and attractive functional domain annotations, functional proteomic mapping of the Smad pathway resulted in validation of eight proteins connected to this pathway. In another approach, the involvement of this set of proteins in Smad signaling was further explored by testing the effect of siRNA duplexes targeting each protein, and these studies showed that knockdown of 7 of the 14 proteins also had a significant effect on the Smad pathway. While their precise role and mechanism of action remain to be determined, this study provides physical and functional evidence for the participation of several proteins in the Smad pathway.

These studies demonstrate the unique facility of the two-hybrid system to target protein–protein interactions in model organisms and in humans as well as the promise this system brings to a more comprehensive understanding of the cell as a molecular system.

EMERGING TECHNOLOGIES

Many of the more recent reports on molecular technology discuss new ways to increase the capacity, simplify the performance, and decrease the cost and time of genetic analysis without sacrificing sensitivity and reliability. A movement toward microfabricated devices capable of analyzing a large number of biologically important molecules has become a dominant theme in the recent literature. The topics in this section represent innovations that are expected to shed light on individual variations in human drug response and provide insights on new diagnostic and therapeutic opportunities of pharmacogenomic importance.

Microfluidics

Interest in the development of microfabricated devices for medical molecular diagnostics has increased notably over the past decade.[135,169–173] Miniaturization of PCR testing has led to the concept of lab-on-a-chip (LOC) or micrototal analysis technologies. Pursuit of this concept has followed two main lines. One concerns development of microarrays[174] (see p. 205) and the other concerns development of microfluidic devices. Microfluidics refers to the flow of fluids in microchannel devices and includes the components (micropumps, valves, microcircuitry, etc.) that are necessary to control the flow. The microfluidic device is based on chips designed to perform all of the analytical steps (separation, amplification, detection) of genotyping analysis. Microfabricated devices offer a number of advantages over macro devices. As currently conceived, integration of all analytical steps within a single device reduces labor and the chance of contamination. Use of very small (nanoliter) quantities reduces the amount of DNA (or RNA) sample, reagents, and costs. Reduction in sample volumes and transport distances also leads to increased efficiency of the biochemical reactions involved. The automation of all steps into a seamless process affords the possibility of portability and will significantly reduce the time to complete analyses and obtain results.

In the main, early work in microfluidics was performed with silicon and glass devices, but polymer-based microchips have emerged recently as inexpensive and disposable alternatives to these materials. These changes in microfabrication methods are adaptable to both prototyping and high-throughput production and they have enhanced the speed and versatility of fabrication. The ease of fabrication with polymer-based materials will also result in the design and creation of integrated systems that will perform with greater efficiency and economy.[175]

To date, microfluidics has been successfully implemented in a variety of biological applications of genomics interest including DNA sequencing, PCR amplification, amino acid, peptide, and protein analysis, immunoassays, cell sorting, and *in vitro* fertilization. In medical diagnostics, microfluidic devices are expected to enhance the prospects of human genotyping in personalized medicine, the efficiency of clinical drug trials, as well as the identification of foodborne pathogens and pathogenic bacteria and viruses. Currently, many companies are exploring the commercial prospects of fully integrated LOC devices that accept a sample, perform a multistep process, and analyze the result.[57,175]

Serial Analysis of Gene Expression on Single Cells

Substantial heterogeneity exists in the drug responsiveness of individual cells, even in the case of a seemingly homogeneous cell population.[176] To understand more fully the manner in which individuals respond to exogenous substances, investigators have sought to develop techniques that can measure specific patterns of gene expression in single cells.

Several methodologies, such as subtractive hybridization, comparative analysis of expressed sequence tags, and differential display, have been used to identify patterns of gene expression. Most of these approaches can be used to assess gene expression in bulk tissue or millions of cells; they cannot analyze expression among transcript populations completely, and they also might not detect transcripts expressed at low levels. Microarrays have also been used to analyze gene expression, but their main strength lies in analyzing transcripts that have been previously identified. On the other hand, the serial analysis of gene expression (SAGE) method[177–179] does provide rapid, comprehensive, and quantitative analysis of gene expression patterns, and modifications of SAGE permit analysis of gene expression on as few as 500–5000 cells.[180] The modifications affect the first few steps of the SAGE procedure, from RNA isolation to PCR, but do not alter the basic principle. Additional modifications of SAGE have now led to techniques capable of exploring gene expression patterns in single cells.[181,182]

Single-Molecule Assays

Most conventional tools for genomics rely on biological propagation to generate large numbers of DNA molecules for analysis. Biological steps such as bacterial cloning that are commonly used to prepare DNA for analysis may introduce errors and distortions. On the other hand, the analysis of single molecules would avoid the need to duplicate and purify selected pieces of DNA, and would also offer the advantages of speed and predictable behavior.[183] Recently, a variety of innovative approaches have been designed to exploit the features of single DNA fragments for genotyping and DNA sequencing.[57]

One group of related methods, collectively referred to as scanning probe microscopy, has been used to image DNA molecules on a subnanometric scale. Specific sequence features can be identified if they are first tagged with a bulky marker. The method uses atomic force microscopy with high-resolution, single-walled carbon nanotube probes to read directly multiple polymorphic sites in DNA fragments containing 100 to 10,000 bases. In an approach developed by Adam Woolley and colleagues, sequence-specific oligonucleotides, tagged with bulky molecules, were allowed to anneal to complementary sequences in denatured DNA.[184] They used this approach to image polymorphic DNA sites and determine haplotypes in DNA fragments by direct visualization. This technique was applied to determine haplotypes on the glucuronosyltransferase-1 locus (*UDP-1A7*) as a risk factor for cancer.[185] This study demonstrated that a considerable portion of the population at risk (15.3%) was homozygous for the low activity allele containing three missense mutations, *UGT1A7*3.*

Rolling circle amplification provides another promising technique sensitive enough to detect a single molecule of DNA.[186–188] This technique uses allele-specific probes (wild-type and mutant) fixed to a solid surface. The 5′- and 3′-end regions of these probes are designed to base pair next to each other on a target strand, and if properly hybridized can be joined by enzymatic ligation. Ligation converts the linear probes to circularly closed molecules that are concatenated to the target DNA sequences. A complex pattern of DNA strand displacement ensues that generates a huge number ($>10^9$) of copies of each circle in 90 minutes. This technique can be coupled to multicolor fluorescent imaging to detect short DNA sequences, point mutations, and haplotypes derived from SNPs.

Other researchers have explored the prospects for ultrarapid sequencing of nucleic acids by nanopore technology. The basic idea is that the sequence of single-stranded DNA or RNA molecules can be determined by fluctuations in current as they are driven very rapidly though a nanopore by a voltage applied to an otherwise insulating membrane.[189] Each base will transiently restrict the flow of current as it passes through the pore, and the sequence can be read off as a series of current fluctuations of different magnitudes. Working with α-hemolysin, a protein that self-assembles in lipid bilayers to form a membrane channel with a relatively large pore (approximately 2 nm in diameter), investigators demonstrated that the duration and extent of current reduction are measurably different for homopolymers of different bases and different lengths.[190] They have also shown that purines and pyrimidines in a synthetic construct could be distinguished as they passed through the pore.[191] If single nucleotide base pair resolution can be achieved, the base sequence in the nucleic acid molecule can be determined at rates between 1000 and 10,000 per second, which would exceed by far the most efficient current sequencing methods ($\sim$30,000 bases per day per instrument).

SNP and Gene Expression Profiling

As knowledge of pharmacogenetic variations accumulates, we see that few if any phenotypic outcomes can be predicted from genetic analysis at a single locus. Recent studies have shown that SNP (DNA) profiling and gene expression (RNA) profiling with microarrays are powerful additions to the tools for analyzing polygenic responses. A novel application of this concept has combined single base primer extension assays (see p. 197) with microarray technology to screen a panel of 74 SNPs of 25 genes encoding proteins involved in blood pressure regulation for their effect on antihypertensive drug treatment.[192] Using this system, combinations of a few SNPs predicted approximately 50% of the variation in individual responsiveness to treatment. As this was a pilot study, it was relatively small and needs to be confirmed in a larger, prospective study. Nevertheless, the results highlight the potential of microarray-based technology for SNP profiling of predictive pharmacogenetic markers.

With advances in microarray technology, an abundance of new and challenging applications has arisen on several other biomedical fronts. For example, in cancer biology, cancer classification has been based historically on morphological appearance. But tumors that are similar in appearance histopathologically can follow significantly different clinical courses and show different responses to therapy. In 1996, Trent's laboratory drew attention to the use of DNA microarrays as a tool to pinpoint gene variants in melanoma cancer cell lines by monitoring gene expression patterns.[23] The potential importance of this technique was brought into sharper focus by Golub and colleagues who used microarrays to classify acute leukemias into distinct subcategories.[154] In a study of a panel of 50 genes most closely correlated with AML–ALL distinction, gene expression patterns in 38 bone marrow samples clearly distinguished acute myelogenous leukemia (AML) from acute lymphoblastic leukemia (ALL). This finding had immediate therapeutic implications because treatment of ALL generally relies on corticosteroids, vincristine, methotrexate, and L-asparaginase, while most AML regimens rely on daunorubicin and cytarabine. Additionally, the distinction between B cell and T cell ALL was discovered.

In a later study of 20 ALL and 17 mixed lineage leukemia (MLL) patients, these investigators demonstrated that acute lymphoblastic leukemias with MLL translocations on chromosome 11 (11q23) specified a distinct gene expression profile that separated them from conventional ALL and AML.[193] Leukemias with a mixed leukemia gene (*MLL, HRX, ALL1*) translocation had a decidedly unfavorable prognosis that did not respond well to standard ALL therapies suggesting that new therapeutic approaches were needed for MLL. This study also noted that *FLT3,* the gene for a tyrosine kinase receptor, was the most differentially expressed gene that distinguished MLL from ALL and AML, and that the FLT3 receptor protein represents an attractive therapeutic target for rational drug development.

As a general approach to a better understanding of the pathogenesis of cancer based on genetically defined molecular markers, gene expression profiling with microarrays has been fruitful for the identification of new classes of cancer (class discovery) and for assigning tumors to known classes (class prediction). Still further, expression profiling has been extended to identify variants that underlie melanoma,[194] lymphoma,[195] and breast cancer.[196–198]

Epigenomic Methodologies

Epigenomic research has demonstrated that stable, reversible alteration of gene expression is mediated by patterns of methylation of cytosines of DNA and of chromatin remodeling resulting from histone modification, the binding of nuclear proteins to chromatin, and interactions between these networks. Many of the basic principles and complexities that underlie epigenetic phenomena have been identified, but the molecular mechanisms by which the DNA methylation patterns and histone modifications are established and maintained are not entirely clear. Nevertheless, rapid progress has been made in the mapping and characterization of DNA methylation patterns and histone modifications, and some of the methodologies that have been used for these purposes are described below.[199,200] Emphasis is placed on newer, automatable techniques that can measure the expression of thousands of genes simultaneously as is needed to establish the diagnostic, prognostic, and therapeutic importance of DNA methylation and histone modifications of emergent candidate genes for cancer and other human disorders.

Older, established methods for measuring the methylation state of DNA include routine chromatographic methods, electromigration methods, and immunoassays.[201] Some of the newer methods reported include semiautomatic detection of methylation at CpG islands,[202] oligonucleotide-based microassays, and tissue microassays.[203–205] Among electromigration methods, multichannel capillary electrophoresis combined with mass spectrometric detection of 5-methylcytosine would appear to provide the potential for a screening method.[61] Pfarr and colleagues describe a method of immunodetection that makes it possible to obtain spatially resolved information on the distribution of 5-methylcytosine on metaphase human chromosomes.[206]

Recently, several microarray methods have been developed to map methyl-cytosine patterns in genomes of interest.[199,200] In one set of methods that uses methylation-sensitive restriction enzymes, Shi and colleagues have measured hypermethylation from various tumor types in defined regions of the genome.[203] DNA samples were first treated with bisulfite and specific genomic regions are then PCR amplified converting the modified UG to TG and conserving the originally methylated dinucleotide as CG. Primers were designed that contained no CpG dinucleotides and were complementary to the flanking sequences of a 200- to 300-bp DNA target. This permitted unbiased amplification of both methylated and unmethylated alleles by PCR. PCR-amplified target DNAs were subsequently purified and labeled with fluorescent dyes (Cy5 or Cy3) for hybridization to the microarray. The fluorescently labeled PCR products were hybridized to arrayed oligonucleotides (affixed to solid supports, e.g., microscope slides) that could discriminate between methylated and unmethylated alleles in regions of interest. Based on the differential methylation profiles of several gene promoters, Shi et al. distinguished two clinical subtypes of non-Hodgkin's lymphomas, mantle cell lymphoma, and grades I/II follicular lymphoma.

Shi's technique can be employed for profiling methylation patterns on DNA microarrays[203] as an approach to discover new classes of cancer in a manner similar to that pioneered by Golub[154,207] and other investigators.[195,197,198,208] This technology can also be used to monitor the effects of new pharmacological agents in patients under treatment and provide valuable information regarding the outcome of epigenetic therapies.

A somewhat different microarray technique for the analysis of hypermethy-lation[204] has been developed by Chen and associates. This approach, which they called methylation target array (MTA), is modeled after the technique that Ko-nonen et al. developed for tissue microarrays.[205] Chen affixed methylation targets to a solid support and hybridized different CpG island probes to the array one at a time. The technique can analyze hypermethylation of CpG islands in hundreds of clinical samples simultaneously. Its applicability to cancer-related problems was demonstrated by determining the hypermethylation profiles of 10 promoter CpG islands in 93 breast tumors, 4 breast cancer cell lines, and 20 normal breast tissues. A panel of 468 MTA amplicons, which represented the whole repertoire of methylated CpG islands in these tissues and cell lines, was arrayed on nylon membrane for probe hybridization. Positive hybridization signals, indicative of DNA methylation, were detected in tumor amplicons, but not in normal ampli-cons, indicating aberrant hypermethylation in tumor samples. The frequencies of hypermethylation were found to correlate significantly with the patient's hormone receptor status, clinical stage, and age at diagnosis. The fact that a single nylon membrane can be used repeatedly for probing with many CpG island loci may be advantageous clinically for the rapid assessment of potential methylation markers that may be useful in predicting treatment outcome.

Recently, two microarray methodologies have been developed for genome-wide mapping of the binding sites of regulatory proteins and the distributions of histone modifications and protein–DNA interactions.[199,200] In one of these, chromatin immunoprecipitation (ChIP) is combined with microarray detection (ChIP-on-chip). Cells are treated with a cross-linking reagent such as formaldehyde, the chromatin is isolated and fragmented, and immunoprecipitation is used to identify the protein of interest along with the attached DNA fragments. To identify the DNA fragments, the cross-links are reversed and the DNA fragments are labeled with a fluorescent dye and hybridized to microarrays with probes corresponding to regions of interest. The second method, called the DamID, utilizes a different principle. In this case, a transcription factor or chromatin-binding protein of interest is fused to DNA adenine methyltransferase (Dam). When this fusion protein is expressed, Dam will be targeted to binding sites of its fusion partner resulting in methylation of adenines in DNA near the binding sites. To identify these sites, the methylated regions are purified or selectively amplified from genomic DNA, fluorescently labeled, and hybridized to a microarray. Because adenine methylation does not occur endogenously in mammals, the binding sites of targeted methylation can be derived from the microarray signals. So far only limited comparisons are available, but studies of one regulatory protein, the GAGA factor, indicate the two methods can yield similar results. However, ChIP-chip requires a highly specific antibody against the protein of interest, while DamID does not. On the other hand, DamID is suited for the detection of histone or other posttranslational modifications. Additional merits and drawbacks of the two methods are noted elsewhere.[199,200]

Knowledge of the binding sites for the transcription factors that regulate genes would appear to be a direct route to understanding regulatory mechanisms. These sites can be determined by ChIP-on-chip and DamID.

High-Throughput Detection of Copy Number Variation

Initial analysis of the human genome suggested that SNPs, estimated to occur on average in 1 of 300 nucleotides within the human genome, were the main source of genetic and phenotypic individual variation. However, with the completion of the primary sequence of the human genome, creation of new strategies and tools for assessing genomic composition such as genome scanning technologies and comparative DNA sequence analyses revealed the large extent of DNA variation involving DNA segments smaller than those recognizable microscopically, but larger that those detected by conventional sequence analysis. These submicroscopic variants ranged from ~1 kilobase to 3 megabases, and comprised deletions, duplications, and large-scale copy number variants. These variants are now collectively referred to as copy number variants (CNVs) or copy number polymorphisms (CNPs). Such variants in some genomic regions have no apparent phenotypic consequences, whereas others influence gene dosage, which might cause disease either alone or in combination with other genetic or environmental factors.

In 2004, two reports using genome-scanning DNA microarray technologies highlighted the widespread nature of normal CNV.[209,210] Other studies have amply confirmed and extended these observations.[211–213] In the initial studies, the key to the identification of the extent of variation was the use of array-based comparative genomic hybridization (array CGH). The microarray that Iafrate et al. used was a commercial BAC array with one clone about every 1 megabase across the genome, while Sebat et al. used long nucleotide arrays with an effective resolution of >90 kb. Both were of limited resolution. While advances in array technology continued to improve resolution, the use of array-CGH was found to be noisy and necessitated averaging of multiple probes to call CNVs.

Recently, Redon, Fieger, and colleagues have described a new tool for high-throughput detection of CNVs in the human genome. These investigators constructed a large-insert clone tiling path resolution DNA array covering the entire human genome,[213] and used it to identify CNVs in human populations.[214] The array consisted of 26,574 clones selected primarily from the "Golden Path" used to generate the reference human sequence[215] covering 93.7% of euchromatic regions. They also developed an algorithm, "CVNfinder," for calling copy number changes. On using CNVfinder to detect CNVs in human populations using DNAs from the 270 cell lines extensively genotyped in the HapMap project, they found that this tool provides accurate, reliable estimates of CNV in the human genome.

SUMMARY

The entire spectrum of modern genetics is closely tied to the analytical and computational technologies that have been developed to understand the composition and function of genomic DNA. Widespread adoption of these technologies, further fueled by the completion of the human genome initiative, made it possible to scan or score the genome for structural and functional polymorphisms relevant to human disease and pharmacogenomic variation. As demands for sequencing, mapping, and identifying human genes have increased, so has the need for efficient means to store, access, and analyze genomic data. Aided by the expertise of scientists outside the immediate realm of biology, new revolutionary tools for the acquisition, analysis, and handling of genomic information were devised as part of a larger attempt to elucidate the relationships between structural and functional changes of the genome. The trend toward miniaturization of analytical technologies for medical diagnostics, led by the development of DNA microarrays and of microfluidic devices, now encompasses many other innovative technologies such as serial analysis of single cells, single-molecule assays, SNP and gene expression profiling, and epigenomic methodologies and is attracting an increasingly larger share of interest.

REFERENCES

1. Southern EM. Detection of specific sequences among DNA fragments separated by gel electrophoresis. J Mol Biol 1975; 98:503–517.
2. Southern E. Tools for genomics. Nat Med 2005; 11(10):1029–1034.
3. Sanger F, Nicklen S, Coulson AR. DNA sequencing with chain-terminating inhibitors. Proc Natl Acad Sci USA 1977; 74(12):5463–5467.
4. Alwine JC, Kemp DJ, Stark GR. Method for detection of specific RNAs in agarose gels by transfer to diazobenzyloxymethyl-paper and hybridization with DNA probes. Proc Natl Acad Sci USA 1977; 74(12):5350–5354.
5. Wyman AR, White R. A highly polymorphic locus in human DNA. Proc Natl Acad Sci USA 1980; 77:6754–6758.
6. Waterman MS. Genomic sequence databases. Genomics 1990; 6(4):700–701.
7. Smith TF. The history of the genetic sequence databases. Genomics 1990; 6(4):701–707.
8. Jeffreys AJ, Wilson V, Thein SL. Individual-specific fingerprints of human DNA. Nature 1985; 316:76–79.
9. Polsky-Cynkin R, Parsons GH, Allerdt L, Landes G, Davis G, Rashtchian A. Use of DNA immobilized on plastic and agarose supports to detect DNA by sandwich hybridization. Clin Chem 1985; 31(9):1438–1443.
10. Lipman DJ, Pearson WR. Rapid and sensitive protein similarity searches. Science 1985; 227(4693):1435–1441.
11. Smith LM, Sanders JZ, Kaiser RJ, Hughes P, Dodd C, Connell CR, et al. Fluorescence detection in automated DNA sequence analysis. Nature 1986; 321(6071):674–679.
12. Mullis KB, Faloona FA. Specific synthesis of DNA in vitro via a polymerase-catalyzed chain reaction. Methods Enzymol 1987; 155:335–350.
13. Rosenthal N. Tools of the trade—recombinant DNA. N Engl J Med 1994; 331(5):315–317.
14. Hillenkamp F, Karas M, Beavis RC, Chait BT. Matrix-assisted laser desorption/ionization mass spectrometry of biopolymers. Anal Chem 1991; 63(24):1193A-1203A.
15. Wheeler DL, Chappey C, Lash AE, Leipe DD, Madden TL, Schuler GD. Database resources of the National Center for Biotechnology Information. Nucleic Acids Res 2000; 28(1):10–14.
16. Ristaldi MS, Piratsu M, Rositelli C, Monni G, Erlich H, Saiki R, et al. Prenatal daignosis of beta-thalaessemia in Mediterranean populations by dot blot analysis with DNA amplification and allele specific oligonucleotide probes. Prenat Diagn 2003; 9:629–638.
17. Wu DY, Nozari G, Schold M, Cooner BJ, Wallace RB. Direct analysis of single nucleotide variation in human DNA and RNA using in situ dot blot hybridization. DNA 1989; 8:135–142.
18. Fields S, Song O. A novel genetic system to detect protein-protein interactions. Nature 1989; 340(6230):245–246.
19. Kawasaki E, Saiki R, Erlich H. Genetic analysis using polymerase chain reaction-amplified DNA and immobilized oligonucleotide probes: Reverse dot-blot typing. Methods Enzymol 1993; 218:369–381.
20. Southern EM, Maskos U. Parallel synthesis and analysis of large numbers of related chemical compounds: Applications to oligonucleotides. J Biotechnol 1994; 35(2–3):217–227.

21. Pease AC, Solas D, Sullivan EJ, Cronin MT, Holmes CP, Fodor SP. Light-generated oligonucleotide arrays for rapid DNA sequence analysis. Proc Natl Acad Sci USA 1994; 91(11):5022–5026.
22. Schena M, Shalon D, Davis RW, Brown PO. Quantitative monitoring of the gene expression patterns with a comprehensive DNA microarray. Science 1995; 270: 467–470.
23. DeRisi J, Penland L, Brown PO, Bittner ML, Melzer PS, Ray M, et al. Use of a cDNA microarray to analyse gene expression patterns in human cancer. Nat Genet 1996; 14:457–460.
24. Ewing B, Hillier L, Wendl MC, Green P. Base-calling of automated sequencer traces using phred. I. Accuracy assessment. Genome Res 1998; 8(3):175–185.
25. Ewing B, Green P. Base-calling of automated sequencer traces using phred. II. Error probabilities. Genome Res 1998; 8(3):186–194.
26. Kirpekar F, Nordhoff E, Larsen LK, Kristiansen K, Roepstorff P, Hillenkamp F. DNA sequence analysis by MALDI mass spectrometry. Nucleic Acids Res 1998; 26(11):2554–2559.
27. von Wintzingerode F, Bocker S, Schlotelburg C, Chiu NH, Storm N, Jurinke C, et al. Base-specific fragmentation of amplified 16S rRNA genes analyzed by mass spectrometry: A tool for rapid bacterial identification. Proc Natl Acad Sci USA 2002; 99(10):7039–7044.
28. Mohlke KL, Erdos MR, Scott LJ, Fingerlin TE, Jackson AU, Silander K, et al. High-throughput screening for evidence of association by using mass spectrometry genotyping on DNA pools. Proc Natl Acad Sci USA 2002; 99(26):16928–16933.
29. Hartmer R, Storm N, Boecker S, Rodi CP, Hillenkamp F, Jurinke C, et al. RNase T1 mediated base-specific cleavage and MALDI-TOF MS for high-throughput comparative sequence analysis. Nucleic Acids Res 2003; 31(9):e47.
30. Vidal M. A biological atlas of functional maps. Cell 2001; 104(3):333–339.
31. Stanssens P, Zabeau M, Meersseman G, Remes G, Gansemans Y, Storm N, et al. High-throughput MALDI-TOF discovery of genomic sequence polymorphisms. Genome Res 2004; 14(1):126–133.
32. Syvanen AC. Toward genome-wide SNP genotyping. Nat Genet 2005; 37 Suppl: S5–10.
33. Jurinke C, Denissenko MF, Oeth P, Ehrich M, van den BD, Cantor CR. A single nucleotide polymorphism based approach for the identification and characterization of gene expression modulation using MassARRAY. Mutat Res 2005; 573(1–2): 83–95.
34. Ehrich M, Nelson MR, Stanssens P, Zabeau M, Liloglou T, Xinarianos G, et al. Quantitative high-throughput analysis of DNA methylation patterns by base-specific cleavage and mass spectrometry. Proc Natl Acad Sci USA 2005; 102(44):15785–15790.
35. Jeffreys AJ. Genetic fingerprinting. Nat Med 2005; 11(10):1035–1039.
36. Sutcharichan P, Saiki R, Huisman TH, Kutlar A, McKie V, Erlich H, et al. Reverse dot blot detection of the African-American beta-thalessaemia mutations. Blood 1995; 86:1580–1585.
37. Erlich H, Bugawan T, Begovich AB, Scharf S, Griffith R, Saiki R, et al. HLA-DR, DQ and DP typing using PCR amplification and immobilized probes. Eur J Immunogenet 1991; 18(1–2):33–55.
38. Grant DM, Phillips MS. Technologies for the analysis of single-nucleotide polymorphisms. In: Kalow W, Meyer UA, Tyndale RF, editors. Pharmacogenomics. New York: Marcel Dekker, 2001: 183–189.

39. Mir KU, Southern EM. Sequence variation in genes and genomic DNA: Methods for large-scale analysis. Annu Rev Genomics Hum Genet 2000; 1(2000):329–360.

40. Stockley TL, Ray PN. Molecular diagnostics and development of biotechnology-based diagnostics. In: Kalow W, Meyer UA, Tyndale RF, editors. Pharmacogenomics. New York: Marcel Dekker, 2001: 169–181.

41. Dovichi NJ. DNA sequencing by capillary electrophoresis. Electrophoresis 1997; 18(12–13):2393–2399.

42. O'Donovan MC, Oefner PJ, Roberts SC, Austin J, Hoogendoorn B, Guy C, et al. Blind analysis of denaturing high-performance liquid chromatography as a tool for mutation detection. Genomics 1998; 52(1):44–49.

43. Cargill M, Altshuler D, Ireland J, Sklar P, Ardlie K, Patil N, et al. Characterization of single-nucleotide polymorphisms in coding regions of human genes. Nat Genet 1999; 22(3):231–238.

44. Bray MS, Boerwinkle E, Doris PA. High-throughput multiplex SNP genotyping with MALDI-TOF mass spectrophotometry: Practice, problems and promise. Human Mut 2001; 17:296–304.

45. Koster H, Tang K, Fu DJ, Braun A, van den BD, Smith CL, et al. A strategy for rapid and efficient DNA sequencing by mass spectrometry. Nat Biotechnol 1996; 14(9):1123–1128.

46. Little DP, Braun A, O'Donnell MJ, Koster H. Mass spectrometry from miniaturized arrays for full comparative DNA analysis. Nat Med 1997; 3(12):1413–1416.

47. Ross PL, Hall L, Haff L, Gravin A. Multiplex genotyping by specialized mass spectrometry. In: Kalow W, Meyer UA, Tyndale RF, editors. Pharmacogenomics. New York: Marcel Dekker, 2001: 201–221.

48. Lockhart DJ, Winzeler EA. Genomics, gene expression and DNA arrays. Nature 2000; 405(6788):827–836.

49. Chen J, Iannone MA, Li MS, Taylor JD, Rivers P, Nelsen AJ, et al. A microsphere-based assay for multiplexed single nucleotide polymorphism analysis using single base chain extension. Genome Res 2000; 10(4):549–557.

50. Stevens PW, Hall JG, Lyamichev V, Neri BP, Lu M, Wang L, et al. Analysis of single nucleotide polymorphisms with solid phase invasive cleavage reactions. Nucleic Acids Res 2001; 29(Online).

51. Grompe M. The rapid detection of unknown mutations in nucleic acids. Nature Genet 1993; 5:111–117.

52. Nollau P, Wagener C. Methods for detection of point mutations: Performance and quality assessment. IFCC Scientific Division, Committee on Molecular Biology Techniques. Clin Chem 1997; 43(7):1114–1128.

53. Schafer AJ, Hawkins JR. DNA variation and the future of human genetics. Nature Biotechnol 1998; 16(1):33–39.

54. Cotton RG. Mutation detection and mutation databases. Clin Chem Lab Med 1998; 36(8):519–522.

55. Sanger F. Sequences, sequences, and sequences. Annu Rev Biochem 1988; 57:1–28.

56. Sanger F, Nicklen S, Coulson AR. DNA sequencing with chain-terminating inhibitors. Proc Natl Acad Sci USA 1977; 74(12):5463–5467.

57. Meldrum D. Automation for genomics, Part One: Preparation for sequencing. Part two: Sequencers, microarrays, and future trends. Genome Res 2000; 10:1081, 1288–1092, 1303.

58. Orita M, Suzuki Y, Sekiya T, Hatashi K. Rapid and sensitive detection of point mutations and DNA polymorphisms using the polymerase chain reaction. Genomics 1989; 5:874–879.

59. Sheffield VC, Beckm JS, Kwitek AE, Sandstrom DW, Stone EM. The sensitivity of single-strand conformation polymorphism analysis for the detection of single base substitutions. Genomics 1993; 16:325–332.

60. Larsen LA, Christiansen M, Vuust J, Andersen PS. High-throughput single-strand conformation polymorphism analysis by automated capillary electrophoresis: Robust multiplex analysis and pattern-based identification of allelic variants. Hum Mut 1999; 13(4):318–327.

61. Larsen LA, Christiansen M, Vuust J, Andersen PS. High throughput mutation screening by automated capillary electrophoresis. Comb Chem High Throughput Screen 2000; 3(5):393–409.

62. Fischer SG, Lerman LS. DNA fragments differing by single base pair substitutions are separated in denaturing gradient gels: Correspondence with melting theory. Proc Natl Acad Sci USA 1983; 80:1579–1583.

63. Myers RM, Maniatis T, Lerman LS. Detection and localization of single base changes by denaturing gradient gel electrophoresis. Methods Enzymol 1987; 155:501–527.

64. Riesner D, Steger G, Zimmat R, Owens RA, Wagenhofer M, Hillen W, et al. Temperature-gradient gel electrophoresis of nucleic acids: Analysis of conformational transtions, sequence variations, and protein-nucleic acid interactions. Electrophoresis 2002; 10(5):377–389.

65. White MB, Carvalho M, Derse D, O'Brien SJ, Dean M. Detecting single base substitutions as heteroduplex polymorphisms. Genomics 1992; 12(2):301–306.

66. Rozycka M, Collins N, Stratton MR, Wooster R. Rapid detection of DNA sequence variants by conformation-sensitive capillary electrophoresis. Genomics 2000; 70(1):34–40.

67. Bolla MK, Wood N, Humphries SE. Rapid determination of apolipoprotein E genotype using a heteroduplex generator. J Lipid Res 1999; 40:2340–2345.

68. Myers RM, Larin Z, Maniatis T. Detection of single base substitutions by ribonuclease cleavage at mismatches in RNA:DNA duplexes. Science 1985; 230:1242–1246.

69. Myers RM, Sheffield SG, Cox DR. Detection of single base changes in DNA: Ribonuclease cleavage and denaturing gradient gel electrophoresis In: Davies KE, editor. Genome Analysis. A Practical Approach. New York: Oxford University Press, 1988: 95–139.

70. Zheng H, Hasty P, Brennaman MA, Grompe M, Gibbs RA, Wilson JH, et al. Fidelity of targeted recombination in human fibroblasts and murine embryonic stem cells. Proc Natl Acad Sci USA 1991; 88(Sep):8067–8071.

71. Mashal RD, Koontz J, Sklar J. Detection of mutations by cleavage of DNA heteroduplexes with bacteriophage resolvases. Nat Genet 1995; 9(Feb):177–183.

72. Youil R, Kemper BW, Cotton RGH. Screening for mutations by enzyme mismatch cleavage with T4 endonuclease VII. Proc Natl Acad Sci USA 1995; 92(Jan):87–91.

73. Del TB Jr, Poff HE III, Novotny MA, Cartledge DM, Walker RI, Earl CD, et al. Automated fluorescent analysis procedure for enzymatic mutation detection. Clin Chem 1998; 44(4):731–739.

74. Multiauthored. The chipping forecast I (1999) and II (2002). Nat Genet 1999; 21 Suppl(1):1–60.

75. Multiauthored. The chipping forecast II. Nature 2002; 32 Suppl(Dec):461–552.

76. Multiauthored. Functional genomics. Nature 2000; 405(15 June):819–865.

77. Hacia JG. Resequencing and mutational analysis using oligonucleotide microarrays. Nat Genet 1999; 21(1 Suppl):42–47.

78. Hacia JG, Brody LC, Chee MS, Fodor SP, Collins FS. Detection of heterozygous mutations in BRCA1 using high density oligonucleotide arrays and two-colour fluorescence analysis. Nat Genet 1996; 14(4):441–447.

79. Southern E, Mir K, Shchepinov M. Molecular interactions on microarrays. Nat Genet Suppl 1999; 21(Jan):5–9.

80. Pastinen T, Syvanen A-C. Minisequencing: A specific tool for DNA analysis and diagnosis on oligonucleotide arrays. Genome Res 1997; 7:606–614.

81. Nikiforov TT, Rendle RB, Goelet P, Rogers YH, Kotewicz ML, Anderson S, et al. Genetic bit analysis: A solid phase method for typing single nucleotide polymorphisms. Nucleic Acids Res 1994; 22(20):4167–4175.

82. Tsujikawa M, Tsujikawa K, Maeda N, Watanabe H, Inoue Y, Mashima Y, et al. Rapid detection of M1S1 mutations by the protein truncation test. Invest Ophthalmol Visual Sci 2000; 41(9):2466–2468.

83. Traverso G, Shuber A, Levin B, Johnson C, Oleson L, Schoetz DJ, et al. Detection of *APC* mutations in fecal DNA from patients with colorectal tumors. N Engl J Med 2002; 346(5):311–320.

84. Cooper DN, Youssoufian H. The CpG dinucleotide and human genetic disease. Hum Genet 1988; 78(2):151–155.

85. Blömeke B, Bennett WP, Harris CC, Shields PG. Serum, plasma, and paraffin-embedded tissues as sources of DNA for studying cancer susceptibility genes. Carcinogenesis 1997; 18(6):1271–1275.

86. Nowell S, Sweeney C, Winters M, Stone A, Lang NP, Hutchins LF, et al. Association between sulfotransferase 1A1 genotype and survival of breast cancer patients receiving tamoxifen therapy. J Natl Cancer Inst 2002; 94(21):1635–1640.

87. Rae JM, Cordero KE, Scheys JO, Lippman ME, Flockhart DA, Johnson MD. Genotyping for polymorphic drug metabolizing enzymes from paraffin-embedded and immunohistochemically stained tumor samples. Pharmacogenetics 2003; 13: 501–507.

88. Day INM, Humphries SE. Electrophoresis for genotyping: Microtiter array diagonal gel electrophoresis on horizontal polyacrylamide gels, hydrolink, or agarose. Anal Biochem 1994; 222:389–395.

89. Nauck M, Hoffmann MM, Wieland H, Marz W. Evaluation of the apo E genotyping kit on the Light-Cycler. Clin Chem 2000; 46(5):722–724.

90. Dahlen P, Carlso J, Liukkonen L, Lilja H, Siitari H, Hurskainen P, et al. Europium-labeled oligonucleotides to detect point mutations: Application to PIZ alpha 1-antitrypsin deficiency. Clin Chem 1993; 39:1626–1631.

91. Newton CR, Graham A, Heptinstall LE, Powell SJ, Summers C, Kalsheker N, et al. Analysis of any point mutation in DNA. The amplification refractory mutation system (ARMS). Nucleic Acids Res 1989; 17:2503–2515.

92. Gibbs RA, Nguyen PN, Caskey CT. Detection of single DNA base differences by competitive oligonucleotide priming. Nucleic Acids Res 1989; 17(7):2437–2448.

93. Gibson NJ, Gillard HL, Whitcombe D, Ferrie RM, Newton CR, Little S. A homogeneous method for genotyping with fluorescence polarization. Clin Chem 1997; 43(8 Pt 1):1336–1341.

94. Zhou G, Kamahori M, Okano K, Chuan G, Harada K, Kambara H. Quantitative detection of single nucleotide polymorphisms for a pooled sample by a bioluminometric assay coupled with modified primer extension reactions (BAMPER). Nucleic Acids Res 2001; 29(19):E93.

95. Landegren U, Kaiser R, Sanders J, Hood L. A ligase-mediated gene detection technique. Science 1988; 241(26 Aug):1077–1080.

96. Nickerson DA, Kaiser R, Lappin S, Stewart J, Hood L, Landegren U. Automated DNA diagnostics using an ELISA-based oligonucleotide ligation assay. Proc Natl Acad Sci USA 1990; 87(Nov):8923–8927.

97. ALves AM, Carr FJ. Dot blot detection of point mutations with adjacently hybridising synthetic oligonucleotide probes. Nucleic Acids Res 1988; 16(17):8723.

98. Baron H, Fung S, Aydin A, Bahring S, Luft FC, Schuster H. Oligonucleotide ligation assay (OLA) for the diagnosis of familial hypercholesterolemia. Nat Biotechnol 1996; 14(10):1279.

99. Hansen TS, Petersen NE, Iitia A, Blaabjerg O, Hyloft-Petersn P, Horder M. Robust nonradioactive oligonucleotide ligation assay to detect a common point mutation in the CYP2D6 gene causing abnormal drug metabolism. Clin Chem 1995; 41:413–418.

100. Foy CA, Parks HC. Emerging homogeneous DNA-based technologies in the clinical laboratory. Clin Chem 2001; 47(6):990–1000.

101. Shi MM. Enabling large-scale pharmacogenetic studies by high-throughput mutation detection and genotyping technologies. Clin Chem 2001; 47(2):164–172.

102. Little MC, Andrews J, Moore R, Bustos S, Jones L, Embres C, et al. Strand displacement amplification and homogeneous real-time detection incorporated in a second-generation DNA probe system, BDProbeTecET. Clin Chem 1999; 45(6): 777–784.

103. Ausina V, Gamboa F, Gazapo E, Manterola JM, Lonca J, Matas L, et al. Evaluation of the semiautomated Abbott LCx Mycobacterium tuberculosis assay for direct detection of Mycobacterium tuberculosis in respiratory specimens. J Clin Microbiol 1997; 35(8):1996–2002.

104. Clegg RM. Fluorescence resonance energy transfer and nucleic acids. Methods Enzymol 1992; 211:353–388.

105. Chen X, Levine L, Kwok PY. Fluorescence polarization in homogeneous nucleic acid analysis. Genome Res 1999; 9(5):492–498.

106. Syvanen AC. From gels to chips: "Minisequencing" primer extension for analysis of point mutations and single nucleotide polymorphisms. Hum Mutat 1999; 13(1): 1–10.

107. Sitbon G, Syvanen AC. Multiplex fluorescent minisequencing applied to the typing of genes encoding drug-metabolizing enzymes. In: Kalow W, Meyer UA, Tyndale RF, editors. Pharmacogenomics. New York: Marcel Dekker, 2001: 191–200.

108. Chen X, Zehnbauer B, Gnirke A, Kwok PY. Fluorescence energy transfer detection as a homogeneous DNA diagnostic method. Proc Natl Acad Sci USA 1997; 94(20):10756–10761.

109. Lovmar L, Syvänen AC. Genotyping single-nucleotide polymorphisms by minisequencing using tag arrays. Methods Mol Med 2005; 114:79–92.

110. Livak KJ. Allelic discrimination using fluorogenic probes and the 5' nuclease assay. Genet Anal 199; 14:143–149.

111. Shi MM, Bleavins MR, de la Iglesia FA. Technologies for detecting genetic polymorphisms in pharmacogenomics. Mol Diagn 1999; 4(4):343–351.

112. Shi MM, Myrand SP, Bleavins MR, de la Iglesia FA. High-throughput genotyping method for glutathione S-transferase T1 and M1 gene deletions using TaqMan probes. Res Commun Mol Pathol Pharmacol 1999; 103(1):3–15.

113. Hiratsuka M, Agatsuma Y, Omori F, Narahara K, Inoue T, Kishikawa Y, et al. High throughput detection of drug-metabolizing enzyme polymorphisms by allele-specific fluorogenic 5' nuclease chain reaction assay. Biol Pharm Bull 2000; 23(10): 1131–1135.

114. Smit ML, Giesendorf BA, Vet JA, Trijbels FJ, Blom HJ. Semiautomated DNA mutation analysis using a robotic workstation and molecular beacons. Clin Chem 2001; 47(4):739–744.

115. Whitcombe D, Theaker J, Guy SP, Brown T, Little S. Detection of PCR products using self-probing amplicons and fluorescence. Nat Biotechnol 1999; 17(Aug): 804–807.

116. Thelwell N, Millington S, Solinas A, Booth J, Brown T. Mode of action and application of Scorpion primers to mutation detection. Nucleic Acids Res 2000; 28(19):3752–3761.

117. Lyamichev V, Mast AL, Hall JG, Prudent JR, Kaiser MW, Takova T, et al. Polymorphism identification and quantitative detection of genomic DNA by invasive cleavage of oligonucleotide probes. Nat Biotechnol 1999; 17(3):292–296.

118. Kwiatkowski RW, Lyamichev V, de Arruda M, Neri B. Clinical, genetic and pharmacogenetic applications of the invader assay. Mol Diagn 1999; 4(4):353–364.

119. Ohnishi Y. [A high-throughput SNP typing system for genome-wide association studies]. Gan To Kagaku Ryoho 2002; 29(11):2031–2036.

120. Staden R. Sequence data handling by computer. Nucleic Acids Res 1977; 4(11): 4037–4051.

121. Schena M. Charting the microarray revolution. Scientist 2004; 18(19 Oct 11): 30–31.

122. Alper J. Weighing DNA for fast genetic diagnosis. Science 2001; 279(27 Mar): 2044–2045.

123. Uetz P. A comprehensive analysis of protein-protein interactions in *Saccharamyces cerevisiae*. Nature 2003; 403(10 Feb):623–627.

124. Sanger F, Air GM, Barrell BG, Brown NL, Coulson AR, Fiddes CA, et al. Nucleotide sequence of bacteriophage phi X174 DNA. Nature 1977; 265(5596): 687–695.

125. Sutcliffe JG. Nucleotide sequence of the ampicillin resistance gene of *Escherichia coli* plasmid pBR322. Proc Natl Acad Sci USA 1978; 75(8):3737–3741.

126. Sutcliffe JG. pBR322 and the advent of rapid DNA sequencing. Trends Biochem Sci 1995; 20(2):87–90.

127. Ambler RP, Scott GK. Partial amino acid sequence of penicillinase coded by *Escherichia coli* plasmid R6K. Proc Natl Acad Sci USA 1978; 75(8):3732–3736.

128. Wilbur WJ, Lipman DJ. Rapid similarity searches of nucleic acid and protein data banks. Proc Natl Acad Sci USA 1983; 80(3):726–730.

129. Waterfield MD, Scrace GT, Whittle N, Stroobant P, Johnsson A, Wasteson A, et al. Platelet-derived growth factor is structurally related to the putative transforming protein p28sis of simian sarcoma virus. Nature 1983; 304(5921):35–39.

130. Pearson WR, Lipman DJ. Improved tools for biological sequence comparison. Proc Natl Acad Sci USA 1988; 85(8):2444–2448.

131. Altschul SF, Gish W, Miller W, Myers EW, Lipman DJ. Basic local alignment search tool. J Mol Biol 1990; 215(3):403–410.

132. Altschul SF, Madden TL, Schaffer AA, Zhang J, Zhang Z, Miller W, et al. Gapped BLAST and PSI-BLAST: A new generation of protein database search programs. Nucleic Acids Res 1997; 25(17):3389–3402.

133. Gallagher R. Seven cheers for technology. Scientist 2005; 19(16):6–51.

134. Rogic S, Mackworth AK, Ouellette FB. Evaluation of gene-finding programs on mammalian sequences. Genome Res 2001; 11(5):817–832.

135. Fickett JW. Finding genes by computer: The state of the art. Trends Genet 1996; 12(8):316–320.

136. Gordon D, Abajian C, Green P. Consed: A graphical tool for sequence finishing. Genome Res 1998; 8(3):195–202.
137. Strausberg RL, Feingold EA, Klausner RD, Collins FS. The mammalian gene collection. Science 1999; 286(5439):455–457.
138. Strausberg RL, Feingold EA, Grouse LH, Derge JG, Klausner RD, Collins FS, et al. Generation and initial analysis of more than 15,000 full-length human and mouse cDNA sequences. Proc Natl Acad Sci USA 2002; 99(26):16899–16903.
139. Lewis EK, Haaland WC, Nguyen F, Heller DA, Allen MJ, MacGregor RR, et al. Color-blind fluorescence detection for four-color DNA sequencing. Proc Natl Acad Sci USA 2005; 102(15):5346–5351.
140. Margulies M, Egholm M, Altman WE, Attiya S, Bader JS, Bemben LA, et al. Genome sequencing in microfabricated high-density picolitre reactors. Nature 2005; 437(7057):376–380.
141. Meinkoth J, Wahl G. Hybridization of nucleic acids immobilized on solid supports. Anal Biochem 1984; 138(2):267–284.
142. Schena M, Heller RA, Theriault TP, Konrad K, Lachenmeier E, Davis RW. Microarrays: Biotechnology's discovery platform for functional genomics. Trends Biotechnol 1998; 16(7):301–306.
143. Maskos U, Southern EM. A novel method for the analysis of multiple sequence variants by hybridisation to oligonucleotides. Nucleic Acids Res 1993; 21:2267–2268.
144. Maskos U, Southern EM. A novel method for the parallel analysis of multiple mutations in multiple samples. Nucleic Acids Res 1993; 21:2269–2270.
145. Blanchard AP, Kaiser RJ, Hood LE. High-density oligonucleotide arrays. Biosens Bioelectron 1996; 11(6–7):687–690.
146. Irizarry RA, Warren D, Spencer F, Kim IF, Biswal S, Frank BC, et al. Multiple-laboratory comparison of microarray platforms. Nat Methods 2005; 2(5):345–350.
147. Larkin JE, Frank BC, Gavras H, Sultana R, Quackenbush J. Independence and reproducibility across microarray platforms. Nat Methods 2005; 2(5):337–344.
148. Bammler T, Beyer RP, Bhattacharya S, Boorman GA, Boyles A, Bradford BU, et al. Standardizing global gene expression analysis between laboratories and across platforms. Nat Methods 2005; 2(5):351–356.
149. Ekins R, Chu FW. Microarrays: Their origins and applications. Trends Biotechnol 1999; 17(6):217–218.
150. Wang DG, Fan JB, Siao CJ, Berno A, Young P, Sapolsky R, et al. Large-scale identification, mapping, and genotyping of single-nucleotide polymorphisms in the human genome. Science 1998; 280(5366):1077–1082.
151. Lockhart DJ, Dong H, Byrne MC, Follettie MT, Gallo MV, Chee MS, et al. Expression monitoring by hybridization to high-density oligonucleotide arrays. Nat Biotechnol 1996; 14(13):1675–1680.
152. Howbrook DN, van der Valk AM, O'Shaughnessy MC, Sraker DK, Baker SC, LLoyd AW. Development in microarray technologies. Drug Discov Today 2003; 8(14):642–651.
153. Fang Y, Lahiri J, Picard L. G protein-coupled receptor microarrays for drug discovery. Drug Discov Today 2003; 8(16):755–761.
154. Golub TR, Slonim DK, Tamayo P, Huard C, Gaasenbeek M, Mesirov JP, et al. Molecular classification of cancer: Class discovery and class prediction by gene expression monitoring. Science 1999; 286(5439):531–537.
155. Multiauthored. The chipping forecast III. Nat Genet Suppl 2005; 37(June):S1–S45.

156. Horning EC, Horning MG, Carroll DI, Dzidic I, Stillwell RN. Chemical ionization mass spectrometry. Adv Biochem Psychopharmacol 1973; 7:15–31.
157. Griffin TJ, Hall JG, Prudent JR, Smith LM. Direct genetic analysis by matrix-assisted laser desorption/ionization mass spectrometry. Proc Natl Acad Sci USA 1999; 96(11):6301–6306.
158. Griffin TJ, Smith LM. Single-nucleotide polymorphism analysis by MALDI/TOF mass spectrometry. Trends Biotechnol 2000; 18(2):77–84.
159. Wu KJ, Steding A, Becker CH. Matrix-assisted laser desorption time-of-flight mass spectrometry of oligonucleotides using 3-hydroxypicolinic acid as an ultraviolet-sensitive matrix. Rapid Commun Mass Spectrom 1993; 7(2):142–146.
160. Hunter JM, Lin H, Becker CH. Cryogenic frozen solution matrixes for analysis of DNA by time-of-flight mass spectrometry. Anal Chem 1997; 69(17):3608–3612.
161. Ding C, Cantor CR. A high-throughput gene expression analysis technique using competitive PCR and matrix-assisted laser desorption ionization time-of-flight MS. Proc Natl Acad Sci USA 2003; 100(6):3059–3064.
162. Rubakhin SS, Jurchen JC, Monroe EB, Sweedler JV. Imaging mass spectrometry: Fundamentals and applications to drug discovery. Drug Discov Today 2005; 10(12): 823–837.
163. Goffeau A, Barrell BG, Bussey H, Davis RW, Dujon B, Feldmann H, et al. Life with 6000 genes. Science 1996; 274(5287):546, 563–567.
164. Ito T, Tashiro K, Muta S, Ozawa R, Chiba T, Nishizawa M, et al. Toward a protein-protein interaction map of the budding yeast: A comprehensive system to examine two-hybrid interactions in all possible combinations between the yeast proteins. Proc Natl Acad Sci USA 2000; 97(3):1143–1147.
165. Ito T, Chiba T, Ozawa R, Yoshida M, Hattori M, Sakaki Y. A comprehensive two-hybrid analysis to explore the yeast protein interactome. Proc Natl Acad Sci USA 2001; 98(8):4569–4574.
166. Giot L, Bader JS, Brouwer C, Chaudhuri A, Kuang B, Li Y, et al. A protein interaction map of *Drosophila melanogaster*. Science 2003; 302(5651):1727–1736.
167. Li S, Armstrong CM, Bertin N, Ge H, Milstein S, Boxem M, et al. A map of the interactome network of the metazoan *C. elegans*. Science 2004; 303(5657):540–543.
168. Colland F, Jacq X, Trouplin V, Mougin C, Groizeleau C, Hamburger A, et al. Functional proteomics mapping of a human signaling pathway. Genome Res 2004; 14(7):1324–1332.
169. McGlennen RC. Miniaturization technologies for molecular diagnostics. Clin Chem 2001; 47(3):393–402.
170. Burns MA, Johnson BN, Brahmasandra SN, Handique K, Webster JR, Krishnan M, et al. An integrated nanoliter DNA analysis device. Science 1998; 282(5388): 484–487.
171. Zhou G, Kamahori M, Okano K, Harada K, Kambara H. Miniaturized pyrosequencer for DNA analysis with capillaries to deliver deoxynucleotides. Electrophoresis 2001; 22(16):3497–3504.
172. Khandurina J, Guttman A. Bioanalysis in microfluidic devices. J Chromatogr A 2002; 943:159–183.
173. Vilkner T, Janasek D, Manz A. Micro total analysis systems. Recent developments. Anal Chem 2004; 76(12):3373–3385.
174. Anderson RC, Su X, Bogdan GJ, Fenton J. A miniature integrated device for automated multistep genetic assays. Nucleic Acids Res 2000; 28(12):E60.

175. Fiorini GS, Chiu DT. Disposable microfluidic devices: Fabrication, function, and application. BioTechniques 2005; 38(3):429–446.

176. Hanash S. Operomics: Molecular analysis of tissues from DNA to RNA to protein. Clin Chem Lab Med 2000; 38(9):805–813.

177. Velculescu V, Zhang L, Vogelstein B, Kinzler KW. Serial analysis of gene expression. Science 1995; 270:484–487.

178. Velculescu VE, Vogelstein B, Kinzler KW. Analysing uncharted transcriptomes with SAGE. Trends Genet 2000; 16(10):423–425.

179. Madden SL, Wang C, Landes G. Serial analysis of gene expression. Transcriptional insights into functional biology. In: Kalow W, Meyer UA, Tyndale RF, editors. Pharmacogenomics. New York: Marcel Dekker, 2001: 223–251.

180. Datson NA, der Perdojong J, van den Berg MP, de Kloet ER, Vreugdenhil E. MicroSAGE: A modified procedure for serial analysis of gene expression in limited amounts of tissue. Nucleic Acids Res 1999; 27(5):1300–1307.

181. Dixon AK, Richardson PJ, Pinnock RD, Lee K. Gene-expression analysis at the single-cell level. Trends Pharmacol Sci 2000; 21(2):65–70.

182. Schober MS, Min Y-N, Chen YQ. Serial analysis of gene expression in a single cell. BioTechniques 2001; 31(6):1240–1242.

183. Dear PH. One by one: Single molecule tools for genomics. Brief Funct Genomic Proteomic 2003; 1(4):397–416.

184. Woolley AT, Guillemette C, Li CC, Housman DE, Lieber CM. Direct haplotyping of kilobase-size DNA using carbon nanotube probes. Nat Biotechnol 2000; 18(7): 760–763.

185. Guillemette C, Ritter JK, Auyeung DJ, Kessler FK, Housman DE. Structural heterogeneity at the UDP-glucuronosyltransferase 1 locus: Functional consequences of three novel missense mutations in the human UGT1A7 gene. Pharmacogenetics 2000; 10(7):629–644.

186. Baner J, Nilsson M, Mendel-Hartvig M, Landgren U. Signal amplification of padlock probes by rolling circle replication. Nucleic Acids Res 1998; 26(22):5073–5078.

187. Lizardi PM, Huang X, Zhu Z, Bray-Ward P, Thomas DC, Ward DC. Mutation detection and using single-molecule counting using isothermal rolling-circle amplification. Nat Genet 1998; 19(Jul):225–232.

188. Zhong X-B, Lizardi PM, Huang X-H, Bray-Ward PL, Ward DC. Visualization of oligonucleotide probes and point mutations in interphase nuclei and DNA fibers using rolling circle DNA amplification. Proc Natl Acad Sci USA 2001; 98(7):3940–3945.

189. Deamer DW, Akeson M. Nanopores and nucleic acids: Prospects for ultrarapid sequencing. Trends Biotechnol 2000; 18:147–151.

190. Kasianowicz JJ, Brandin E, Branton D, Deamer DW. Characterization of individual polynucleotide molecules using a membrane channel. Proc Natl Acad Sci USA 1996; 93(24):13770–13773.

191. Akeson M, Branton D, Kasianowicz JJ, Brandin E, Deamer DW. Microsecond time-scale discrimination among polycytidylic acid, polyadenylic acid, and polyuridylic acid as homopolymers or as segments within single RNA molecules. Biophys J 1999; 77(6):3227–3233.

192. Liljedahl U, Karlsson J, Melhus H, Kurland L, Lindersson M, Kahan T, et al. A microarray minisequencing system for pharmacogenetic profiling of antihypertensive drug response. Pharmacogenetics 2003; 13(1):7–17.

193. ARmstrong SA, Staunton JE, Silverman LB, Pieters R, den Boer ML, Minden MD, et al. *MLL* translocations specify a distinct gene expression profile that distinguishes a unique leukemia. Nat Genet 2002; 30(Jan):41–47.

194. Bittner M, Meltzer P, Chen Y, Jiang Y, Seftor E, Hendrix M, et al. Molecular classification of cutaneous malignant melanoma by gene expression profiling. Nature 2000; 406(6795):536–540.

195. Alizadeh AA, Eisen MB, Davis RE, Ma C, Lossos IS, Rosenwald A, et al. Distinct types of diffuse large B-cell lymphoma identified by gene expression profiling. Nature 2000; 403(6769):503–511.

196. Hedenfalk I, Duggan D, Chen Y, Radmacher M, Bittner M, Simon R, et al. Gene-expression profiles in hereditary breast cancer. N Engl J Med 2001; 344(8):539–548.

197. van't Veer LJ, Dai H, van de Vijver MJ, He YD, Hart AA, Mao M, et al. Gene expression profiling predicts clinical outcome of breast cancer. Nature 2002; 415(6871):530–536.

198. van de Vijver MJ, He YD, van't Veer LJ, Dai H, Hart AA, Voskuil DW, et al. A gene-expression signature as a predictor of survival in breast cancer. N Engl J Med 2002; 347(25):1999–2009.

199. van Steensel B, Henikoff S. Epigenomic profiling using microarrays. BioTechniques 2003; 35(2):346–4, 356.

200. van Steensel B. Mapping of genetic and epigenetic regulatory networks using microarrays. Nat Genet 2005; 37(6 Suppl):S18–S24.

201. Havlis J, Trbusek M. 5-Methylcytosine as a marker for the monitoring of DNA methylation. J Chromatogr B Analyt Technol Biomed Life Sci 2002; 781(1–2):373–392.

202. Hong KM, Yang SH, Guo M, Herman JG, Jen J. Semiautomatic detection of DNA methylation at CpG islands. BioTechniques 2005; 38(3):354, 356, 358.

203. Shi H, Maier S, Nimmrich I, Yan PS, Caldwell CW, Olek A, et al. Oligonucleotide-based microarray for DNA methylation analysis: Principles and applications. J Cell Biochem 2003; 88(1):138–143.

204. Chen CM, Chen HL, Hsiau TH, Hsiau AH, Shi H, Brock GJ, et al. Methylation target array for rapid analysis of CpG island hypermethylation in multiple tissue genomes. Am J Pathol 2003; 163(1):37–45.

205. Kononen J, Bubendorf L, Kallioniemi A, Barlund M, Schraml P, Leighton S, et al. Tissue microarrays for high-throughput molecular profiling of tumor specimens. Nat Med 1998; 4(7):844–847.

206. Pfarr W, Webersinke G, Paar C, Wechselberger C. Immunodetection of 5'-methylcytosine on Giemsa-stained chromosomes. BioTechniques 2005; 38(4):527–528, 530.

207. Golub TR. Genome-wide views of cancer. N Engl J Med 2001; 344(8):601–602.

208. Camp RL, Dolled-Filhart M, King BL, Rimm DL. Quantitative analysis of breast cancer tissue microarrays shows that both high and normal levels of HER2 expression are associated with poor outcome. Cancer Res 2003; 63(7):1445–1448.

209. Iafrate AJ, Feuk L, Rivera MN, Listewnik ML, Donahoe PK, Qi Y, et al. Detection of large-scale variation in the human genome. Nat Genet 2004; 36(9):949–951.

210. Sebat J, Lakshmi B, Troge J, Alexander J, Young J, Lundin P, et al. Large-scale copy number polymorphism in the human genome. Science 2004; 305(5683):525–528.

211. Feuk L, Carson AR, Scherer SW. Structural variation in the human genome. Nat Rev Genet 2006; 7(2):85–97.
212. Freeman JL, Perry GH, Feuk L, Redon R, McCarroll SA, Altshuler DM, et al. Copy number variation: New insights in genome diversity. Genome Res 2006; 16(8): 949–961.
213. Redon R, Ishikawa S, Fitch KR, Feuk L, Perry GH, Andrews TD, et al. Global variation in copy number in the human genome. Nature 2006; 444(7118):444–454.
214. Fiegler H, Redon R, Andrews D, Scott C, Andrews R, Carder C, et al. Accurate and reliable high-throughput detection of copy number variation in the human genome. Genome Res 2006.
215. Lander ES, Linton LM, Birren B, Nusbaum C, Zody MC, Baldwin J, et al. Initial sequencing and analysis of the human genome. Nature 2001; 409(6822):860–921.

8

Ethnic Pharmacogenetics

Individuals of different ethnic or raciogeographic origin are important sources of information on variations in response to drugs and other exogenous substances. Prior to the 1920s, such variations were reported very infrequently in the medical literature. In one early study, Marshall and colleagues found that blacks were much more resistant than whites to the blistering of skin by mustard gas caused by exposure to this biological weapon during World War I.[1] In other reports, blacks were found to be less susceptible to slowing of the pulse than whites by small doses of atropine. Several investigators published observations that ephedrine and various other mydriatic agents such as cocaine and pseudoephedrine dilated the pupils of Chinese and African blacks only slightly compared with those of whites. During the 1930s, ethnic studies of "taste blindness," a hereditary deficit in sensory perception, showed that the frequency of nontasters in European populations was appreciably higher (35–40%) than that in African subpopulations, Chinese, Japanese, South Amerinds, and Lapps (<10%).[2]

The association of race or ethnicity with human responsiveness to so few drugs and other chemicals suggested this phenomenon might be of more general significance. Because researchers located at different raciogeographic sites around the world examined pharmacogenetic phenomena among local subjects, a number of striking ethnic specificities were soon observed. Since then, the study of ethnogeographic variation has been regarded as an important part of any comprehensive pharmacogenetic study.

MARRYING RACE AND ETHNICITY TO GENETIC VARIATION

Biologists have long tussled with the meaning of race and ethnicity. Studies of these concepts can be traced to the beginning of recorded history and numerous efforts have been made at their classification. Initially, skin color and other conspicuous differences between populations were used for this purpose, but no serious attempts at classification could be made until the eighteenth century when greater geographic knowledge of the earth became available. Then, lists of human races, or "varieties" as Linneaus called them, were made, and classification was based on anthropomorphic traits, such as the cephalic index, stature, and limb measurements. But Darwin argued it was hardly possible to accept any of these as clear-cut distinctions because they were subject to rapid changes induced by the environment, and graduated into each other.[3]

As modern humans (*Homo sapiens*) spread around the world, naturalists were prompted to classify them into three groups, Negroids, Mongoloids, and Caucasoids. But this classification has not always been applied consistently because two smaller groups, the Capoids (Bushmen and Hottentots) and Australoids, are sometimes added to these three major races, and as recent as the year 2000, five major groups—black or African-American, white, Asian, native Hawaiian or other Pacific Islander, and American Indian or Alaska native—were used in the U.S. census for that year.[4] Broadly speaking, four descriptive criteria have been used to specify races: (1) *geographic,* which is founded on the idea that the exchange of genes is reduced as the distance between populations increases (until 150 years ago, most movements covered distances of no more than 150 miles and only rarely did people venture beyond this short range); (2) a*nthropologic,* which focuses on similarity of height, weight, body build, and facial features as traits that could be easily perceived; (3) *linguistic,* which takes account of the relationships between 4736 languages of the world (interestingly the evolution of linguistic and genetic trees tend to parallel each other); and (4) *ethnic,* which attempts to take account of social, behavioral, and cultural characteristics. Historically, geography appears to be the greatest force affecting genetic differentiation among humans, and the order of importance of these criteria for racial classification diminishes from *geographic* to *ethnic*.[3] For the past two decades, the greatest genetic differentiation has occurred between continentally separated groups.[4]

GRAPPLING WITH RACE AND ETHNICITY DURING THE TWENTIETH CENTURY

Two perspectives dominated the study of race and ethnicity well into the twentieth century. One view, rooted in the eugenics movement, treated racial and ethnic categories as meaningful biological classifications and attempted to specify biological differences between socially labeled populations; the other, opposing, view, derived mainly from works in physical anthropology and social science, treated race and ethnicity as cultural and historical constructs of little biological significance.

Ethnically related variations in the action of genes was an outgrowth of observations by L. Hirschfeld and H. Hirschfeld first reported in 1919. The Hirschfelds were army physicians in the Balkans, and they used this opportunity to determine the blood groups of soldiers of various races and nationalities brought together as an accident of World War I. They found significant differences in the frequencies of the four *ABO* blood groups in the 16 nationalities studied.[5]

Within a brief span during the early 1930s, R.A. Fisher, Sewall Wright, and J.B.S. Haldane wrote books and delivered lectures that gave a new impetus to Darwin's theory of evolution. Before 1930, most biologists accepted evolution as a given, but many of them doubted the power of natural selection to account for observed degrees of individual adaptation. It is necessary to consider the works of Fisher and Wright immediately preceding those of Haldane to see how they contributed to an understanding of race and ethnicity. Fisher constructed a systematic, testable hypothesis of evolution to determine whether natural selection of random mutations could and did account for observed degrees of adaptation. His results predicted that even slight selective differentials, particularly in large populations, were sufficient to substitute a favored gene for a less advantageous one. He concluded that most organisms were precisely adapted to circumstances in their lives. Wright then questioned what circumstances best favored the spread of new adaptations throughout a population, and argued that adaptive evolution was favored in species composed of many small subpopulations. In such a species, more different gene combinations would arise, primarily by chance, and a really advantageous gene combination could multiply under the additional force of natural selection and spread through the whole species. In his book on the *Causes of Evolution* that grew out of a series of lectures he delivered in 1931 at the National University of Wales, Haldane foresaw many of the modern issues of evolutionary theory and attempted to explain events of the remote past in terms of the new science of genetics. Focusing on differences between individuals of the same species, he divided the causes of variation into those that operated before and those that began during the life of the individual. He noted that differences between (and within) species could be explained in terms of differences between individual genes at comparable loci, differences between the arrangement of genes on chromosomes, and differences in number, either of individual chromosomes (aneuploidy) or of whole sets of chromosomes (polyploidy). The ideas of Fisher, Wright, and Haldane were based mainly on variation in plants and animals, but it seems evident that they, taken together, would apply equally well to humans and their subdivision into racial and ethnic groups.

But the significance of these observations and the actual extent of human variation were not fully appreciated until protein polymorphism was detected with the aid of electrophoresis in the 1950s and 1960s.[6–9] In 1951, Laurence Snyder,* one of the first presidents of the American Society of Human Genetics, stated that "human populations differ one from another almost entirely in the varying *proportions* of the allelic genes of the various sets of hereditary factors, and not in the *kinds* of genes they contain. The extreme positions held by those who on the one hand maintain that there are no significant genetic differences between human races, and those who on the other hand hold that certain races were 'superior' and others 'inferior,' require drastic modification in the light of the accumulated data on the gene frequency dynamics of human

---

*Laurence Snyder was the first to describe the genetics and recessive character of taste blindness in the 1930s (see Chapter 1).

populations."[10] Snyder's statement largely captured the consensus of geneticists at that time.

The introduction of genetic markers followed more recently by the discovery of DNA polymorphism further solidified the study of human variation. During the 1960s and early 1970s, databases of genetic information on protein sequence and structure and computer analysis systems for retrieval and analysis of data became available online. In 1972, Lewontin used a sample of data collected on 15 protein loci to assess human genetic diversity at the protein level. His analysis showed that 85% of human genetic diversity was represented by individual diversity within populations, whereas differences among seven racial groups accounted for less than 7% of the total. Studies of populations on three continents by other investigators reached a similar conclusion. These results were confirmed repeatedly by additional studies of protein markers, but the idea persisted that the human species was deeply divided into races. In 1997, Barbujani and colleagues analyzed the distribution of DNA variation at 109 markers at 30 microsatellite loci and 79 restriction fragment length polymorphism (RFLP) sites in 16 populations of the world.[11] They too found that differences between members of the same population accounted for 84.4% of the total variation. They concluded that racial subdivision of the human species failed to reflect any major discontinuity in the human genome.

The simplistic interpretation of race and ethnicity associated with the eugenics movement has been discredited for decades, but today, despite an extensive collection of data on allelic distributions within and between human populations, there are still tensions between social and biological interpretations of race and ethnicity. However, the tone of the debates surrounding these issues has changed. Genetic criteria are used in evolutionary studies to reconstruct human phylogeny and in clinical and population genetic studies to identify and characterize differences between and within contemporary racial, ethnic, and geographic communities. In 1998, the American Anthropological Association stated that "human populations are not unambiguous, clearly demarcated, biologically distinct groups," and "any attempt to establish lines of division among biological populations is both arbitrary and subjective."[12] In the present context, race is defined genetically as a large group of individuals that has a significant fraction of its genes in common and can be distinguished by its gene pool. It is also clear that Snyder's comment of more than 50 years ago closely resembles current views on race and ethnicity.

Genoscoping the Time Scale of Racial Diversity

According to the most commonly accepted estimate, modern humans (*Homo*) originated in Africa about 2 million years ago. The first efforts at reconstructing human evolution from genetic data were made by Cavalli-Sforza and colleagues in 1964 from data on nuclear genes; DNA collected from 15 populations on five blood group genes (ABO, MN, Rh, Diego, and Duffy) comprising a total of 20 alleles was used for this purpose.[3] This study and later research indicated a greater number of genes and a more balanced sample of populations that was as

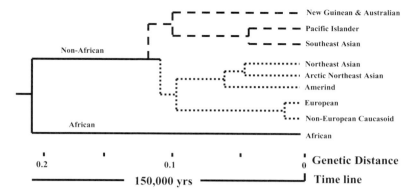

Figure 8.1 Human phylogenetic tree. With permission from Princeton University Press.

close as possible to what may have been the aboriginal set of populations were necessary for evolutionary analysis. In another study in 1988 by Cavalli-Sforza and associates, these shortcomings were eliminated; 42 aboriginal populations incorporating 120 alleles grouped into "clusters" representing nine populations were drawn from the literature for analysis at the world level. The final sample, which was obtained on data culled from 1950 populations, yielded the human phylogenetic tree shown in Figure 8.1.[13] This analysis placed the separation of African from non-African populations at about 150,000 years ago. Estimates based on other criteria vary somewhat. Thus an estimate based on 30 autosomal microsatellite polymorphisms placed the major split in human phylogeny at about 156,000 years ago,[14] whereas comparisons of genetic distances[†] (Figure 8.1) and archeological time data suggest that Africans separated from non-Africans about 92,000 years ago, and the next major split, separating Northeurasians from Southeast Asians, occurred about 40,000 years ago. Approximately 35,000 years ago Caucasoids split off from a cluster that included Northeast Asians and Amerinds.[13]

It is notable that Chinese populations are clustered with Mainland and Southeast Asians while Japanese and Korean populations cluster with Northeast Asians; hence the gene pool of Japanese and Korean populations would probably resemble each other more closely than Chinese. Additionally, there are

[†]Cavalli-Sforza et al.[3] refers to D as the genetic distance used in all phylogenetic analyses. D is defined by the following equation:

$$D = -\log(1-d) = -t/2N$$

where t is time in generations, N is effective population size, and

$$d = (x - y)^2/[2P(1 - P)]$$

where x and y are gene frequencies and P is the ancestral gene frequency estimated by the mean gene frequency for all populations being considered.

Table 8.1 Racial Variation of Taste Blindness: Frequency of Phenylthiourea Nonstasters[15]

Population	Number tested	Nontasters (%)
Hindus	489	33.7
Danish	251	32.7
English	441	31.5
Spanish	203	25.6
Portuguese	454	24.0
Negritos (Malaya)	50	18.0
Malays	237	16.0
Japanese	295	7.1
Lapps	140	6.4
West Africans	74	2.7
Chinese	50	2.0
South Amerinds (Brazil)	163	1.2

indications that some populations may have received contributions from other clusters. In Europe, Lapps, Sardinians, Basques, and Icelanders are four major outliers in order of divergence on the basis of genetic and historical information, and Lapps join more closely with Asian Arctic populations than Europeans.[3] In this connection it is interesting that the frequency of nontasters among Lapps, a Scandinavian population, is much closer to that of Japanese and Chinese than to Europeans (Table 8.1).

ETHNIC SPECIFICITY IN DRUG RESPONSE

The importance of racial and ethnic classification in biomedical research continues to be a contentious issue,[4,10,12,15–22] but the considerable evidence in the pharmacogenetics literature points to the importance of racial and ethnic categories for generating and exploring hypotheses about genetic and environmental risks posed by exposure to drugs and other exogenous substances.

"Primaquine sensitivity" was one of the first, and ranks as one of the best-known examples of ethnic variation in drug response. As a sex-linked trait that is due to deficiency of the housekeeping enzyme, glucose-6-phosphate dehydrogenase (G6PD), it occurs primarily among males of African, Mediterranean, and Southeast Asian descent who reside in tropical and semitropical regions of the Earth. Numerous adverse drug reactions and interactions attributable to drug-metabolizing enzyme traits vary greatly from one population to another. One important example of this type concerns the sensitivity of Japanese to the aversive effects of alcohol compared to Caucasians. This example of ethnic variation in drug response is attributed to variant forms of alcohol dehydrogenase (ALDH2). Another well-known set of reactions accompanies the administration of drugs that are eliminated by variant forms of acetyltransferase, an enzyme that encodes for genetically slow and rapid acetylation. Slow acetylators are predisposed to isoniazid-induced neuropathy; they, particularly those in older age groups, are also predisposed to isoniazid-induced hepatitis. Slow acetylators make up about 50% (40–60%) of many Caucasian populations and about 80% of certain Middle Eastern populations compared to fewer than 20% of Japanese. Hence, for patients administered isoniazid in the treatment of tuberculosis, the predisposition of Caucasians and Middle Easterners to peripheral neuropathy and to isoniazid-induced liver damage is likely greater than that of Japanese.

Many unanticipated reactions to drugs have been associated with variant forms of P450 enzymes that encode for genetically poor metabolism such as CYP2D6 and CYP2C19.[23] The frequency of CYP2D6 poor metabolism may vary from about 1 in 8 in certain African populations to about 1 in 10 in Caucasians, but is much lower among Japanese at less than 1 in 100. The risk of such reactions to drugs that are eliminated by CYP2C19, on the other hand, trends in the opposite direction, being about six to seven times greater among Asians (Japanese, Chinese, and Korean) (13–23%) than in Caucasians.

Ethnic specificities in human response to drugs and other exogenous substances raise a number of questions. How frequent are ethnic specificities of pharmacogenetic interest? Might they suggest a starting point for further investigations of drugs, carcinogens, and other environmental chemicals? Would such differences be important in the development and clinical trials of new drugs? Do they occur frequently enough to affect the clinical care of patients? And does the use of this information clinically improve patient care significantly?

FREQUENCY OF PHARMACOGENETIC ETHNIC SPECIFICITIES

Many of these questions are answerable, at least in part, from current knowledge of various pharmacogenetic traits, as discussed below.

Glucose-6-Phosphate Dehydrogenase Deficiency

It was recognized in the 1930s and 1940s that sudden hemolytic anemia induced by sulfanilamide and primaquine occurs preferentially in black males and other dark-skinned persons.[24–26] The cause of this trait, G6PD deficiency, was discovered in World War II servicemen exposed to preventive and therapeutic treatment with a number of antimalarial drugs (primaquine, pamaquine, pentoquine, and isopentoquine). More than 400 million people worldwide are affected. Those of African, Mediterranean, and Southeast Asian descent are particularly susceptible to this trait; in some populations between 10% and 60% of males are affected.

The biochemical basis of drug-induced hemolytic anemia was defined as G6PD deficiency in the 1950s[27–29] and a biochemical test devised to detect this trait prior to drug exposure was developed in 1957.[30] Hemolytic reactions that occur at such a high frequency in dark-skinned races are rare among whites and are brought about by a different panel of drugs.[31]

In Africans, two types of variants are found by biochemical analysis: G6PD A and G6PD A-. The first produces normal levels of red cell activity and the second is unstable *in vivo,* yielding only about 10% of normal activity levels. Recombinant DNA analysis indicates that the enzyme that characterizes G6PD deficiency, G6PD A-, is caused by a Val → Met substitution at codon 68 ($G^{202}A$).[32] A second mutation that causes G6PD deficiency, A → T at nt 542, is found in another African variant, G6PD Santamaria. This mutation causes an Asp → Val substitution at codon 181. In Mediterranean peoples, a C → T change at nt 563 results in a Ser → Phe substitution at codon 188. Less is known about deficiency mutations in Orientals than in Mediterraneans, but one of the more common Oriental variants, G6PD Canton, has an Arg → Leu substitution at codon 459. Thus, the ethnic specificities in G6PD deficiency are due to different molecular causes.[33]

More than 30 different mutations in G6PD are listed in Beutler's review of the molecular biology of G6PD variants. Most of these produce a phenotypically altered enzyme, having abnormal activity, quantity, properties, or a combination of these properties.[33]

NAT2 Polymorphism

Acetylation polymorphism confers rapid or slow acetylator status on individuals, and is widely acknowledged as a reliable prognosticator of individual susceptibility to effective and safe use of numerous drugs (isoniazid, sulfonamides, procainamide, hydralazine, sulfasalazine, etc.), to toxicity from industrial/ occupational chemicals with carcinogenic potential, and possibly to dietary mutagens. Studies of the global distribution of acetylator gene frequencies encompass measurements on more 10,000 individuals in dozens of different populations since the trait was discovered in the 1950s.[34] The percentage of slow acetylators ranges from 80% or more in Egyptians and certain other Middle Eastern populations to 20% or less of Japanese and Canadian Eskimos. Populations of Europeans and African origin have, with few exceptions, intermediate percentages of slow acetylators (Figure 8.2).

The "cline" in slow acetylator frequencies among populations of the Northern hemisphere provides one of the most dramatic illustrations of ethnic variation for any human trait described so far (Figure 8.3). Population surveys of slow acetylator allelic frequencies conducted by Sunahara et al.[35] initially disclosed a trend of increasing slow acetylator allelic frequencies from northern to southern latitudes among Japanese. Estimates of ethnic variation in acetylator allelic frequencies based on global observations by Karim et al.[36] fully bear out Sunahara's idea of a relationship between latitude and acetylator status and extend them to a number of other populations of the Northern hemisphere. The occurrence of such a trend in the frequency of hereditary traits is a perplexing phenomenon in population and evolutionary genetics. Such phenomena are well known in wild plant and animal populations[37] but such relationships are much less numerous between human gene frequencies and the environment.[38] We do not know the natural or endogenous substrate for *N*-acetyltransferase (later shown to be NAT2), so we do not understand the origin of this relationship. Lacking this information, speculation suggests that rapid acetylation may have conferred a selective advantage to

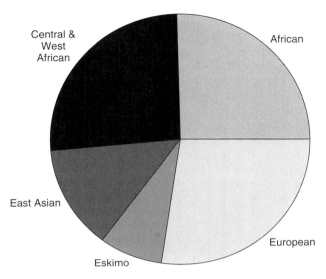

Figure 8.2 Racial differences among the slow acetylator (NAT2) phenotype in various ethnic populations.

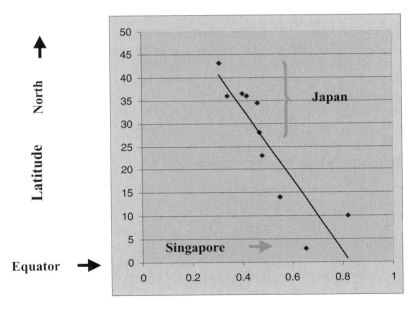

Slow NAT2 allele frequency

Figure 8.3 A cline of slow NAT2 acetylator phenotypes among North Pacific Asian coastal populations.

survival among populations in more northerly latitudes, perhaps through differences in the dietary habits of people evolving in these regions or in their chemical or physical environment.

DNA analysis of the acetylation polymorphism revealed that humans encode two functional N-acetyltransferases (NATs), NAT1 and NAT2. Both of these loci, *NAT1** and *NAT2**, are polymorphic,[39] and NAT1* and NAT2* are both implicated in the disposition of numerous therapeutic agents and various environmental/occupational chemicals, but the data on ethnicity concern *NAT2** genotypes and phenotypes. Some background and a few remarks about the allelic variation at the human *NAT2** locus are in order.

More than 20 alleles for *NAT2** have been reported. The coding region of the gene is the site of multiple mutations, but analysis of regions upstream and downstream are very limited. At least nine nucleotide changes in the coding region occur singly or in combinations of two and three to yield at least 20 distinct alleles. Seven of the nucleotide changes result in changes in the deduced amino acid, some of which strongly affect acetylating activity. The *NAT2*4* allele is taken as the "wild type" since it is found in individuals phenotyped as rapid acetylators. The other alleles are associated with slow acetylation when any two are paired in an individual.[40]

Ethnicity data indicate the distribution patterns of *NAT2** allelic frequencies across different populations are neither uniformly nor randomly distributed. Among North American and European Caucasians, the frequency of the rapid *NAT2*4* allele is 20–25%, among African-Americans, 36%, and among Hispanics, 42%. Among Asiatics, the frequency is 66% among Hong Kong Chinese, 66% among Koreans in America, and >70% among native Japanese. The distribution of slow *NAT2** alleles shows that for Caucasians three alleles (4, 5B, and 6A) account for about 95% of all *NAT2** alleles. In Oriental populations, the 5B allele becomes rare (5% in Hong Kong Chinese to <1% in Japanese) and 6A (20–30%) and 7A/7B (7–16%) are most frequent.[40]

CYP2D6 and CYP2C19 Polymorphisms

The *CYP2D6** (debrisoquine/sparteine oxidation) polymorphism results in four separable phenotypes: poor metabolizers, extensive and heterozygous metabolizers, and ultrarapid metabolizers. Poor metabolizers are homozygous for an inactive or deficient CYP2D6 enzyme due to truncation or missense mutations of the *CYP2D6** gene, while ultrarapid metabolizers possess an enhanced capacity to metabolize due to multiple copies of an amplified gene (*CYP2D6L**).[41,42] Up to 20% of widely used therapeutic agents including β-adrenergic blockers, antidepressants, antiarrhythmics, neuroleptics, and various miscellaneous drugs such as phenformin, dextromethorphan, and codeine are subject to these polymorphisms.[43] Among Northern European populations, more than 95% of the deficient alleles responsible for CYP2D6* poor metabolizers have been identified.[44] Ultrarapid metabolizers may fail to respond to drugs that are inactivated by CYP2D6* (e.g., the antianxiety agent nortryptiline) or may exhibit

Table 8.2 Polymorphisms in Cytochrome CYP2D6[a]

CYP2D6 allele[b]	Nucleotide changes and their locations											People from
	C→T	C→A	A→G	C→G	C→T	C→T	G→C	G→C	G→A	C→T	G→C	
2							1749		2938		4268	Europe
4A	188	1062	1072	1085			1749	1934			4268	Europe
4B	188	1062	1072	1085				1934			4268	Europe
10A	188						1749				4268	Japan
10B	188			1127			1749				4268	China
10C	188			1127			1749				4268	China
17					1111	1726			2938		4268	Africa

[a]Compiled from data in (45) and (46) by W. Kalow (private communication).
[b]The variants 4A and 4B represent enzymes without activity. All others have reduced activity compared to the wild type.

exaggerated toxicity to agents that are activated by CYP2D6* (e.g., the analgesic codeine).

Population studies have been performed on more than 10,000 subjects since the discovery of the *CYP2D6** polymorphism in the 1970s. Table 8.2 (W. Kalow, private communication) concisely describes the extent of ethnic variation of people from Africa, Asia, and Europe with 11 nucleotide changes belonging to 7 CYP2D6 allelic variants.[45,46] Certain mutations (G → C at nt 4268) are shared by people from all three continental regions suggesting the mutation probably occurred before evolutionary separation. Other mutations occur in people within particular regions such as the C → T at nt 1127 in China, or the G → C at nt 1726 in Africa suggesting that these mutations probably occurred after evolutionary separation.

The prevalence of CYP2D6 poor metabolizers, phenotypes (Figure 8.4)[47] and ultrarapid metabolizers (Figure 8.5)[48] varies considerably from one population, and subpopulation, to another. The frequency of the poor metabolizers varies from about 0.1% in Japanese and Egyptians and up 10% in Caucasians of Europe and North America, and one study reported an absence of this phenotype in Cunas Amerindians of Panama.[42] In Europeans, poor metabolizers of debrisoquine are also poor metabolizers of sparteine, but among Ghanians, poor metabolizers of debrisoquine (and phenformin) are not poor metabolizers of sparteine.[49] The reason for this lack of concordance has not been determined.

Individuals of the ultrarapid metabolizer phenotype possess *CYP2D6L** 2, 3, 4, 5, and 13 copies of the *CYP2D6L* gene in one allele.[50] The ethnic distribution of ultrarapid metabolizer phenotypes in Northern European populations summarized in Table 8.3[51] shows that Swedes and Germans possess 1–2% of the CYP2D6L ultrarapid phenotype, whereas the frequency of ultrarapid carriers in Ethiopia[52] and in Saudi Arabia (20%) (not shown in Table 8.3)[48] is much higher. Spaniards also have a high proportion of individuals carrying amplified *CYP2D6L** genes, presumably due to the admixture of African genes.[53,54]

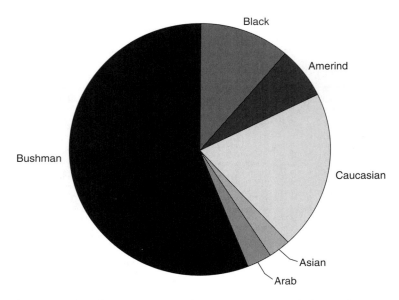

Figure 8.4 Racial differences among CYP2D6 poor metabolizer phenotypes in various ethnic populations.

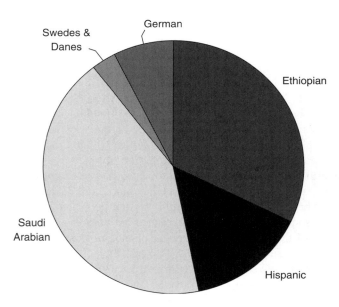

Figure 8.5 Racial differences in CYP2D6 ultrarapid metabolizer phenotypes among various ethnic populations.

Table 8.3 Ethnic Distribution of CYP2D6 Ultrarapid Metabolizers[51]

CYP2D6 Allele	Allele frequency (%)			
	Swedes	Germans	Spaniards	Ethiopians
1×2	0	0.5	nd	nd
2×2	1.5	1.3	3.5–5	13
2×3	0.2	0	nd	1.6
2×4	0	0	nd	0.8
2×5	0	0	nd	0.4
2×13	0.1	0	nd	0

Ingelman-Sundberg proposed that certain dietary components may have exerted selective pressure to explain the preservation of alleles with multiple CYP2D6* copies.[51,55] He suggested that the presence of CYP2D6* alleles, which have a very high affinity for various plant-derived alkaloids, could provide a high detoxification potential for individuals exposed to diets containing these substances. In support of this hypothesis he notes that very few CYP2D6* with inactivating mutations are found in Ethiopia and Saudi Arabia.

Polymorphic variants of CYP2C19* also exhibit significant ethnic variation. The CYP2C19* polymorphism, originally identified as the mephenytoin polymorphism, is a recessively (codominantly) inherited trait that is important because it determines the metabolic elimination of at least 15% of prescribed drugs, including antiulcer proton pump inhibitors such as omeprazole and pantoprazole, the antimalarial proguanil, and a number of barbiturate hypnotics. The frequency of CYP2C19* poor metabolizers is 2–5% in Caucasians but is much higher in Oriental populations (13–23%). The data on specific CYP2C19 variants indicate the frequency of poor metabolizers with the m1 (CYP2C19*2) variant is high in Japanese compared to Caucasians. Another variant, m2 (CYP2C19*3), occurs in Japanese and Africans but has not been detected in Caucasians. The wt, m1, and m2 variants account for almost 100% of the variation in Chinese and Japanese poor metabolizers, but these and additional allelic variants account for only about 92% of the variation in Caucasians.[56]

Two other features regarding ethnic variation in CYP2D6 and CYP2C19 are brought out by the study of Evans and colleagues. They determined the frequencies of these polymorphisms in Filipinos in Bombay and Saudi Arabians in Riyadh and compared them with historical frequencies in Asian and Caucasian populations.[57] Saudi Arabians and other Middle Easterners resemble Europeans in the frequency of CYP2C19 poor metabolizers, but resemble Asians in the frequency of CYP2D6 poor metabolizers. Because of these findings, Middle Eastern populations should be relatively well protected from adverse drug reactions associated with both these recessive phenotypes. Moreover, the distribution of the frequency of the recessive CYP2C19 allele controlling poor metabolism as measured in 18 populations residing at various longitudes is related to longitude. Thus, there is a longitudinal cline that contains an apparent discontinuity between Riyadh and Bombay.

Potassium Channel Polymorphisms and the Long QT Syndrome

Ackerman and colleagues have shown that there are striking differences in risk of sudden death among various ethnic groups that are predisposed to the long QT syndrome (LQTS).[58] The LQTS is recognized as a primary channelopathy caused by mutations in five genes that encode cardiac channel subunits. To determine the spectrum, frequency, and ethnic sensitivity of channel variants genomic DNA from 744 apparently healthy subjects was subjected to comprehensive mutational analysis—305 blacks, 187 whites, 134 Asians, and 118 Hispanics were included. Overall, 49 distinct amino acid-altering variants, 36 new, were identified. Two known common polymorphisms, *K897T-HERG* and *G38S-minK,* were identified in all four ethnic groups. Excluding the common polymorphisms, 25% of black subjects had at least one nonsynonymous potassium channel variant compared with 14% of white subjects ($p < 0.01$).

Interestingly, 86% (42/49) of the variants were ethnic specific, with 26 variants found in blacks only, 12 in whites, 2 in Asians, and 2 in Hispanics only. Every variant identified in white, Asian, and Hispanic subjects was confined to the cytoplasmic N- and C-terminal domains of the channel subunits. Of the 11 *KVLQT1* variants found in blacks, four were localized to key structural (transmembrane-spanning) domains.

This study shows that after excluding the common polymorphisms, approximately one in three black subjects and one in seven white subjects harbor one or more potassium channel variants. Thus, functionally relevant variants in cardiac channels are significantly more frequent in blacks than in other ethnic groups, and are of greater channel diversity in black subjects. Whether individuals harboring such channel variants are at greater risk of lethal arrhythmias is not known but warrants careful scrutiny.

CCR5Δ32 Polymorphism

The chemokine coreceptor CCR5 is required for attachment and infectivity of HIV-1. A 32-base pair deletion of this receptor gene, *CCR5Δ32,* yields a nonfunctional receptor that blocks entry of HIV-1 and slows progression of AIDS in adult patients.[59–61] A genotype survey of 38 ethnic populations including 4166 individuals revealed a cline of CCR5Δ32 allele frequencies of 0–14% across Eurasia but the variant is absent in African, American Indian, and East Indian ethnic groups.[62] Its rarity or absence in non-Caucasian populations led to the speculation that the mutation occurred only once in the ancestry of Caucasians, subsequent to the separation of Caucasians from African ancestors estimated to be 150,000–200,000 years ago. Based on haplotype analysis combined with linkage analysis to two microsatellite loci, the origin of the CCR5Δ32-containing ancestral haplotype was estimated to be ~700 years ago (range 275–1875 years). The geographic cline and its recent emergence suggested a historic event, possibly a widespread fatal epidemic of a pathogen such as HIV-1 or another infectious agent such as *Shigella, Salmonella,* or *Mycobacterium tuberculosis* that utilizes CCR5, elevating its frequency in ancestral Caucasian populations. An alternative hypothesis suggests that epidemics of bubonic plague or smallpox may provide a better explanation for its prevalence in Caucasian populations.[63]

ETHNICITY AS A STARTING POINT FOR PHARMACOGENETIC INVESTIGATION

It follows from the preceding discussion that extrapolation across different ethnogeographic groups for a given trait and a given drug may not be permissible. On the other hand, observations on ethnic specificity may be useful in other ways, e.g., to improve the diagnosis and clinical care of patients or to provide a fuller understanding of a given trait. For example, African, Mediterranean, and Oriental males affected by G6PD deficiency may be more susceptible to hemolysis induced by exposure to more than 200 therapeutics, but the potential to cause clinically significant hemolysis of drugs and other agents may differ from that among Caucasians. Thus, several agents (e.g., trinitrotoluene, quinidine, nitrofurazone, chloramphenicol) are capable of inducing hemolytic reactions of greater severity and of longer duration among Caucasians than among G6PD-deficient African-Americans.[31]

Another example concerns ethnic differences in response to alcohol. Screening of various populations indicates that an alcohol dehydrogenase (ALDH2) deficiency occurs at varying frequencies (8–45%) in populations of Mongoloid origin but is not found in Caucasian or Negroid populations. Facial flushing, an acute vasomotor dilation in response to ethanol, has attracted attention by its association with variant forms of ALDH2. Among Japanese, homozygotes and most heterozygotes for the atypical ("Asian") ALDH2 are flushers, while those homozygous for the usual ALDH2 are nonflushers. Nearly 86% of Japanese subjects who always experienced facial flushing have inactive ALDH2, whereas infrequent flushing or an absence of flushing is associated with active ALDH2.[64] As a consequence of the aversive vascular effects of ethanol, Japanese men and women with the "Asian" form of ALDH2 drink significantly less alcohol than those with the "Caucasian" form, and are more highly protected from alcoholism.[65] Thus, ethnic variations have shown that flushing may act as a deterrent to ethanol abuse, but may also serve as a useful biomarker of the "Asian" ALDH2 phenotype that is easily perceived by patients and physicians.

A patient who exhibits an unexpected clinical response to a drug whose disposition and metabolism are dependent on a known pharmacogenetic trait characterized by ethnic specificities poses another situation of therapeutic interest. It should raise the question of whether the ethnicity of the patient suggests a basis for the response. Consider the *CYP2D6** polymorphism as the trait of interest. As already mentioned, the disposition of many commonly used therapeutic agents is subject to control by this polymorphism, and differences in response to medicines between the extreme CYP2D6* phenotypes, the poor and ultrarapid phenotypes, can be quite dramatic (see Chapter 2). Since the frequency of *CYP2D6** poor metabolizers is significantly higher among Africans and Caucasians compared to

Asians, an unexpected response to any given drug might be expected to occur more frequently among the former populations. Thus, the failure of poor metabolizers to experience analgesia from codeine[66,68] and to be protected against dependence on the oral opiates would be more likely to occur among Africans and Caucasians than among Asian patients.[69] Since poor metabolizers are more likely to experience interactions with other drugs[70] and to experience the neurotoxic effects of amphetamine analogs such as 3,4-methylenedioxymethamphetamine (MDMA, also referred to as "Ecstasy"),[71] these unexpected responses would also be expected to occur more frequently among Africans and Caucasians than among Asians. Similar considerations may apply to the analysis of the basis for an unexpected response to a given drug in connection with ethnic differences in the ultrarapid metabolizer phenotype. Accordingly, the unexpected failure to respond to nortriptyline,[41] or of an unexpected exaggerated response of *CYP2D6** ultrarapid metabolizers to codeine,[66] would be expected to occur more frequently among African or Saudi Arabian patients than among Asian patients. Consequently, when a patient experiences an unexpected response to a given drug, the physician should consider whether the ethnic or geographic origin of the patient suggests a basis for the response.

The use of probe substrates alone or in various combinations to assess the contribution is noted in Appendix B, but caution should be observed in the selection of probe drugs for phenotyping in different ethnic populations. Wennerholm and colleagues evaluated four different CYP2D6 probes (codeine, debrisoquine, dextromethorphan, and metoprolol) in whites and in black Tanzanian subjects carrying the African-specific *CYP2D6*17* and *29* alleles.[68] The data showed that *CYP2D6*17* has altered substrate specificity *in vivo* compared with the common CYP2D6 variants in white subjects, and that the *CYP2D6*29* variant contributes to slower metabolism of some CYP2D6 substrates in black Tanzanians.

Further study of genetically variable phenotypes exhibiting ethnic specificity may also provide new information about the structures of the genes and regulatory pathways that may be responsible for unexpected or unusual drug responses. Thus, ethnic specificity due to inactive or low activity enzymes, or to other defective protein variants, may be explained alternatively as a deletion of an entire gene,[72,73] as truncated genes,[74,75] and as missense mutations of the coding region.[76,77] Consider, for example, differences at the CYP2D locus between Chinese and Caucasians.[78] Up to 50% of CYP2D6 alleles are accounted for by a variant in which a mutation at residue 34 replaces serine with proline. This substitution results in an unstable enzyme with lower mean CYP2D6 activity in Chinese persons compared to that in Caucasians, which explains the relatively slower metabolism of drug substrates for CYP2D6 and the lower doses of antidepressant and neuroleptic drugs that are used among Chinese. Examples involving interethnic variation in which phenotypes are due to high activity enzymes may be explained as regulatory variants,[79] as kinetic variants,[80,81] and as duplicated genes.[50,82]

Another excellent example to illustrate how ethnic differences in dietary habits may provide a starting point for pharmacogenetic investigation of evolutionary issues is provided by the analysis of lactase nonpersistence (lactose intolerance). Lactase nonpersistence is a genetically unusual autosomal recessive trait that is determined by a polymorphic gene (LCT) as described in Appendix A. LCT is located on chromosome 2q21.[83,84] For many years efforts to find LCT variants responsible for lactase persistence proved fruitless; but it was suggested that a *cis*-acting element contributed to this phenotype.[85,86] In 2002 a breakthrough occurred when a C/T single nucleotide polymorphism (SNP) located in the 13th intron of a completely different gene, MCM6, was found to be strongly associated with the trait in Finnish families.[84] Sequence analysis of the complete 47-kb region of interest and association analysis revealed that a SNP DNA variant, C/T–13910, approximately 14 kb upstream of but separate from the LCT locus, was completely associated with lactase nonpersistence. A second variant, G/A–22018, 8 kb telomeric to C/T-13910 was also associated with the trait.[84] Tissue-based and *in vitro* functional assays met the requirement that the variant had a *cis*-acting effect on LCT promoter activity, and the occurrence of the variant C/T-13910 in distantly related populations indicated that it was very old. However, follow-up studies showed that while this SNP was a good predictor of lactase persistence in Europeans, it was a poor predictor in Africans even though they harbored what appeared to be lactase nonpersistent alleles.[87] Pursuit of the possibility that African populations must harbor one or more additional variants that confer a similar lactase-persistence phenotype resulted in a second breakthrough by Tishkoff and colleagues.[88] They sampled patterns of variation in 43 African ethnic populations, including dairying and nondairying groups, and discovered a new SNP, G/C-14010, that was also located in intron 13 of MCM6, and was significantly associated with lactase persistence. And like the C/T–13910 variant, it seemed to affect LCT promoter activity. Thus, Africans and Finns show similar patterns of lactase persistence but composed of different genetic variants.

In commenting on the discoveries of Enattah et al.[84] and Tishkoff et al.,[88] Wooding draws attention to the extraordinary evolutionary significance that attaches to these findings.[89] Taken together, they tell us that divergent human populations have been under similar pressures involving milk, the main source of dietary carbohydrate, and have converged on the same solution of prolonging lactase phlorizin hydrolase (LPH) expression into adulthood. Not only are they a testament to the powerful evolutionary influence culture can exert on our genes, but they show it has done so at least twice in different regions of the world.

Ethnic Differences in Quantitative Gene Expression

The discovery of racial differences in phenylthiocarbamide (PTC) taste sensitivity in the 1930s and 1940s first alerted biologists to population variations in the human drug response (see Figure 1.3). Since the demonstration of raciogeographic variation in polymorphisms of G6PD and isoniazid (NAT2) acetylation in the 1950s, allele-specific differences in gene expression between ethnic populations has been an important part of pharmacogenetic analysis. Originally, allele-specific differences in levels of gene expression were primarily associated with epigenetic phenomena during development, with genomic X-inactivation and genomic imprinting being notable examples (see Chapter 6). More recent studies have shown that differences in allele-specific gene expression among nonimprinted autosomal genes are also relatively common.[90,91] Such differences have also been shown to be heritable,[92] and can be mapped as quantitative traits.[90,93]

Extensive pharmacogenetic studies of numerous metabolic and receptor traits, including G6PD deficiency and isoniazid acetylation (NAT2), have shown that nonsynonymous, allele-specific, coding sequence polymorphisms capable of modifying protein structure and function account for the ethnic variation in human drug response that has been identified. However, the proportion of the total variation in human genetic diversity for which such variations account is unclear. In contrast to coding sequence polymorphisms where the consequences of nonsynonymous polymorphisms can be identified at the level of the protein phenotype, the genetic cause or causes of quantitative variation are more difficult to define. More than 30 years ago, shortly after the discovery of the genetic code and before the invention of recombinant DNA technologies, Mary-Claire King and Allan Wilson performed a study to determine the genetic distance between humans and chimpanzees from comparisons of human and chimpanzee proteins. Of particular interest to this discussion were the conclusions that a relatively small number of genetic changes in gene expression systems, which they ascribed to redundancies in the genetic code or to differences in nontranscribed regions of the genome, were more likely to account for the major organismal differences between humans and chimpanzees than changes in amino acid sequences. Today, there is growing evidence at experimental and population levels that genetic variations in nontranscribed regions of the genome, as in regulatory sequences of the 5' and 3' untranslated regions, may underlie a substantial fraction of complex human disorders including ethnic variations of human drug responses.[90,93] Other recent studies point to the possibility that synonymous polymorphisms, in contrast to nonsynonymous polymorphisms, may account, in part, for quantitative variations in protein phenotypes[94–96] (see pp. 35 and 363).

Spielman et al.[97] recently extended the genetic analysis of population differences from qualitative phenotypes to the quantitative expression level of genes. They determined the proportion of gene expression phenotypes that differed significantly between populations and the extent to which the phenotypic differences were attributable to specific genetic polymorphisms. Measurements of gene expression were made with the Affymetrix Genome Focus Array on annotated genes expressed in transformed lymphoblastoid cell lines from 142 persons of three populations taken from the International HapMap Project.[98] Among 1097 gene expression phenotypes, 35 genes whose mean expression differed by 2-fold or more were identified from a total of 4197 genes expressed in the lymphoblastoid cell lines. Among the 1097 expression phenotypes, about 25% of those tested, there were marked differences in allele frequencies between populations. For the phenotypes with the strongest evidence of *cis* determinants, most of the variation was due to allele frequency differences at *cis*-linked regulators. Overall, Spielman et al. found that at least 25% of the gene expression phenotypes differed significantly between major population groups, and that specific genetic variations in allele frequency accounted for the difference in the most significant instances among the phenotypes that were *cis* regulated. In 11 phenotypes studied in detail, expression phenotypes were also largely attributable to frequency differences at the DNA level. They note that variants in coding regions of candidate genes do not account for a large proportion of disease susceptibility,[91] and they speculate, but do not demonstrate, that quantitative variations in gene expression are responsible instead.

In his review of regulatory polymorphisms underlying complex disease traits, Knight shows that allele-specific effects on gene expression are relatively common, are typically of modest magnitude, and are context specific.[91] To date, most research has focused on the modulation of expression of regulatory polymorphisms by the process of transcriptional initiation. The functional characterization of such polymorphisms is problematic because of the many potential confounders of commonly used functional assays, and because many of the studies on allele-specific transcription factor binding and promoter analysis demonstrate no definitive mechanism beyond relative allelic differences in levels of transcription. Ways in which regulatory polymorphisms may act to alter gene expression are shown by modulation of transcriptional regulation of the Duffy binding protein, by modulation of alternative splicing at *CTLA4* encoding cytotoxic T lymphocyte antigen, and by modulation of translational efficiency by the serine protease factor, *F12* (XII). To advance further our understanding of regulatory polymorphisms on gene expression, the role of DNA sequence polymorphisms will need to be considered more broadly in modulating gene expression.

ETHNIC SPECIFICITY IN DRUG DEVELOPMENT

The ultimate purpose of pharmacogenetic investigation is to gather information that provides clues to the basis for an unexpected drug response and enables the expression of a given trait in susceptible persons to be avoided or managed safely and effectively. In essence, the genetics (mode of inheritance, allelic frequencies, ethnic and geographic specificities) and molecular basis (genes responsible and their mutation spectrum) constitute the information that characterizes a given pharmacogenetic trait. Clearly, information on ethnogeographic variations in response of individuals contributes to these categories of information and lacking such global information could severely compromise efforts to optimize the development and clinical testing of new drugs.

CULTURALLY SPECIFIC RISKS OF ETHNIC RESEARCH

The potential risks that genetic studies pose for individual participants are commonly required in informed consent documents by funding agencies and institutional ethics review boards charged with protecting human subjects. For this reason, most experienced investigators are familiar with them. However, these risks are to be contrasted with culturally specific risks that include discrimination or stigmatization of a study population, as well as adverse associations that may be detrimental to the population. Comprehensive consideration of these matters is beyond the primary scope of this book, but they should be addressed because of their importance to the assessment of the effect of ethnogeographic factors on human drug response. The brief comments that follow rely mainly on the writings and recommendations of authors whose primary expertise concerns these issues.[10,19,99,100]

Various types of culturally specific risks should be distinguished. They include what have been termed "external" risks, that is, harms that are inflicted by individuals who are not members of the study population. Perhaps the most important of these is overt racism. Populations with unique legal and political status might also be challenged by genetic findings. Genetic information might also undermine a group's ability to assert legal claims for land or for items of cultural inheritance based on oral history or tradition. Such information can also be interpreted by members of a study population in a manner that can disrupt the established social order of their shared community. Moreover, certain targeted genetic screening programs have raised concerns that can present barriers to broad participation in beneficial tests. Because they are culturally defined, outsiders may not be able to anticipate such risks.

Another type of risk involves the potential for disruption of existing relationships within families or between social groups that may arise from recruitment of community members for any purpose as part of a study, but particularly for matters relating to health. Additionally, genetic tests that are meant to identify predisposition to disease may be viewed as interfering with or usurping traditional functions for prevention in the community. The modification of research designs may be necessary to accommodate specific concerns.

Publication of genetic findings can also disrupt existing social arrangements, especially if the study populations are powerless to contest claims made about them. To suggest, for example, that a socially homogeneous population is biologically, and hence ancestrally more heterogeneous than previously thought could affect the social standing of an entire community. In one study, genealogical research combined with linkage analysis indicated a significantly greater admixture of European heritage that was acknowledged by the study participants. Claims to Native ancestry were thereby reduced, which in turn threatened opportunities for leadership in the community.

Investigators with experience in working with indigenous communities have learned that a research study that bypasses a community's decision-making process by relying solely on individual informed consent presents a risk that may undermine moral authority within the community. Individuals who decide to participate in a study on this basis may invite problems where a process of collective decision making is customary prior to individual choice. If individuals voice their opinions before a community consensus emerges, it may call into question both the authority of that consensus and the collective decision-making process that produced it. On the other hand, decisions by outsiders or by arbitrarily selected local representatives can be equally hazardous to the performance of the study.

Researchers who engage constituents of a prospective study population in a more thorough discussion of a proposed study than is gained by a standard informed consent statement can be helpful in clarifying the goals and approaches to the study. Members of the population to be studied may help to identify and minimize risks that may not be obvious to outsiders. Unarticulated concerns and fears may come to light that can lead to controversy and undermine recruitment participants, or their willingness to embrace diagnostic and therapeutic methods developed from the study. By learning how members of diverse study populations perceive risk, investigators will improve their chances of assessing specific benefits that information on human genetic variation offers and of communicating risks that may be associated with such variation.

SUMMARY

Africa is believed to be the cradle of the most recent ancient ancestors of modern humans and estimates indicate their expansion out of Africa began about 92,000 to 156,000 years ago. Based on geographic, anthropological, linguistic, and ethnic criteria, evolutionists divide human populations into Negroid, Mongoloid, and Caucasoid races where race is defined as a large group of individuals that has a significant fraction of its genes in common and can be distinguished by its gene pool. Population frequencies of many pharmacogenetic traits depend on race or ethnic specificity and may differ greatly within and between raciogeographic groups. Pharmacogenetic variants may be shared by different populations if they occurred before evolutionary separation, but may be specific for a population if they occurred after separation. Person-to-person differences in drug disposition, efficacy, and toxicity across ethnogeographic populations are closely associated with differences in allelic frequencies of genes that determine these events. These differences are valuable as starting points for pharmacogenetic research, for individualization of drug therapy, and for improving the efficiency of development and clinical trials of new drugs. Culturally specific risks may be encountered in diverse study populations in conducting research to discover ethnic variation, and investigators will improve their chances of assessing specific benefits if they are prepared to modify their research design and conduct to accommodate them.

REFERENCES

1. Marshall EK, Lynch V, Smith HW. On dichloroethylsulfide (Mustard gas). II. Variation in susceptibility of the skin to dichloroethylsulfide. JPET 1918; 12: 291–301.
2. Weber WW. Populations and genetic polymorphisms. Molec Diagnosis 1999; 4(4):299–307.

3. Cavalli-Sforza LL, Menozzi C, Piazza A. The History and Geography of Human Genes, 1st ed. Princeton, NJ: Princeton University Press, 1994.

4. Burchard EG, Ziv E, Coyle N, Gomez SL, Tang H, Karter AJ, et al. The importance of race and ethnic background in biomedical research and clinical practice. N Engl J Med 2003; 348(12):1170–1175.

5. Hirschfeld L, Hirschfeld H. Serological differences between the blood of different races. Lancet 1919; 2(Oct 18):675–679.

6. Itano H, Robinson ER. Genetic control of the α- and β-chains of hemoglobin. Proc Natl Acad Sci USA 2004; 46(11):1492–1501.

7. Ingram VM. Gene evolution and the haemoglobins. Nature 1961; 189:704–708.

8. Smithies O, Connell GE, Dixon GH. Chromosomal rearrangements and the evolution of haptoglobin genes. Nature 1962; 196:232–236.

9. Baglioni C. The fusion of two peptide chains in hemoglobin Lepore and its interpretation as a genetic deletion. Proc Natl Acad Sci USA 1962; 48:1880–1886.

10. Foster MW, Sharp RR. Race, ethnicity, and genomics: Social classifications as proxies of biological heterogeneity. Genome Res 2002; 12(6):844–850.

11. Barbujani G, Magagni A, Minch E, Cavalli-Sforza LL. An apportionment of human DNA diversity. Proc Natl Acad Sci USA 1997; 94(9, Apr 29):4516–4519.

12. Schwartz RS. Racial profiling in medical research. N Engl J Med 2001; 344(18): 1392–1393.

13. Cavalli-Sforza LL, Piazza A, Menozzi P, Mountain J. Reconstruction of human evolution: Bringing together genetic, archaeological, and linguistic data. Proc Natl Acad Sci USA 1988; 85(16):6002–6006.

14. Goldstein DB, Ruiz LA, Cavalli-Sforza LL, Feldman MW. Genetic absolute dating based on microsatellites and the origin of modern humans. Proc Natl Acad Sci USA 1995; 92(15):6723–6727.

15. Exner DV, Dries DL, Domanski MJ, Cohn JN. Lesser response to angiotensin-converting-enzyme inhibitor therapy in black as compared with white patients with left ventricular dysfunction. N Engl J Med 2001; 344(18):1351–1357.

16. Yancy CW, Fowler MB, Colucci WS, Gilbert EM, Bristow MR, Cohn JN, et al. Race and the response to adrenergic blockade with carvedilol in patients with chronic heart failure. N Engl J Med 2001; 344(18):1358–1365.

17. Wood AJ. Racial differences in the response to drugs—pointers to genetic differences. N Engl J Med 2001; 344(18):1394–1396.

18. Wilson JF, Weale ME, Smith AC, Gratrix F, Fletcher B, Thomas MG, et al. Population genetic structure of variable drug response. Nat Genet 2001; 29(3): 265–269.

19. Kaplan JB, Bennett T. Use of race and ethnicity in biomedical publication. JAMA 2003; 289(20):2709–2716.

20. Cooper RS, Kaufman JS, Ward R. Race and genomics. N Engl J Med 2003; 348(12):1166–1170.

21. Mamiya K, Kojima K, Yukawa E, Higuchi S, Ieiri I, Ninomiya H, et al. Phenytoin intoxication induced by fluvoxamine. Ther Drug Monit 2001; 23(1):75–77.

22. Taylor AL, Ziesche S, Yancy C, Carson P, D'Agostino R Jr, Ferdinand K, et al. Combination of isosorbide dinitrate and hydralazine in blacks with heart failure. N Engl J Med 2004; 351(20):2049–2057.

23. Xie H-G, Kim RB, Wood AJJ, Stein CM. Molecular basis of ethnic differences in drug disposition and response. Annu Rev Pharmacol Toxicol 2001; 41:815–850.

24. Wood Jr WB. Anemia during sulfanilamide therapy. JAMA 1938; 111(Nov 19): 1916–1919.

25. Earle DP, Bigelow FS, Zubrod CG, Kane CA. Studies on the chemotherapy of the human malarias. IX. Effect of pamaquine on the blood cells of man. J Clin Invest 1948; 27:121–129.

26. Hockwald RS, Arnold J, Clayman CB. Toxicity of primaquine in negroes. JAMA 1952; 149:1568–1570.

27. Dern RJ, Weinstein IM, Leroy GV, Talmage DW, Alving AS. The hemolytic effect of primaquine. I. The localization of the drug-induced hemolytic defect in primaquine-sensitive individuals. J Lab Clin Med 1954; 43(2):303–309.

28. Flanagan CL, Beutler E, Dern RJ, Alving AS. Biochemical changes in erythrocytes during hemolysis induced by aniline derivatives. J Lab Clin Med 1954; 46:814.

29. Beutler E, Dern RJ, Flanagan CL, Alving AS. The hemolytic effect of primaquine. VII. Biochemical studies of drug-sensitive erythrocytes. J Lab Clin Med 1955; 45(2):286–295.

30. Beutler E. The glutathione instability of drug-sensitive red cells; a new method for the in vitro detection of drug sensitivity. J Lab Clin Med 1957; 49(1):84–95.

31. Kirkman HN. Glucose-6-phosphate dehydrogenase variants and drug-induced hemolysis. Ann NY Acad Sci 1968; 151(2):753–764.

32. Hirono A, Beutler E. Molecular cloning and nucleotide sequence of cDNA for human glucose-6-phosphate dehydrogenase variant A(-). Proc Natl Acad Sci USA 1988; 85(11):3951–3954.

33. Beutler E. The molecular biology of G6PD variants and other red cell enzyme defects. Annu Rev Med 1992; 43:47–59.

34. Weber WW. The acetylator genes and drug response. New York: Oxford University Press, 1987.

35. Sunahara S, Urano M, Ogawa M. Genetical and geographic studies on isoniazid inactivation. Science 1961; 134:1530–1531.

36. Karim AK, Elfellah MS, Evans DA. Human acetylator polymorphism: Estimate of allele frequency in Libya and details of global distribution. J Med Genet 1981; 18(5):325–330.

37. Lewontin RC. The Genetic Basis of Evolutionary Change. New York: Columbia University Press, 1974.

38. Cavalli-Sforza LL, Bodmer WF. The Genetics of Human Populations. San Francisco: W.H. Freeman, 1971.

39. Grant DM, Hughes NC, Janezic SA, Goodfellow GH, Chen HJ, Gaedigk A, et al. Human acetyltransferase polymorphisms. Mutat Res 1997; 376(1–2):61–70.

40. Levy GG, Weber WW. Interindividual variability of arylamine acetyltransferases. In: Pacifici G, Pelkonen O, editors. Interindividual variability in drug metabolism in man. London: Taylor & Francis, 2001: 333–357.

41. Bertilsson L, Aberg-Wistedt A, Gustafsson LL, Nordin C. Extremely rapid hydroxylation of debrisoquine: A case report with implication for treatment with nortriptyline and other tricyclic antidepressants. Ther Drug Monit 1985; 7(4):478–480.

42. Arias TD, Jorge LF, Inaba T. No evidence for the presence of poor metabolizers of sparteine in an Amerindian group: The Cunas of Panama. Br J Clin Pharmacol 1986; 21(5):547–548.

43. Zanger UM, Raimundo S, Eichelbaum M. Cytochrome P450 2D6: Overview and update on pharmacology, genetics, biochemistry. Naunyn Schmiedebergs Arch Pharmacol 2004; 369(1):23–37.

44. Dahl ML, Johansson I, Bertilsson L, Ingelman-Sundberg M, Sjoqvist F. Ultrarapid hydroxylation of debrisoquine in a Swedish population. Analysis of the molecular genetic basis. J Pharmacol Exp Ther 1995; 274(1):516–520.

45. Daly AK, Brockmoller J, Broly F, Eichelbaum M, Evans WE, Gonzalez FJ, et al. Nomenclature for human CYP2D6 alleles. Pharmacogenetics 1996; 6(3):193–201.
46. Marez D, Legrand M, Sabbagh N, Guidice JM, Spire C, Lafitte JJ, et al. Polymorphism of the cytochrome P450 CYP2D6 gene in a European population: Characterization of 48 mutations and 53 alleles, their frequencies and evolution. Pharmacogenetics 1997; 7(3):193–202.
47. Kalow W. Interethnic variation of drug metabolism. Trends Pharmacol Sci 1991; 12:102–107.
48. McLellan RA, Oscarson M, Seidegard J, Evans DA, Ingelman-Sundberg M. Frequent occurrence of CYP2D6 gene duplication in Saudi Arabians. Pharmacogenetics 1997; 7(3):187–191.
49. Woolhouse NM, Eichelbaum M, Oates NS, Idle JR, Smith RL. Dissociation of co-regulatory control of debrisoquin/phenformin and sparteine oxidation in Ghanaians. Clin Pharmacol Ther 1985; 37(5):512–521.
50. Johansson I, Lundqvist E, Bertilsson L, Dahl ML, Sjoqvist F, Ingelman-Sundberg M. Inherited amplification of an active gene in the cytochrome P450 CYP2D locus as a cause of ultrarapid metabolism of debrisoquine. Proc Natl Acad Sci USA 1993; 90(24):11825–11829.
51. Ingelman-Sundberg M. The Gerhard Zbinden Memorial Lecture. Genetic polymorphism of drug metabolizing enzymes. Implications for toxicity of drugs and other xenobiotics. Arch Toxicol Suppl 1997; 19:3–13.
52. Aklillu E, Persson I, Bertilsson L, Johansson I, Rodrigues F, Ingelman-Sundberg M. Frequent distribution of ultrarapid metabolizers of debrisoquine in an Ethiopian population carrying duplicated and multiduplicated functional CYP2D6 alleles. J Pharmacol Exp Ther 1996; 278(1):441–446.
53. Agundez JA, Ledesma MC, Ladero JM, Benitez J. Prevalence of CYP2D6 gene duplication and its repercussion on the oxidative phenotype in a white population. Clin Pharmacol Ther 1995; 57(3):265–269.
54. Bernal ML, Sinues B, Johansson I, McLellan RA, Wennerholm A, Dahl ML, et al. Ten percent of North Spanish individuals carry duplicated or triplicated CYP2D6 genes associated with ultrarapid metabolism of debrisoquine. Pharmacogenetics 1999; 9(5):657–660.
55. Ingelman-Sundberg M. The human genome project and novel aspects of cytochrome P450 research. Toxicol Appl Pharmacol 2005; 207(2 Suppl):52–56.
56. Ibeanu GC, Blaisdell J, Ghanayem BI, Beyeler C, Benhamou S, Bouchardy C, et al. An additional defective allele, CYP2C19*5, contributes to the S-mephenytoin poor metabolizer phenotype in Caucasians. Pharmacogenetics 1998; 8(2):129–135.
57. Evans DA, Krahn P, Narayanan N. The mephenytoin (cytochrome P450 2C 19) and dextromethorphan (cytochrome P450 2D6) polymorphisms in Saudi Arabians and Filipinos. Pharmacogenetics 1995; 5(2):64–71.
58. Ackerman MJ, Tester DJ, Jones GS, Will ML, Burrow CR, Curran ME. Ethnic differences in cardiac potassium channel variants: Implications for genetic susceptibility to sudden cardiac death and genetic testing for congenital long QT syndrome. Mayo Clin Proc 2003; 78(12):1479–1487.
59. Liu R, Paxton WA, Choe S, Ceradini D, Martin SR, Horuk R, et al. Homozygous defect in HIV-1 coreceptor accounts for resistance of some multiply-exposed individuals to HIV-1 infection. Cell 1996; 86(3):367–377.
60. Samson M, Libert F, Doranz BJ, Rucker J, Liesnard C, Farber CM, et al. Resistance to HIV-1 infection in Caucasian individuals bearing mutant alleles of the CCR-5 chemokine receptor gene. Nature 1996; 382(6593):722–725.

61. Dean M, Carrington M, Winkler C, Huttley GA, Smith MW, Allikmets R, et al. Genetic restriction of HIV-1 infection and progression to AIDS by a deletion allele of the CKR5 structural gene. Hemophilia Growth and Development Study, Multicenter AIDS Cohort Study, Multicenter Hemophilia Cohort Study, San Francisco City Cohort, ALIVE Study. Science 1996; 273(5283):1856–1862.

62. Chen Q, Kirsch GE, Zhang D, Brugada R, Brugada J, Brugada P, et al. Genetic basis and molecular mechanism for idiopathic ventricular fibrillation. Nature 1998; 392(6673):293–296.

63. Galvani AP, Slatkin M. Evaluating plague and smallpox as historical selective pressures for the CCR5-delta 32 HIV-resistance allele. Proc Natl Acad Sci USA 2003; 100(25):15276–15279.

64. Shibuya A, Yasunami M, Yoshida A. Genotype of alcohol dehydrogenase and aldehyde dehydrogenase loci in Japanese alcohol flushers and nonflushers. Hum Genet 1989; 82(1):14–16.

65. Higuchi S, Muramatsu T, Shigemori K, Saito M, Kono H, Dufour MC, et al. The relationship between low Km aldehyde dehydrogenase phenotype and drinking behavior in Japanese. J Stud Alcohol 1992; 53(2):170–175.

66. Dalen P, Frengell C, Dahl ML, Sjoqvist F. Quick onset of severe abdominal pain after codeine in an ultrarapid metabolizer of debrisoquine. Ther Drug Monit 1997; 19(5):543–544.

67. Gasche Y, Daali Y, Fathi M, Chiappe A, Cottini S, Dayer P, et al. Codeine intoxication associated with ultrarapid CYP2D6 metabolism. N Engl J Med 2004; 351(27):2827–2831.

68. Wennerholm A, Dandara C, Sayi J, Svensson JO, Abdi YA, Ingelman-Sundberg M, et al. The African-specific CYP2D617 allele encodes an enzyme with changed substrate specificity. Clin Pharmacol Ther 2002; 71(1):77–88.

69. Tyndale RF, Droll KP, Sellers EM. Genetically deficient CYP2D6 metabolism provides protection against oral opiate dependence. Pharmacogenetics 1997; 7(5): 375–379.

70. Ozdemir V, Naranjo CA, Herrmann N, Reed K, Sellers EM, Kalow W. Paroxetine potentiates the central nervous system side effects of perphenazine: Contribution of cytochrome P4502D6 inhibition in vivo. Clin Pharmacol Ther 1997; 62(3):334–347.

71. Wu D, Otton SV, Inaba T, Kalow W, Sellers EM. Interactions of amphetamine analogs with human liver CYP2D6. Biochem Pharmacol 1997; 53(11):1605–1612.

72. Gaedigk A, Blum M, Gaedigk R, Eichelbaum M, Meyer UA. Deletion of the entire cytochrome P450 CYP2D6 gene as a cause of impaired drug metabolism in poor metabolizers of the debrisoquine/sparteine polymorphism. Am J Hum Genet 1991; 48(5):943–950.

73. Oscarson M, McLellan RA, Gullsten H, Yue QY, Lang MA, Bernal ML, et al. Characterisation and PCR-based detection of a CYP2A6 gene deletion found at a high frequency in a Chinese population. FEBS Lett 1999; 448(1):105–110.

74. Gonzalez FJ, Skoda RC, Kimura S, Umeno M, Zanger UM, Nebert DW, et al. Characterization of the common genetic defect in humans deficient in debrisoquine metabolism. Nature 1988; 331(6155):442–446.

75. Goldstein JA, de Morais SM. Biochemistry and molecular biology of the human CYP2C subfamily. Pharmacogenetics 1994; 4(6):285–299.

76. Bertina RM, Koeleman BP, Koster T, Rosendaal FR, Dirven RJ, de Ronde H, et al. Mutation in blood coagulation factor V associated with resistance to activated protein C. Nature 1994; 369(6475):64–67.

77. Feder JN, Gnirke A, Thomas W, Tsuchihashi Z, Ruddy DA, Basava A, et al. A novel MHC class I-like gene is mutated in patients with hereditary haemochromatosis. Nat Genet 1996; 13(4):399–408.

78. Johansson I, Oscarson M, Yue QY, Bertilsson L, Sjoqvist F, Ingelman-Sundberg M. Genetic analysis of the Chinese cytochrome P4502D locus: Characterization of variant CYP2D6 genes present in subjects with diminished capacity for debrisoquine hydroxylation. Mol Pharmacol 1994; 46(3):452–459.

79. McCarver DG, Byun R, Hines RN, Hichme M, Wegenek W. A genetic polymorphism in the regulatory sequences of human CYP2E1: Association with increased chlorzoxazone hydroxylation in the presence of obesity and ethanol intake. Toxicol Appl Pharmacol 1998; 152(1):276–281.

80. Buhler R, Hempel J, Von Wartburg JP, Jornvall H. Human liver alcohol dehydrogenase: The unique properties of the "atypical" isoenzyme beta 2 beta 2-Bern can be explained by a single base mutation. Alcohol 1985; 2(1):47–51.

81. McCarver DG, Thomasson HR, Martier SS, Sokol RJ, Li T. Alcohol dehydrogenase-2*3 allele protects against alcohol-related birth defects among African Americans. J Pharmacol Exp Ther 1997; 283(3):1095–1101.

82. McLellan RA, Oscarson M, Alexandrie AK, Seidegard J, Evans DA, Rannug A, et al. Characterization of a human glutathione S-transferase mu cluster containing a duplicated GSTM1 gene that causes ultrarapid enzyme activity. Mol Pharmacol 1997; 52(6):958–965.

83. Kruse TA, Bolund L, Grzeschik KH, Ropers HH, Sjostrom H, Noren O, et al. The human lactase-phlorizin hydrolase gene is located on chromosome 2. FEBS Lett 1988; 240(1–2):123–126.

84. Enattah NS, Sahi T, Savilahti E, Terwilliger JD, Peltonen L, Jarvela I. Identification of a variant associated with adult-type hypolactasia. Nat Genet 2002; 30(2): 233–237.

85. Wang Y, Harvey CB, Pratt WS, Sams VR, Sarner M, Rossi M, et al. The lactase persistence/non-persistence polymorphism is controlled by a cis-acting element. Hum Mol Genet 1995; 4(4):657–662.

86. Harvey CB, Pratt WS, Islam I, Whitehouse DB, Swallow DM. DNA polymorphisms in the lactase gene. Linkage disequilibrium across the 70-kb region. Eur J Hum Genet 1995; 3(1):27–41.

87. Mulcare CA, Weale ME, Jones AL, Connell B, Zeitlyn D, Tarekegn A, et al. The T allele of a single-nucleotide polymorphism 13.9 kb upstream of the lactase gene (LCT) (C-13.9kbT) does not predict or cause the lactase-persistence phenotype in Africans. Am J Hum Genet 2004; 74(6):1102–1110.

88. Tishkoff SA, Reed FA, Ranciaro A, Voight BF, Babbitt CC, Silverman JS, et al. Convergent adaptation of human lactase persistence in Africa and Europe. Nat Genet 2007; 39(1):31–40.

89. Wooding SP. Following the herd. Nat Genet 2007; 39(1):7–8.

90. Knight JC. Allele-specific gene expression uncovered. Trends Genet 2004; 20(3):113–116.

91. Knight JC. Regulatory polymorphisms underlying complex disease traits. J Mol Med 2005; 83(2):97–109.

92. Wilson W III, Pardo-Manuel d V, Lyn-Cook BD, Chatterjee PK, Bell TA, Detwiler DA, et al. Characterization of a common deletion polymorphism of the UGT2B17 gene linked to UGT2B15. Genomics 2004; 84(4):707–714.

93. King MC, Wilson AC. Evolution at two levels in humans and chimpanzees. Science 1975; 188(4184):107–116.

94. Nackley AG, Shabalina SA, Tchivileva IE, Satterfield K, Korchynskyi O, Makarov SS, et al. Human catechol-O-methyltransferase haplotypes modulate protein expression by altering mRNA secondary structure. Science 2006; 314(5807):1930–1933.

95. Kimchi-Sarfaty C, Oh JM, Kim IW, Sauna ZE, Calcagno AM, Ambudkar SV, et al. A "silent" polymorphism in the MDR1 gene changes substrate specificity. Science 2007; 315(5811):525–528.

96. Komar AA. Genetics. SNPs, silent but not invisible. Science 2007; 315(5811): 466–467.

97. Spielman RS, Bastone LA, Burdick JT, Morley M, Ewens WJ, Cheung VG. Common genetic variants account for differences in gene expression among ethnic groups. Nat Genet 2007; 39:226–231.

98. The International HapMap Consortium. The International HapMap Project. Nature 2003; 426(18/25 Dec):789–796.

99. Foster MW, Sharp RR. Genetic research and culturally specific risks: One size does not fit all. Trends Genet 2000; 16(2):93–95.

100. Andrews L, Nelkin D. Whose body is it anyway? Disputes over body tissue in a biotechnology age. Lancet 1998; 351(9095):53–57.

9

Modeling Human Drug Response

In humans, any approach to assess genetic causation of a pharmacogeneic trait is necessarily indirect. However, a convincing experimental model can often help dissect the genetic basis of the trait, or provide insight into mechanisms responsible for the trait, and may disclose its biological significance under experimental conditions that cannot be met in human experimentation for ethical or methodological reasons. Responders of known genotypes and phenotypes to a toxic chemical can be examined under carefully controlled conditions that reveal the pharmacological and toxicological consequences of a given trait. Even models that may be unsuitable for assessing new drug therapy may yet be excellent for elucidating the molecular basis and physiological mechanisms of human traits. Such studies can turn our thinking toward previously unsuspected pathways and mechanisms, and thereby direct attention toward the acquisition of information that advances our understanding of the human condition. Of course, the findings in any nonhuman model system must be assessed in humans to assess their applicability to the human condition.

Until recently, chance observations of spontaneous mutations in naturally occurring populations of domesticated species or laboratory stocks were the primary source of animal models for genetic research. But there are several disadvantages associated with naturally occurring models of human genetic traits that limit their usefulness for genetic analysis. Frequently, the mutation is rare, making it difficult to find the appropriate model, and the specific genetic defect may be difficult to identify and compare with its human counterpart. Because many domesticated species as well as some of the laboratory species are difficult to breed, and because maturation times may be lengthy, they become very expensive to maintain.

Some of these problems can be avoided by a proper choice of species and strains of laboratory animals to find traits that mimic those of humans. For many years, geneticists have relied mainly on inbred strains, including recombinant, congenic, and recombinant congenic strains for the development of genetic models of human hereditary traits because of the long-term stability of strain characteristics, genetic authenticity, phenotypic uniformity, and the unique combinations of genetic material that occur in individual strains. Most of these desirable features are a result of the homozygosity and isogenicity that is achieved at nearly every gene locus through prolonged inbreeding. Moreover, inbred strains can provide an unlimited supply of replicate genotypes and can be bred to yield new combinations of genes that do not occur in nature.

Many highly inbred strains of mice, rats, hamsters, guinea pigs, and pigeons are commercially available. Additional inbred stocks of laboratory species are maintained independently at universities, research institutes, and governmental laboratories by investigators who are usually willing to supply mating pairs of specialized strains on request at no charge or at nominal cost. Although human and mouse genomes have dominated genome science, the annotation of genomic sequences of several nonmammalian eukaryotic organisms (yeast, fruit fly, nematode, zebrafish) provides additional opportunities to use comparative genomics for pharmacogenomics analysis and therapeutics.

MOUSE MODELS OF PHARMACOGENETIC TRAITS

Modern mouse genetics started around 1900 when Lucien Cuenot in France and William Castle and Abbie Lathrop in the United States generated colonies of mice to study the inheritance of coat color and tumor development. These investigators and their students recognized the relevance of homozygous mice to inheritance studies and Castle and Lathrop established the first inbred strains by brother–sister matings. Many of the more than 450 inbred strains now available are derived from founder populations in the laboratories of these investigators. Subsequently, information on the origin and genetic similarities of these strains was assembled and first charted by Joan Staats.[1] New models are continually being generated and the various techniques and genetic resources that have facilitated their development are reviewed by Bedell and associates[2]; in a companion paper these authors present a status report on the progress that had been made in mouse model development as of 1997 and discuss areas where these models are likely to contribute in the future.[3] Recent compilations of genealogical and genetic data on inbred strains are available at the website (http://www .informatics.jax.org/external/festing/search_form.cgi) and in other electronic sources (see Table 1, http://genetics.nature.com/mouse/).[4]

Several factors favor the mouse as an ideal model for human disease.[2] (1) Mice are cheaper to house and easier to handle than other mammals. (2) Mouse development, and its body plan, physiology, behavior, and diseases have much in common with those of humans. (3) At least 99% of mouse genes are orthologous to human genes. (4) Mouse strains present unequaled opportunities for manipulating mouse genes orthologous to human genes involved in disease or in the disposition of drugs and other exogenous substances through construction of recombinant and congenic inbred strains. Additionally, the mouse genome supports targeted mutagenesis of specific genes by homologous recombination, permitting genes to be altered efficiently and precisely. The tools for the creation of targeted null ("knockout") mutants and transgenic lines are applicable not only to single loci, but to multiple members of gene families and to larger mutational events. The availability of strategies for inducing the tissue-specific expression and temporal manipulation of gene expression has broadened further the landscape for the creation of designer mice. (5) Extensive genetic resources for mice are available. When the human genome initiative was organized, the mouse was chosen as one of five model organisms targeted for the creation of genetic, physical, and sequence maps. By 2002, members of the Mouse International Sequencing Consortium had completed the initial draft of the sequence and a comparative analysis of the mouse genome[5]; at the same time, investigators had created a dense genetic map including more than 12,000 polymorphic markers[6] and a physical map consisting of 16,992 unique simple sequence length polymorphisms (SSLPs, also called microsatellites).[7] In addition, a consensus is being sought to create a publicly available resource of knockout mice and phenotypic data. Currently, information about the Mouse Knockout and Mutation Database is available at http://research.bmn.com/mkmd/ and about the Mouse Genome Database is available at http://www.informatics.jax.org/.[8]

Comparative analysis revealed that the mouse genome is about 14% smaller than the human genome (2.5 gigabases compared to 2.9 gigabases), a difference that is believed to reflect a higher rate of deletion from the mouse genome. It also showed that over 90% of the mouse and human genomes could be partitioned into corresponding conserved regions, and at the nucleotide level, approximately 40% of the human genome could be aligned with the mouse genome representing orthologous sequences that remain in both lineages from the common ancestor. The physical map of the mouse genome constructed by Simon Gregory and colleagues serves as a guide for navigation around the mouse genome.[7] In a separate study, Claire Wade and colleagues demonstrated that genetic variations between strains occur in a pattern of alternating blocks of either a high or low single-nucleotide polymorphism (SNP) rate, typically extending more than 1 megabase. Detailed knowledge of these blocks permits reconstruction of the molecular history and relationships among existing mouse strains and this information can be used to perform association studies by correlating the underlying block structure of genetic variation with differences in phenotype across multiple strains. Wade and her collaborators also note that their study on the mosaic structure of variation in the genome of the laboratory mouse has important implications for the design and interpretation of positional cloning experiments.[9]

The laboratory mouse has thus become a prototype for experimental approaches to the whole of mammalian biology and the leading mammalian system for modeling genetic research on human physiology and disease.[4]

CONSTRUCTING INBRED MOUSE MODELS

Development of tools for the analysis of genetic variation dates back to the tumor transplantation studies conducted by Jensen and Loeb around 1900.[10] These early observations, especially the hunt for histocompatibility genes during the 1940s, revealed a surprising amount of genetic variation in common mouse stocks. Discovery of this variation led to the large collection of inbred strains, the basis of all mouse genetics. In the introductory chapter to his classic book on *The Origins of Inbred Mice*, Herbert Morse quotes Hans Gruneberg, another mouse geneticist of repute, who said "The introduction of inbred strains into biology is probably comparable in importance with that of the analytical balance in chemistry." The concept of congenic strains was conceived by George Snell at the Jackson Laboratory in the 1940s as a tool to dissect histocompatability genes, and recombinant inbred strains were developed in the 1970s by Don Bailey and Ben Taylor, also at the Jackson laboratory, as a further tool for unraveling complex traits in mice.

Recombinant Strains

Recombinant inbred (RI) strains are a set of strains that has been derived from the cross of two unrelated but highly inbred progenitor strains and maintained independently under a regimen of strict inbreeding since the F_2 generation. After 20 generations of systematic brother–sister inbreeding, each new inbred strain that is established contains a unique mixture of the genes of the two parental strains. Once inbred, a given RI strain represents a stable population in which all of the alleles are homozygous. Unlinked genes are randomly distributed in the F_2 generation, while linked genes will tend to become fixed in the same combinations as they were in the parental strains. A set of RI strains derived in this way from the same pair of parental strains as shown in Figure 9.1 provides the tools for genetic analysis of traits.

On reflection, it will be seen that the common inbred strains represent collectively a large set of RI strains.

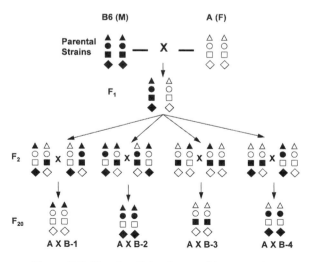

Figure 9.1 Construction of recombinant strains.

Individual strains within a set are customarily named by an abbreviation for the maternal parent strains followed by a capital X followed by the abbreviation for the paternal strain. For instance, in the set derived from maternal A strain mice and paternal C57BL/6 mice, the abbreviations are A and B, and the individual RI strains are designated AXB-1, AXB-2, AXB-3, etc., while those created from maternal B6 and paternal A mice are designated BXA-1, BXA-2, BXA-3, etc.

A long list of studies demonstrates the usefulness of RI strains in single-gene analysis, gene linkage, and gene mapping. An individual RI strain can be typed for specific differences that distinguish the parental strains, and all loci in a given set have a particular pattern called the strain distribution pattern (SDP). Typing of individual strains indicates which of the alleles from the parental strains is fixed in a given strain, and it need be done only once for a particular locus. In a typical analysis of a new genetic variant, the RI set then needs to be typed only for the new locus. Linked loci will often have SDPs that are similar or identical and they then become candidates for conventional methods of linkage analysis. If no linkage is detected, it may be necessary to await the identification of additional differential markers that may reveal linkage.

Once the SDP of an RI set has been determined, linkage of new loci to known loci can be sought by comparisons of their SDPs. Collation of SDPs for many loci for established RI sets was initiated long ago. The fact that the data on SDPs obtained are cumulative affords RI sets an enormous advantage over conventional crosses for mapping and linkage analysis. There is one major drawback of RI strain analysis, namely that only loci that differ in the parental strains can be analyzed. However, the rapidity with which strain differences are being reported at the DNA level by the application of molecular biological and related techniques makes it possible to recognize differences that heretofore were inaccessible.

Congenic Strains

The concept of congenic strains was conceived and developed in the 1940s and 1950s by George Snell as an experimental method by which he sought to reveal the individuality of genes.[11] Congenic strains are genetically identical except for a short chromosomal segment, and hence these strains enable the effects of particular genes to be studied as free as possible from the effects of background genes.

A congenic strain is created by crosses between an inbred partner strain that donates the genetic background and another inbred strain that donates the chromosomal segment followed by a succession of backcrosses. Construction of a congenic strain is illustrated for the A.B6-*Nat^r* rapid acetylator congenic strain (abbreviated A.B6) in Figure 9.2. In accord with the protocol shown there, A and B6 inbred mice are crossed and the heterozygous F1 progeny are crossed back to A (background strain) mice. This scheme is repeated for 12 generations; the heterozygous (rs) progeny are selected from each generation for the next backcross, and the homozygous (ss) progeny are discarded. Theoretically, one-half of the B6 genes are lost at each backcross, and at the 12th generation $\frac{1}{2}^{12}$, or less than

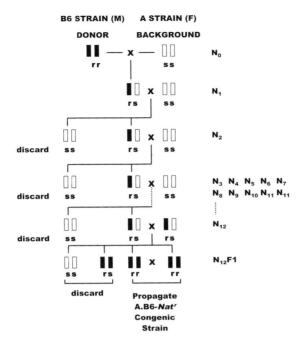

Figure 9.2 Construction of congenic mouse strains.

0.0005 (0.05%) of the B6 genome remains. After the 12th backcross generation, heterozygous (rs) sibling pairs are interbred, and homozygous rapid (rr) acetylator progeny are selected and used to found the A.B6 congenic line. A mirror image procedure can be used to produce the reciprocal slow acetylator congenic line, B6.A-Nat^s, or B6.A for short.

The average length of the chromosomal segment that is donated to the background can be calculated. An approximation of the length in centiMorgans is given by $200/n$ where n is the number of backcross generations, and for a congenic strain created by 12 backcross generations, the inbred partner and its congenic differ by 15–20 cM.

Other methods can be used to create a congenic line; the method chosen depends on the characteristics of the differential allele and whether it affects survival and fertility. The backcross method schematized in Figure 9.2 is applicable when the allele contributed by the donor strain is transmitted as an autosomal dominant or codominant character. The cross–intercross system, which involves a somewhat more complicated mating system, is used when the differential allele is recessive and undetectable in the heterozygous state. Details of this system are given by Flaherty.[12]

Recently, with the advent of complete genetic linkage maps, Lander and Schork proposed a strategy to construct "speed congenics" in only 3–4 generations instead of 12 or more generations according to the standard protocol described above by using marker breeding.[13] Yui et al.[14] and Monel et al.[15] have applied this strategy to the construction of mouse congenic strains while Jeffs et al. have applied a similar strategy to the construction of rat congenic strains.[16]

The vocabulary and symbols customarily applied to congenic strains are set forth by Snell.[11] Individual congenic strains are named by an abbreviation of the background strain (also called the "inbred partner") followed by a period followed by an abbreviation of the donor strain. The rapid acetylator congenic strain diagrammed in Figure 9.2 would be called A.B6-Nat^r where Nat^r is the name of the differential allele contributed by the donor strain. The reciprocal congenic slow acetylator strain, in which B6 is the background strain and A is the donor strain, would be designated B6.A-Nat^s where Nat^s represents the differential slow N-acetyltransferase allele.

The availability of "quartets" provides a tool well suited to the search for the effects of background genes on the expression of a differential allele. The quartet consists of the two parental strains and the reciprocal congenic partner strains derived from them. In the specific illustration referred to earlier, A and B6 are the parental strains while A.B6 and B6.A are the reciprocal congenic strains (Figure 9.2). Differences among various quartet members reveal the background effects that influence the expression of either allele at the differential locus. In this example, comparison of strains A and B6 reveals the effects of the background genes plus the effects of the differential allele (upper and lower panels of Figure 9.3), whereas the comparison of the strains in the column on the left (A and A.B6) or of the column on the right (B6 and B6.A) reveals the effects of allelic differences expressed on different backgrounds. Cross comparisons, as for A vs. B6.A or B6 vs. A.B6, reveals the influence of background differences on the differential alleles.

Other crosses between different quartet members can yield additional information of interest. For instance, comparison of parental (say strain A) mice with the hybrid animals resulting from the cross A × B6.A reveals the influence of the F_1 background relative to that of the inbred background on the expression of the differential allele. And finally, since the chromosomal segments introduced in reciprocal congenic strains are almost inevitably of different lengths, comparison of the F_1 offspring of the parental strains (A × B6) with the F_1s from the reciprocal congenic strains (A.B6 × B6.A) affords a way of assessing the influence of the nonidentical regions that immediately surround the differential allele on its expression.

It is intuitively evident that congenic strains provide a versatile and very powerful method for the analysis of genetic variation.

Double Congenic Mouse Strains

A double congenic strain differs from its inbred background partner at two loci. The two loci are usually unlinked and they may be derived from the same second (donor) strain or different second strains. A double congenic line is created from crosses between two congenic inbred strains. The F_1 progeny are then interbred and the F_2 offspring are typed for both loci. With two unlinked loci, 16 combinations of gametes are possible among F_2 progeny (Figure 9.4). One in 16 offspring

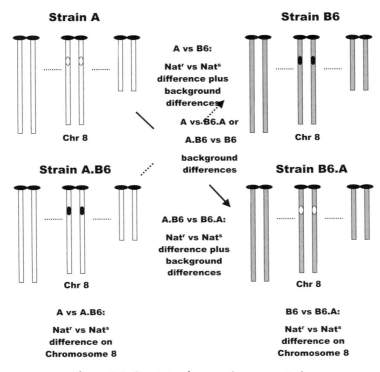

Figure 9.3 Quartets of congenic mouse strains.

has the desired genotype with homozygosity at both loci (ssdd) of interest; sibling pairs with this genotype are selected to found the double congenic strain. Notice that in contrast to the creation of the inbred strain congenic at a single locus described in Figure 9.2, the creation of the double congenic strain requires only four additional generations.

The naming of double congenic strains follows guidelines similar to those given above for lines congenic at a single genetic locus. Consider the double congenic strain for the *Nat* locus on chromosome 8 and the *Ahr* receptor locus on chromosome 12, both placed on the B6 background. This strain has been used to investigate the effects of genetic interactions between the acetylation and *Ahr* receptor polymorphisms (see pp. 271 and 274). The B6.A-Nat^s congenic strain is created from B6 as the normally rapid acetylator background strain and A as the donor strain for the slow acetylator locus, Nat^s according to the protocol described above (see Figure 9.2). The B6.D-Ahr^d congenic strain is created by a similar protocol from B6, a normally high-affinity *Ahr* receptor background strain and DBA/2 as the donor strain for the low-affinity form of the Ahr^d locus. The double congenic line that is created is designated as B6.A-Nat^s.D-Ahr^d, abbreviated B6.A.D.

The quartet of strains consisting of the background strain (B6), each of the single congenic strains (B6.A and B6.D), and the double congenic strain (B6.A.D)

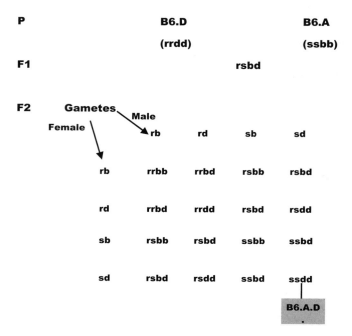

Figure 9.4 Construction of double congenic mouse strains.

is used to assess the effects of one genetic region on another as illustrated in Figure 9.5. Thus, differences between B6 and B6.A.D compared to those between B6 and B6.A will disclose the effect of a segment of chromosome 12 on the expression of the differential *Nat* allele on chromosome 8. Conversely, differences between B6 and B6.A.D compared to those between B6 and B6.D will disclose the effect of a segment on chromosome 8 on the expression of the differential *Ahr* receptor allele on chromosome 12.

Recombinant inbred strains together with congenic strains have been used with great success to investigate a number of qualitative and some quantitative genetically polymorphic traits. These systems are most effective for analysis of traits whose characteristics are determined primarily by a single gene. They can help determine whether more than one gene is involved, and the minimal number that is involved, but cannot identify these loci. Hence they are less effective in studying multifactorial traits.

Recombinant Congenic Strains

In more complex systems, additive and interactive effects obscure or disrupt the association of genotype and phenotype that is required to interpret observed SDPs of recombinant inbred lines. As a means of mapping and investigating the individuality of genes that play a role in multifactorial traits, recombinant congenic strains were developed. In this system, nonlinked genes are sep-

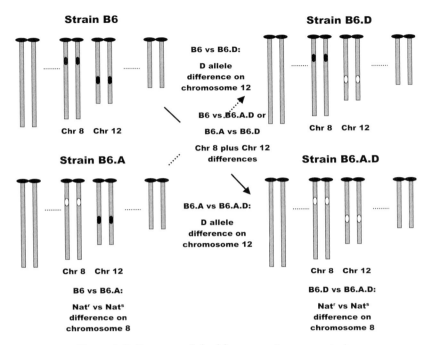

Figure 9.5 Quartets of double congenic mouse strains.

arated in different recombinant congenic strains and are then more accessible to study.

The procedure for producing recombinant congenic strains combines the approaches described above for the construction of recombinant inbred strains and congenic strains. By limited backcrossing of two selected strains and subsequent brother–sister mating, a set of 15–20 strains is produced. Each of the individual strains carries a small fraction of the genome of the donor strain on the genome of the background strain. The number of backcross generations used, unlike that for the production of strains congenic at a single locus, depends on the degree of genetic resolution called for to separate the genes of interest that are transferred. For example, two backcross generations yield an average of 12.5% of the donor genome transferred and 87.5% of the background genome retained, while three backcrosses result in the transfer of 6.25% of the donor genome. Consequently, genes from the donor that are unlinked are likely to be redistributed into different strains. A multigene trait that depends on differential alleles at multiple loci is thereby transformed into a set of single gene differences between the background strain and individual recombinant congenic strains.

Recombinant congenic strains provide a versatile experimental system for separating unlinked loci affecting a given trait, for establishing new linkage relationships for any trait with genes that can be assayed, and if appropriate crosses are made between recombinant congenic strains carrying different genes, they can provide a flexible system for evaluating gene interactions. When recombinant congenic strains are used in combination with mice created by gene targeting (see p. 278), they can be used to assess the influence of the rest of the genome on the expression and function of the targeted gene. In this way, recombinant congenic strains and strains created by gene targeting complement each other. The primary disadvantage of recombinant congenic strains is the same as that for recombinant inbred strains—they can be used to analyze only genes that possess differential alleles at loci of interest.

A considerable amount of information can be collected by polymerase chain reaction in a short time for SSLPs. The SDPs of SSLPs in a set of recombinant congenic strains can then be used to search the mouse genome for new genes involved in the control of polygenic traits. For example, the SDPs of SSLPs in a CcS/Dem set of recombinant congenic strains have been used to search for genes that are involved in the genetic control of colon cancer. The parental strains of the CcS/Dem set, BALB/cHea (background strain) and STS/A (donor strain), differ in the number of colon tumors induced by the carcinogen 1,2-dimethylhydrazine: BALB/c mice are relatively resistant and STS mice are highly sensitive to tumor induction by this agent. Among the set of 20 CcS/Dem recombinant congenic strains created from these parental lines, several were highly sensitive and several were resistant. Each CcS/Dem strain carries a unique subset of about 12.5% of the genes derived from the STS strain on the BALB/c background, and individual STS susceptibility genes are segregated into different recombinant congenic strains. To map the susceptibility of gene(s) present in one of the highly susceptible strains, CcS-19, BALB/c × (BALB/c × CcS-19) F_1 backcross mice were treated with 1,2-dimethylhydrazine. After 6 weeks, the number and size of colon tumors were recorded, and linkage of the susceptibility to the battery of SSLP markers for the STS allele A was tested. A new susceptibility gene (Scc-1) for colon tumors was mapped to chromosome 2 in the vicinity of the SSLP marker. CD44. Scc-1 differs from the oncogenes and tumor suppressor genes known to be involved in colon tumorigenesis. Because the colon tumors induced were significantly larger than those in BALB/c mice, and because the size of the tumors did not segregate with CD44, the investigators also concluded that the number and size of the tumors are controlled by different genes.

Chromosome Substitution Strains (CSSs)

CSSs were originally proposed as an approach to gene identification of complex traits by quantitative trait locus (QTL) analysis[17] (see p. 282). A CSS is an inbred strain in which one chromosome has been substituted from a different inbred strain by repeated backcrossing. The CSS A.B-Chr(i) is thus defined as an inbred strain that is identical to strain A except that chromosome "i" has been substituted by the corresponding chromosome from strain B. In the mouse, a CSS panel consists of 21 strains, corresponding to the 19 autosomes and two sex chromosomes.

The strategy for constructing a CSS as described by Nadeau et al.[17] is shown in Figure 9.6. As a pilot project to test the usefulness of CSSs to dissect genetic factors affecting complex traits, these investigators constructed a complete CSS panel

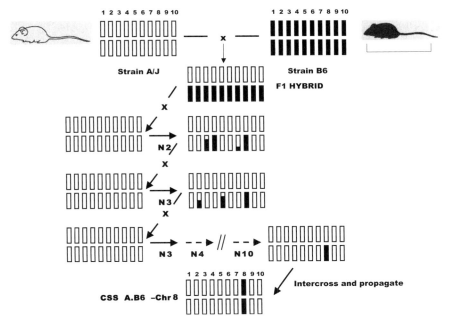

Figure 9.6 Construction of chromosome substitution mouse strains.

using A/J as the donor strain and C57BL/6 as the host strain. A survey conducted to test the ability of the panel to dissect genetic factors affecting representative complex traits revealed evidence for 150 QTLs affecting traits that affected the levels of sterols and amino acids, diet-induced obesity, and anxiety.

This program was not a small task as it required production of about 17,000 mice and about 7 years, although it could perhaps be shortened to about 4 years as a more efficient methodology for selective breeding and genotyping was developed over time. The complete panel, which consists of 21 strains, has been provided to the Jackson Laboratory for preservation and distribution as a research resource.[18]

MOUSE MODELS OF THE ARYLHYDROCARBON RECEPTOR AND N-ACETYLTRANSFERASE POLYMORPHISMS

Interest in the arylhydrocarbon receptor and N-acetyltransferase polymorphisms stems from their roles in toxicity from environmental chemicals. Variant forms of the Ah-receptor protein and of N-acetyltransferase, a drug-metabolizing enzyme protein, are encoded by the responsible genes. The polymorphisms at these loci influence individual variations at pharmacodynamic and pharmacokinetic levels of drug response, respectively. The Ah locus is located on mouse chromosome 12 and the N-acetyltransferase loci are on mouse chromosome 8; hence they are not linked. The nomenclatures for the Ah locus, *Ahr* (formerly *Ah*), and for *N*-acetyltransferase, *Nat**, are used in this discussion.

Arylhydrocarbon Receptor Polymorphism

The *Ahr* receptor is a ligand-activated transcription factor that regulates a large number of biological responses to planar aromatic hydrocarbons such as benzo[*a*]pyrene, 3-methylcholanthrene, and 2,3,7,8-tetrachlorodibenzo-*p*-dioxin (TCDD). It is best known for its role in mediating biological responses to halogenated dioxins and related toxic and carcinogenic environmental chemicals. A series of observations in rats, mice, and various other species had indicated that 3-methylcholanthrene is a potent inducer (i.e., causes increased synthesis) of arylhydrocarbon hydroxylase as well as other xenobiotic metabolizing enzymes. A mouse strain survey revealed the locus was polymorphic, that is some mouse strains such as B6 and C3H were responsive to induction while other strains such as DBA and AKR were unresponsive. Responsiveness segregated as a simple autosomal dominant Mendelian character and the responsible locus was named the *Ah* (renamed *Ahr*) locus. Strains carrying the "responsive" allele were designated Ahr^b (from B6 mice) and the "nonresponsive" allele was designated Ahr^d (from DBA mice).[19,20]

Experimental proof that the *Ahr* locus encodes a receptor came from efforts of many laboratories that began in the 1960s and spanned more than two decades. Formal proof of this concept is based on the demonstration of high- and low-affinity binding sites that segregate with responsiveness and nonresponsiveness, and the demonstration that hydrocarbon ligands cause an increased affinity of the receptor for DNA and its redistribution from the cytosolic compartment of the cell to the nuclear compartment. Further investigation revealed that responsive mice possess receptors having apparent molecular weights of 94 kDa (Ahr^{b-1}), 104 kDa (Ahr^{b-2}), and 105 kDa (Ahr^{b-3}), whereas nonresponsive mice possess receptors having a molecular weight of 104 kDa (Ahr^d).[21,22]

The concept that the Ah receptor is a ligand-activated transcription factor evolved from experiments in mice that demonstrated that induction of arylhydrocarbon hydroxylase activity was blocked by inhibitors of transcription or translation, and that on binding the agonist the Ah receptor develops a high affinity for the cell nucleus and for DNA. Agonist-dependent up-regulation of the receptor comes about because of increased transcriptional initiation. Evidence from deletion analysis indicated the presence of regulatory domains located in the 5' region of genes that respond to ligand (TCDD)-induced induction, such as the P450 gene, *Cyp1A1*. The mouse TCDD-responsive domain possesses the characteristics of a typical enhancer element, that is, it activates transcription at a distance from the promoter in an orientation-independent manner. For *Cyp1A1*, enhancer activity is the sum of effects of at least six distinct responsive elements acting independently in some cases and cooperatively in others. These elements are designated by different groups as dioxin-responsive, or xenobiotic-responsive, or Ah-responsive receptor elements and are abbreviated as DREs,

XREs, and AHREs, respectively. Direct sequencing, footprinting, and mutational analysis of these elements defined the core recognition sequence, GCGTG, as that essential for receptor interaction and enhancer function; outside this core the sequence TNGCGTG corresponds to a site with the highest affinity.

A number of genes that may be upregulated in response to arylhydrocarbons such as TCDD have been identified and referred to as members of the "Ah gene battery." As a group, they are characterized by rapid increases in protein and mRNA levels after exposure to the agonist. For example, Ah receptor DRE-mediated increases in *Cyp1A1* mRNA are observed within 30 minutes of exposure to TCDD. Genes for a number of drug-metabolizing enzymes are assigned to this gene battery, and several additional genes as yet to be identified appear to be regulated by the Ah receptor gene.

Somatic cell genetics carried out on mouse-derived cell lines proved to be a fruitful way to identify additional genes involved in the Ah receptor signaling pathways that lead to induction of arylhydrocarbon hydroxylase activity (largely Cyp1A1 activity). Complementation studies have revealed that mutations at four distinct loci can generate resistant phenotypes: (1) mutations that inactivate the responsive gene, *Cyp1A1*, (2) those that have approximately 10-fold lower cytosolic receptor concentrations, (3) those that have wild-type receptor concentrations but the receptor fails to show increased nuclear affinity on agonist binding, and (4) those that appear to exhibit both of the latter defects—i.e., a low receptor number and decreased nuclear affinity of the ligand-bound receptor. Rescuing experiments of the decreased nuclear affinity mutants demonstrated that the Ah receptor required a dimeric partner to bind the DREs. This protein became known as ARNT because its absence correlated with decreased affinity of the Ah receptor for the nuclear compartment. Apart from their value in identifying additional genes involved in Ah receptor pathways, the complementation pattern of somatic cell mutants and the importance of the ARNT protein were some of the first indicators to distinguish the Ah receptor from the steroid/thyroid receptor supergene family and prove it to be a unique signaling molecule.

The Ah receptor and ARNT molecules had sequence identity with the Per and Sim proteins of *Drosophila*, proteins of a family of transmission factors. This family is characterized by a motif referred to as the "PAS" domain, which harbors sequences in the Ah receptor involved in the formation of a hydrophilic pocket that binds the arylhydrocarbon agonist. Adjacent to the PAS domain is a basic/helix–loop–helix (bHLH) domain that is believed to mediate heterodimerization and sequence-specific DNA-binding properties. The domain map is consistent with the observation that the Ah receptor and ARNT proteins are heterodimeric partners that activate gene expression. A hypothetical model of the receptor based on putative functional domains observed in mice has been proposed by Hollie Swanson and Christopher Bradfield.[23] Older versions of a molecular model of the mechanism by the Ah receptor transduce the signal of arylhydrocarbon agonists and thus have been revised because they were based incorrectly on the premise that the Ah receptor was a member of the steroid/thyroxine gene family.

Several studies have been performed in congenic mouse strains differing in their *Ahr* receptor responsiveness. The acute toxicity of TCDD, a potent inducer of the Ah receptor, has been examined in male mice differing only at the *Ahr* locus. In a study by Birnbaum and colleagues, the LD_{50} values were 159 and 3351 μg/kg body weight for responders and nonresponders, respectively, although the mean time of death (22 days) was independent of dose and *Ahr* receptor genotype.[24] Among various anatomical and biochemical signs of dose-related acute toxicity that were observed, necrosis of germinal epithelium in the testes occurred at doses 8–24 times greater in nonresponsive than in responsive mice. The spectrum of toxicity was found to be dependent on the *Ahr* genotype, but the relative doses required to bring about acute responses to TCDD are much greater in congenic mice homozygous for the nonresponsive allele than for mice homozygous for the responsive *Ahr* allele.

The pathogenesis of hexachlorobenzene-induced porphyria was investigated in female B6.*Ahr*[b] (responsive) and B6.*Ahr*[d] (nonresponsive) congenic strains.[25] TCDD led to urinary excretion of porphyrins that was 200 times greater in untreated responsive control mice compared to only 6 times greater in untreated nonresponsive control females. The hepatic accumulation of hexachlorobenzene was also greater in responsive than in nonresponsive mice and was associated with greater hepatic lipid levels in the former strain. These findings as well as other biochemical indices indicated that the *Ahr* locus influences the susceptibility of mice to hexachlorobenzene-induced porphyria, and further studies showed that specific P450 isoforms that are members of the *Ahr* gene battery are likely causative factors in the development of this disorder.

The effect of 3-methylcholanthrene on atherosclerosis has also been examined in congenic mouse strains that differ in Ah responsiveness.[26] The effect of 3-methylcholanthrene was found to be greater in responsive mice receiving an atherogenic diet than in nonresponsive mice treated similarly. Thus, exposure to 3-methylcholanthrene increased the area of atherosclerotic lesions in both congenic strains, but the magnitude of the increase was significantly greater in *Ahr*-responsive than nonresponsive mice even though the high-density lipoprotein levels were not significantly altered by such treatment or by the *Ahr* receptor genotype. The study of the F_1 progeny of responsive (AKXL-38a) and nonresponsive (AKXL-38) mice backcrossed to the nonresponsive parent revealed that increased susceptibility to 3-methylcholanthrene-induced atherosclerosis segregated with the *Ahr* receptor locus.

A developmental role for the Ahr locus was indicated by the observation that mice congenic to the C57BK/6 strain harboring a null allele show a portocaval vascular shunt throughout life.[27] Three-dimensional (3D) visualization at various developmental times indicated that the shunt is an embryonic remnant acquired before birth. The ontogeny of the shunt plus its 3D position suggested that the shunt is due to a patent ductus arteriosus. During the first 48 hours, most major hepatic veins including the portal and umbilical veins usually decrease in diameter but do not change in Ahr null mice. In searching for its physiological cause, it appears that failure of the ductus to close may be a consequence of increased blood pressure or a failure in vasoconstriction in the developing liver.

Acetylation Polymorphism

The hereditary variability in the acetylation of an array of chemicals with arylamine and hydrazine moieties is a well-known trait that occurs in humans (see Appendix A), mice, and several other mammalian laboratory animal species. This trait is determined by significant differences in N-acetyltransferase (NAT2) activity in liver and several other tissues, and it is referred to as the N-acetyltransferase polymorphism.

A survey of inbred mouse strains identified 17 with rapid acetylator phenotypes and 3 with slow phenotypes. Studies in two representative strains, C57BL/6 mice representing rapid acetylation and A/J mice (henceforth referred to as B6 and A mice, respectively) representing slow acetylation, have repeatedly demonstrated that the polymorphism observed in Nat activity in the liver of mice also occurs in kidney, urinary bladder, blood, colon, and other tissues. These mice were chosen because they differ in many physiological, anatomical, behavioral, and oncological traits including important models of birth defects and adult diseases in humans.[28] Further studies of A and B6 mice by standard intercross and backcross matings demonstrated that a single gene with two major codominant alleles accounted for the differences in Nat activity. Studies in recombinant inbred strains derived from B6 and A parental mice confirmed the Mendelian inheritance of NAT activity and also revealed significant background gene effects on the differential *Nat* allele. The metabolic, molecular genetic, and toxicological aspects of the acetylation polymorphism summarized below are reviewed by Levy and colleagues.[29]

Biochemical studies with prototypical substrates for Nat, p-aminobenzoate (PABA), and the arylamine carcinogen, 2-aminofluorene (AF), showed tissue-specific variations in Nat activity ranging from 1.5-fold to 20-fold *in vitro* for liver and 21 other tissues. In agreement with these observations, the elimination of AF from blood was two to three times higher for B6 than A mice and for B6 and A hepatocytes isolated in primary culture. On the other hand, no differences in rates of isoniazid N-acetylation *in vitro* or *in vivo* were detected in urine of B6 and A mice.

The large difference in blood PABA N-acetylating activity between B6 and A phenotypes (up to 20-fold), and the ability to discriminate heterozygote animals from homozygous rapid and slow phenotypes by assaying blood were exploited to construct two acetylator congenic lines, A.B6 and B6.A, as explained in Figure 9.2 and the previous section. The availability of quartets shown in Figure 9.3 provided the means to test for the effects of background genes on NAT activity for various substrates and on the role of acetylation polymorphism on individual susceptibility to arylamine carcinogenesis. The background effect on NAT activity with AF, for example, indicated that the A background contributed a factor that increased the phenotypic difference in NAT activity with, for example, AF or conversely that the B6 background reduced the phenotypic difference in NAT activity.

Acetylator congenic lines were used to evaluate the role of acetylation polymorphism on individual susceptibility to arylamine carcinogenesis as measured over a short term (3 hours) by AF-induced hepatic DNA-adduct formation. Differences in the acetylator phenotype caused differences in the formation of DNA-AF adducts; for hepatic DNA, adduct formation in B6 mice was about twice that of A mice. The comparisons of parental to congenic mice were also revealing because the A.B6 mice had about 4-fold (for females) and 10-fold (for males) more hepatic DNA-AF adducts than A mice. The difference on the B6 background was somewhat less: B6 mice had 2.7-fold (females) and 1.4-fold (males) more hepatic DNA adducts than B6.A mice. These experiments indicated that differences in acetylator phenotype do contribute to differences in AF-induced DNA damage, and show that mouse gender can influence tissue-specific arylamine-induced DNA damage even though no gender-related differences in hepatic NAT activity have been found.

Another (subchronic 28 day) study of arylamine exposure and acetylator phenotype was also performed using B6 and B6.A mice exposed to 4-aminobiphenyl, another arylamine with carcinogenic potential. Little or no relationship was observed between acetylator phenotype and liver damage, but in the urinary bladder, one of the major targets for arylamine carcinogens, rapid acetylator females had more adducts than slow acetylator females. However, slow acetylator males had higher bladder adducts than rapid acetylator males. Both the 28-day study with 4-aminobiphenyl and the short-term (3-hour exposure) tests with AF show higher adduct formation in liver for females compared to males and higher adduct formation in bladder for males compared to females. The relationship of sex to organ site of arylamine carcinogenesis indicated by both 3-hour and 28-day exposures is the same as has been observed in lifetime feeding studies. This observation suggests that measurement of DNA-carcinogen adducts may be an acceptable adjunct to lifetime tumor production in assessing carcinogenicity.

Another example of the use of the A.B6 and B6.A acetylator congenic mice in toxicology focused on the study of cleft palate (CP) and cleft lip with and without cleft palate [CL(P)].[29] A mice are more susceptible to teratogen-induced and spontaneous CP than B6 mice. Using conventional genetic analysis of a number of AXB and BXA recombinant inbred lines, a few genetic markers including *Nat* on chromosome 8 were found for increased sensitivity to the teratogens phenytoin, glucocorticoids, and 6-aminonicotinamide. Refinement of these experiments through the use of acetylator congenic mice showed that the sensitivity to glucocorticoid-induced cleft palate was high in A and B6.A mice whereas B6 and A.B6 mice were resistant to the teratogenic effects. While *Nat* is considered unlikely to be the cause of the teratogenesis, the results indicate that the gene responsible for teratogen sensitivity is quite near *Nat* on mouse chromosome 8. Given the high degree of homology existing between the *Nat*-containing region of mouse chromosome 8 and human chromosome 8, the *NAT** genes may also be useful markers for the study of CP and [CP(P)] in humans.

While these toxicological studies with congenic mice were in progress, recombinant DNA studies of *Nat* were advancing in another direction. Molecular biological techniques had shown that several mammalian species including humans are characterized by at least two genes that encode two very similar NAT proteins expressed in liver and other tissues. For the mouse, recombinant and heterologous expression studies revealed several points of interest. First, three *Nat* genes *Nat1*, Nat2*, and Nat3** are present, one of which (*Nat2**) is polymorphic. The coding region sequences of *Nat1** for A and B6 mice are identical, while that for *Nat2** from the slow acetylator A mice contains a single base missense mutation that is accompanied by replacement of asparagine by isoleucine at position 99 in the coding region. Second, recombinant studies provide an explanation for the genetically variant patterns of N-acetylation of PABA, AF, and isoniazid. The *Nat** genes transiently expressed in COS-1 cells showed that Nat1 has selectivity for acetylation of isoniazid, Nat2 has absolute specificity for PABA, and Nat1 and Nat2 have overlapping specificities for AF. Mutant Nat2 from A mice with the N99I amino acid substitution is less active than its counterpart in B6 mice in the acetylation of PABA and AF, but the rates of isoniazid acetylation with Nat1 from A and B6 mice are comparable.

Molecular genetic and biochemical studies of B6 and A mice and congenic acetylator lines have provided insight into the mechanism for genetic slow acetylation. The evidence indicates that defective acetylation in slow acetylator mice is caused by a conformationally modified Nat2 enzyme (*Nat2*9*) with markedly reduced stability and with decreased affinity for the substrate.[30] The missense mutation has no effect on the amount of Nat2 transcript or protein and the mouse mutant *Nat2*9*, unlike mutant *Nat2* in human liver or in mammalian expression systems, is not subject to degradation by hepatic proteases. These mouse studies suggest that proteolytic processing of structurally altered proteins is not a universal phenomenon but more likely the type and extent of conformational modification introduced may dictate whether proteolysis takes place.

Further investigations of congenic mice and double congenic mice have revealed interactions between the polymorphisms of the Ah receptor and acetyltransferases that affect the extent of DNA damage induced by exposure to arylamine carcinogens.[31,32] A critical step in hepatic metabolic activation of arylamines appears to be N-oxidation catalyzed by the cytochrome P450, CYP1A2. This isozyme has been associated with arylamine metabolism in both mice and humans. In mice, *CYP1A2* is a member of the gene battery controlled by the *Ahr* receptor locus, and hence differences in inducibility of such a key P450 enzyme might lead to differences in susceptibility to arylamine-induced cancer. The likelihood that both acetylation polymorphism and Ah receptor polymorphism could play an interactive role in the early stages of arylamine carcinogenesis led to the construction of the double congenic line, B6.A.D, a mouse line that is both a slow acetylator and a nonresponder. The quartet of lines on the B6 background, B6, B6.A, B6.D, and B6.A.D, was studied to examine the effect of induction of the Ah receptor by β-naphthoflavone on arylamine-induced hepatic DNA damage (Figure 9.5). The results were in agreement with previous observations on noninduced mice: rapid acetylators had more hepatic DNA-AF adducts than males, and females had a greater adduct burden than males. The greater adduct burden in livers of females of all strains was also found after induction, although since male mice responded to induction to a greater extent than did females, the differences in adduct formation between males and females after β-naphthoflavone treatment was reduced in lines that had a significant response to induction. This study demonstrated differences in arylamine-induced hepatic DNA damage in mice of differing acetylator status and *Ahr* responsiveness. Since all four lines tested shared the B6 genetic background, differences in DNA damage that were found can be attributed only to differences in responsiveness to the inducer and/or to differences in acetylation capacity. Other differences between the mice in this study arise from gender-related effects, and therefore results for males and females are considered separately.

A similar type of study using the same four lines of congenic and double congenic mice was performed to examine the effects of both polymorphisms on the effects arising from exposure to food mutagens (heterocyclic arylamines) derived from cooked meats and suspected of being cancer initiators.[32] The results of these studies are complex, but in sum they confirm that *Ahr* and *Nat* genotypes and coexposure to an Ah agonist (such as β-naphthoflavone) contribute significantly in a tissue-specific way to the amount and profile of DNA-amine adducts formed in several organs, which in humans are target organs for the food mutagens.

CREATING MOUSE MODELS BY GENE TARGETING

In 2001, Martin Evans of the United Kingdom and Mario Capecchi and Oliver Smithies of the United States were honored for developing "gene targeting," a technology that allows the creation of "knockout" and other designer strains of mice in which almost any gene can be disabled and its function probed.[6,33–35] Two principal conceptual advances in the 1980s, comparable in inventiveness and impact to other revolutionary biological innovations including recombinant DNA, DNA sequencing, polymerase chain reaction, and monoclonal antibodies, led to this breakthrough. The first was the development of stem cell methods to culture embryonic stem (ES) cells by Evans and the second was the development of the method of homologous recombination by Capecchi and Smithies independently. Homologous recombination occurs between a native target chromosomal gene and exogenous DNA to modify a specific target locus. The combination of the Evans technique with the Capecchi–Smithies technique led to construction of the first "knockout" mice in 1989, an advance that provided an efficient means of producing laboratory models of human disease in a predictable manner by making it possible to evaluate the function of almost any single gene. By 2001, well over 7000 genes of approximately 30,000 mouse genes had been analyzed with gene targeting.[35]

The gene-targeting protocol for generating chimeric mice from embryonic stem cells containing a targeted mutation, outlined in Figure 9.7, as it is now performed is as follows:[35]

The desired sequence modification is introduced into a cloned copy of the chosen gene by standard recombinant DNA technology. Then, the modification is transferred, by means of homologous recombination, the cognate genomic locus in ES cells and the ES cell lines carrying the desired alteration are selected. Finally, ES cells containing the altered genetic

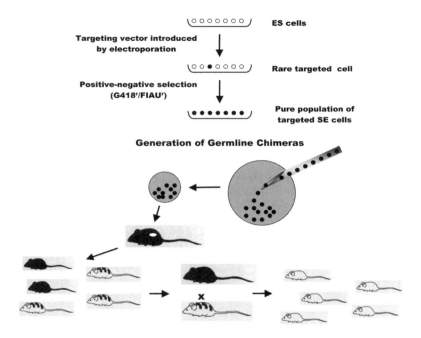

Figure 9.7 Generation of mouse germline chimeras.

locus are injected into mouse blastocysts, which are in turn brought to term by surgical transfer to foster mothers, generating chimeric mice that are capable of transmitting the modified genetic locus to their offspring.

Embryonic stem cells that contain the targeted mutation are enriched (if necessary) by a procedure involving *positive selection* for cells that have incorporated the targeting construct anywhere within the stem cell genome, followed by *negative selection* against the cells that have integrated the construct randomly into their genome. Homologous recombination between the targeting vector and chromosomal copy of the targeted gene results in disruption of one copy of the target gene and loss of the *HSV-tk* sequence. The vector is designed so that transfer of the *HSV-tk* gene does not accompany replacement of the endogenous gene. *HSV-tk* is excluded because it represents a discontinuity between homology and nonhomology with the target sequence. The genotype of the embryonic stem cells in which targeting has occurred will be *Gene X^+, neo^{r+}, $HSV\text{-}tk^-$*, whereas the genotype of the cells in which random integration of the vector has occurred should be *Gene X^+, neo^{r+}, $HSV\text{-}tk^+$*. At the concentration used for negative selection, gancyclovir is not toxic to parental embryonic stem cells but selectively kills cells containing the viral thymidine kinase gene. By selecting for cells containing a functional *neo^r* gene with G418, and against cells containing a functional *HSV-tk* gene with gancyclovir, the net effect is to enrich cells containing the targeted mutation.

The replacement vector used in gene targeting typically contains 10–15 kb of DNA homologous to the target gene, say *Gene X,* followed by a neomycin-resistant gene (*neo^r*) and a herpes simplex thymidine kinase gene (*HSV-tk*) adjacent to the target homology (Figure 9.8). The *neo^r* gene disrupts the coding sequence of the target gene and acts as a marker conferring resistance to a neomycin-like drug (G418) that is used for selecting cells that contain a copy of the recombinant vector. The pMC1 NEO *neo^r* vector is used in these constructs because it maximized the expression efficiency of the DNA integrated into the stem cells. The *HSV-tk* gene is used to negatively select for nonhomologous events. Nonhomologous events will lead to the insertion of *tk* and the resultant clone can be selected against with gancyclovir. In the more recent protocol, a nucleoside analog, FIAU (that specifically kills cells with functional *HSV-tk* genes, but is not toxic to cells with only cellular Tk), replaces gancyclovir.

Gene targeting has been used to generate animals with null ("knockout") alleles, overexpressed alleles, and "humanized" transgenic animals, that is, mice that have been modified by replacing a native mouse gene with its human counterpart. In fact, this technique can be used to modify the pattern of any property of a given gene including its transcription, mRNA, development, or the capacity of its gene products to interact with the products of other genes. The possibility of engineering large-scale changes such as chromosomal translocation or deletions into the mouse germ line by gene targeting has been demonstrated, which would facilitate creation of mouse models with chromosomal rearrangements that are associated with human cancers (see, for example, Appendix A). Even though transgenesis and gene targeting are often directed toward different ends, the former toward the gain of new functions and the latter toward augmenting or generating a loss of existing functions, the technique of gene targeting is applicable to the creation of animals of either type. Additional strategies have made possible the creation of mice with mutations that can be targeted to specific cells and tissues[36] and timed to specific developmental stages.[37]

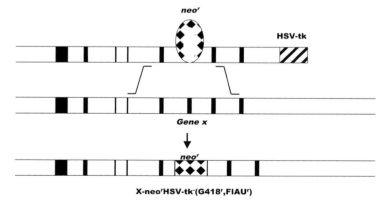

Figure 9.8 A sequence replacement vector.

MOUSE MODELS OF HUMAN DISORDERS
CREATED BY GENE TARGETING

The capacity to produce mice with null alleles or transgenes as well as other kinds of variant genes by targeting genes of the mouse germline is of monumental importance to human genetic analysis. The popularity of this approach is evident from the number and variety of experimental models of human disease that have been created to elucidate the role of specific human genes in normal and pathological states. Some specific examples of models that have been constructed, many of which are relevant to pharmacogenomics, are described in Table 9.1.

QUANTITATIVE TRAIT LOCUS (QTL) ANALYSIS

The first step in classical (Mendelian) genetic analysis is to identify the subset of genes that accounts for the genetic variation in a specific trait, and to locate these genes on a genetic map of the genome. While a measure of success has been achieved in associating genotype with phenotype for so-called monogenic traits, major problems remain to be resolved even for disorders caused by mutations in a single gene, and the challenge for dissecting the causes of complex traits is far greater.[38] Complex traits are biological phenotypes that arise from variations at a number of genetic loci, and the genes responsible for these variations are termed quantitative trait loci.

Historically, genetic mapping of trait-causing genes to chromosomal locations dates back to the work of Morgan and Sturtevant on fruit flies in 1913 (see p. 5). Genetic mapping has since become a mainstay of experimental studies to track the heritability of any chromosomal region in a controlled mating of fruit flies, nematode worms, yeast, rodents, and humans. Following the development of automated sequencing of whole genomes in 1986, genome-wide QTL analysis was first applied to fruiting characteristics in the tomato in 1988[39] and soon the technique was applied to mammalian disorders.[13] As an analytical tool for the dissection of complex genetic traits,[13] QTL mapping is performed with the purpose of localizing genes affecting quantitative or continuously distributed traits to broad chromosomal regions.[40] Only recently, with the construction of dense genetic linkage maps for mouse[5] and rat,[41] and the development of "interval mapping" as a tool for searching the whole genome,[42] has QTL mapping become a realistic possibility.

"Interval mapping" refers to the estimation of the probable genotype and most likely the QTL effect at every point in the genome from phenotypic and genetic marker information. The most satisfactory general approach to these analyses is by way of the method of maximum likelihood. Each possible linkage map constructed by this technique consists of an order for the loci and the recombination fractions between them. Available computer programs enable the probability that a given map would have given rise to the observed data to be computed. The computed probability is referred to as the "likelihood" of the map, and the "best"

Table 9.1 Mouse Models Created by Gene Targeting*

Disorder modeled	System	Gene targeted	Description
Defective B6 metabolism	Knockout mouse	Tissue alkaline phosphatase *TNAP*	Mice lacking tissue nonspecific alkaline phosphatase (*TNAP*) develop seizures that are subsequently fatal approximately 2 weeks after birth. Defective metabolism of pyridoxal 5′-phosphate (PLP), characterized by elevated serum PLP levels, results in reduced levels of the inhibitory neurotransmitter γ-aminobutyric acid (GABA) in the brain. The mutant seizure phenotype can be rescued by the administration of pyridoxal and a semisolid diet.[1]
Heart defects	Knockout mouse	Gap junctions *Gja1Cx43*	Mice lacking a gene-encoding connexin43, a member of a family of proteins that forms gap junctions between cells, were constructed by creating a null mutation in the gene *Gja1* providing a model for understanding the causes of congenital heart defects and pulmonary stenosis.[2] Study of the model suggests that connexins may play an essential role in heart development and that human patients with congenital cardiac malformations may be missing certain connexins.
Hemophilia A	Knockout mouse	Factor VIII	The factor VIII gene is 186 kb long, contains 26 exons, and encodes a mature protein of 2332 amino acids. Disruption of exon 16 by gene targeting provided the first genetically engineered small animal model of hemophilia A that is desirable for studies of factor VIII deficiency. Factor VIII activity was <1% of normal and indistinguishable from zero, and two male F_2 mice both of whom carried the exon 16 disruption bled excessively and died within 12 hours.[3]

*See Appendix C for table references.

Table 9.1 (*continued*)

Disorder modeled	System	Gene targeted	Description
Benzo[*a*]pyrene-induced teratogenesis	Transgenic mouse	Tumor suppressor *p53*	Investigation of the teratologic suppressor role of *p53*, a gene that facilitates DNA repair, was used to examine the effects of benzo[*a*]pyrene treatment in a p53-deficient transgenic mouse model. The findings demonstrated that benzo[*a*]pyrene-treated heterozygous dams were two to four times more susceptible to embryotoxicity and teratogenicity than normal *p53* controls. Fetal resorptions reflecting *in utero* death were increased 2.6-fold and 3.6-fold, respectively, with heterozygous and homozygous p53-deficient embryos. The findings in this model indicate that *p53* may be an important suppressor gene that protects the embryo from DNA-damaging chemicals and developmental oxidative stress.[4]
Blood pressure regulation	Knockout mouse	Endothelial nitric oxide synthase *eNOS*	Nitric oxide (NO), a potent vasodilator produced by endothelial cells, acts as a "relaxing factor" (EDRF) that mediates vascular relaxation in many vascular beds and regulates blood pressure and regional blood flow; abnormalities in its production are associated with atherosclerosis, diabetes, and hypertension. Homozygous endothelial nitric oxide synthase (eNOS) mutant mice generated by gene targeting are viable, fertile, and indistinguishable from wild-type and heterozygous littermates but their mean blood pressure is 35% higher than in control littermates (110 vs. 81 mm Hg), confirming that endothelial nitric oxide plays a role in normal blood pressure regulation, and in fact may be a primary

(*continued*)

Table 9.1 (*continued*)

Disorder modeled	System	Gene targeted	Description
			determinant of physiological blood pressure as a vasodilator. Studies in this model raise questions as to whether subpopulations of humans with hypertension have defects in eNOS expression and of the development of more specific inhibitors of various NOS isoforms.[5]
Hepatic porphyria	Knockout mouse	Porphobilinogen deaminase *Pgbd*	Acute intermittent porphyria (AIP) is a human disease resulting from a dominantly inherited partial deficiency of the heme biosynthetic enzyme, porphobilinogen deaminase (PBGD). The clinical expression of this disorder is characterized by acute, life-threatening attacks of "porphyric neuropathy" that include abdominal pain, motor and sensory neurological deficits, and psychiatric symptoms. Identical symptoms occur in other hepatic porphyrias. Attacks are frequently precipitated by drugs, alcohol, and low caloric intake. To study the pathogenesis of the neurological symptoms of acute intermittent porphyria, Pbgd-deficient mice were generated by gene targeting. These mice exhibit the typical biochemical characteristics of human AIP, notably, decreased hepatic Pbgd activity, increased δ-aminolevulinic acid synthase activity, and massively increased urinary excretion of the heme precursor, δ-aminolevulinic acid, after treatment with drugs such as phenobarbital. Behavioral tests reveal decreased motor function and histopathological findings that include axonal neuropathy and neurological muscle atrophy.[6]

Table 9.1 (*continued*)

Disorder modeled	System	Gene targeted	Description
Resistance to intestinal tumorigenesis	Transgenic mouse	Phospholipase *Pla2g2a*	A mapping study suggested the secretory phospholipase gene, *Pla2g2a*, located on chromosome 4 as a potential candidate for *Mom1*, a strong modifier locus found in the same region of that chromosome. To test this hypothesis more directly, a transgenic mouse carrying a functional overexpressed *Pla2g2a* allele was constructed on a B6 background. This transgene caused a reduction in tumor multiplicity and size comparable to that conferred by a single copy of *Mom1* indicating that this phospholipase can provide active resistance to intestinal tumorigenesis.[7]
Resistance to cholera toxin	Knockout mouse	Cystic fibrosis transmembrane conductance regulator *Cftr*	The effect of the number of cystic fibrosis alleles on cholera toxin-induced intestinal secretion was examined in a knockout mouse model.[8] Homozygous knockout mice did not secrete any fluid in response to cholera toxin, while heterozygous mice expressed 50% of the CFTR protein and secreted 50% of the normal fluid and chloride ion in response to cholera toxin. This correlation suggests that cystic fibrosis might possess a selective advantage of resistance to cholera.
Susceptibility to organophosphate insecticides and atherosclerosis	Knockout mouse	Paraoxonase *Pon1*	*Paraoxonase (PON1)* knockout mice were produced by targeted disruption of exon 1 of the PON1 gene. Results with these *PON1* null mice show their ability to inactivate organophosphate poisons was severely compromised, and when fed a high-fat, high-cholesterol diet were more susceptible to atherosclerosis than their intact littermates.[9]

(continued)

Table 9.1 (*continued*)

Disorder modeled	System	Gene targeted	Description
Obesity	Human knockin transgenic mouse	Human leptin aP2 promoter fragment	Mice carrying a weakly expressed human leptin transgene indicated that dysfunctional regulation of the leptin gene can result in obesity with relatively normal levels of leptin, and that this form of obesity is responsive to leptin treatment.[10]
Aberrant cardiac development and pulmonary hypertension	Knockout mouse	Serotonin receptor 5-HT$_{2B}$	Studies of serotonin receptor (5-HT$_{2B}$) knockout mice show that 5-HT$_{2B}$ is an important regulator of cardiac development. Mutant embryos exhibit lack of trabeculae in the heart and a specific reduction in expression levels of a tyrosine kinase receptor, Erb-2, leading to midgestation lethality.[11] Using the chronic hypoxic mouse model of pulmonary hypertension, Launay and co-workers showed that the hypoxia-dependent increase in pulmonary blood pressure and lung remodeling was associated with vascular proliferation, elastase activity, and transforming growth factor-β levels, and that these parameters were potentiated by dexfenfluramine treatment. In contrast, hypoxic knockout mice manifested no change in any of these parameters[12] (see also p. 373).
Long QT syndrome	Knockin mouse	KPQ deletion $SCN5A^{\Delta/+}$	*Cre/loxP*-mediated targeting was used to create mutant mice heterozygous for a knockin KPQ deletion ($SCN5A^{\Delta/+}$) in the cardiac sodium channel. Mice with deletion of amino acid residues 1505–1507 (lysine–proline–glutamine, KPQ) show the features of LQT3. A sudden acceleration in heart rate or premature beats caused lengthening of the action potential with early afterdepolarization and triggered ventricular arrhythmias in Scn5a$^{\Delta/+}$ mice. Adrenergic agonists (mexilitine) suppressed arrhythmias upon premature stimulation, suggesting

Table 9.1 (*continued*)

Disorder modeled	System	Gene targeted	Description
			that this mouse model may be useful for the development of new treatments for the LQT3 syndrome.[13]
Acute promyelocytic leukemia suppression	Human transgenic mouse	PML$^{-/-}$ mutant mice crossed with human cathepsin G (*hCG*)-*PMLRARα* transgenic mice	A mouse model was constructed to determine whether promyelocytic leukemia protein acts as a tumor suppressor. This model was constructed by crossing PML$^{-/-}$ mice with human cathepsin G (hCG)-PMLRARα transgenic mice. In this model, a progressive reduction of the dose of PML resulted in a dramatic increase in the incidence of leukemia, and an acceleration of the onset of leukemia in PMLRARα transgenic mice. These results demonstrate that PML acted as a tumor suppressor rendering cells resistant to proapoptotic and differentiating stimuli.[14]
Lethal seizures due to deficient GABA degradation	Knockout mouse	Succinic semialdehyde dehydrogenase *Aldh5a1*	Succinic semialdehyde dehydrogenase (*ALDH5A1*, encoding SSADH) deficiency is a defect in GABA degradation that manifests itself as 4-hydroxybutyric (γ-hydroxybutyric acid, GHB) aciduria. Aldh5a1-deficient mice constructed by gene targeting displayed ataxia and developed generalized seizures rapidly leading to death.[15] Therapeutic intervention with phenobarbital or phenytoin was ineffective, whereas intervention with vigabatrin, or the GABA receptor antagonist CGP 35348, prevented convulsions and significantly enhanced survival in mutant mice. This model may provide insight into the pathological mechanisms of SSADH deficiency and may have therapeutic relevance for the human condition.

(*continued*)

Table 9.1 (*continued*)

Disorder modeled	System	Gene targeted	Description
Organic cation transporter (Oct) defect	Knockout mouse	Organic cation transporter defect	The effect of knocking out the organic cation transporter gene (*Oct1*) was explored in a mouse model.[16] Results show that Oct1 in itself is not essential for normal health and fertility of mice, but that it has an important role in the uptake and excretion of several organic cationic drugs and toxins by the liver and intestine.[17] This model may contribute to our understanding of the mechanisms of drug transport and elimination, and provide insights for the prevention of the adverse effects of these substances.
Acetylcholinesterase deficiency	Knockout mouse	Acetylcholinesterase *Ache*	The acetylcholinesterase knockout mouse was constructed to explore the role of acetylcholinesterase in neural development.[18] Observations on these mice show that nullizygous mice were born alive and survived up to 21 days, but that physical development was delayed. The generally high levels of butyrylcholinesterase in tissues of nullizygous mice, including the motor endplate, and additional observations suggest that butyrylcholinesterase plays an essential role in these animals.
Pregnenolone xenobiotic receptor	Human transgenic mouse	Pregnenolone xenobiotic receptor *PXR*	To examine the significance of the pregnenolone xenobiotic nuclear receptor on the disposition of drugs subject to metabolism by CYP3A enzymes, transgenic mice containing a humanized form of the PXR mouse receptor were generated.[19] These mice were responsive to human-specific inducers of CYP3A such as the antibiotic rifampin. The exclusive profile of CYP3A inducibility exhibited by these mice suggests their potential usage in pharmacological studies and drug development.

map is the one with the maximum likelihood; the ratio of the probabilities for two maps is a measure of how well one fits the data compared to the other.

Traditional QTL Mapping Studies

The basic idea of QTL mapping involves following the inheritance of restriction fragment length polymorphisms (RFLPs) in appropriate pedigrees.[42] The mouse and rat are particularly advantageous for systematic QTL mapping because of the availability of inbred lines and large families. The most efficient approach to this end is to study F_2 generations derived from two inbred lines through the use of progeny testing, recombinant inbred strains, and recombinant congenic strains. Accurate construction of such maps requires multipoint linkage analysis of particular pedigrees, and computer packages specifically designed for this purpose have been described.[43] However, the difficulty of QTL analysis is much greater than for a Mendelian disorder because the responsible genomic intervals are much greater and more difficult to define and the responsible variant is more subtle to detect.

Overall, QTL mapping is a tedious process, requiring 10–15 generations of linkage mapping and congenic construction, corresponding to 3–5 years for the mouse and longer for the rat. Traditional QTL analysis consists of three steps. The first requires large crosses between at least two strains producing and assaying relevant phenotypes and genotypes for polymorphic markers in hundreds or thousands of offspring with the purpose of localizing QTLs to large chromosomal regions. This step results in chromosomal localization but with relatively poor resolution, typically about 20 cM, or about 25% of a mouse chromosome. The second step involves molecular identification of the individual genes responsible for each QTL. In experimental animals such as mice and rats, one solution is to construct congenic strains that differ only in the region of a single locus. Construction of congenic strains by the traditional protocol requires up to 12 generations of inbreeding as discussed above (see p. 262); with the advent of complete genetic linkage maps, however, "speed congenics" can be constructed in only three to four generations as described by Lander and Schork.[13] Jeff et al.[16] demonstrated how they used the "speed congenic" strategy to dissect blood pressure quantitative trait loci on rat chromosome 2. The strategy enabled them to verify the existence of a QTL on chromosome 2, and to reduce the size of the chromosomal region to one applicable to positional cloning of the causal gene. The third step is to identify the QTL by fine structure mapping, usually by standard genetic mapping or positional cloning.

Traditional QTL mapping has been used to identify and map the chromosomal loci of mouse and rat genes relevant to a number of pharmacogenomic traits. Among these are QTL studies of genes that control the susceptibility to hypertension in the stroke-prone spontaneously hypertensive rat,[16,44] susceptibility to intestinal neoplasia,[45] morphine preference,[46] airway hyperresponsiveness,[47] morphine antinociceptive sensitivity,[48] and susceptibility to butylated hydroxytoluene-induced lung tumor production and pulmonary inflammation.[49] In their study of substance abuse in mice, Berritini and colleagues[46] compared the morphine preference of B6 mice to that of DBA/2 mice. Animals from an F_2 intercross between these two inbred strains were phenotyped for morphine preference; mice demonstrating extreme values for morphine consumption were then genotyped for 157 microsatellite polymorphisms (SSLPs). Maximum likelihood estimates indicated that a major part (85%) of the genetic variance was associated with chromosomal loci on proximal chromosome 10, on the middle of chromosome 6, and on distal chromosome 1. The B6 strain consumed 200–300 mg/kg/day of morphine whereas the DBA/2 strain consumed only 1/20th as much under the same experimental conditions. In addition, unlike B6, DBA/2 mice showed neither opiate-induced tail (Straub) contraction nor severe withdrawal symptoms. No genes were immediately evident as candidates to explain the association with differences in morphine consumption, and the investigators suggested that congenic mice might prove useful for refining further the genetic loci responsible for this trait. They proposed that these mice be constructed by direct backcross of B6-DBA/2 F_1 progeny onto a DBA/2 background. Progeny could be selected for the presence of the B6 alleles from relevant chromosomes, and they could be tested with morphine to determine whether they possess the B6 phenotype. Mice that possessed the B6 phenotype could be studied further with microsatellite markers (SSLPs) localized to the relevant chromosomes to identify responsible loci.

Chromosome Substitution Strains Applied to QTL Mapping

Limitations of time and the expense of traditional QTL mapping spurred the development of alternative approaches to QTL analysis.[50] Construction of chromosome substitution strains (CSSs) for this purpose has recently been described by Nadeau and colleagues (see p. 268).[17,51]

Several advantages accrue to the CSS approach for QTL detection and mapping. This approach is more efficient than the traditional approach in that it requires fewer animals to detect a given effect, or permits detection of smaller effects with a given number of animals.[50,51] CSS models are also advantageous for detecting a given QTL in the presence of many other QTLs. In comparing results of published mapping studies, as many, and usually substantially more, QTLs were detected with CSSs than with F_2 intercrosses of comparable size.[51] CSSs greatly simplify the subsequent work of fine structure mapping and molecular identification of the QTL. Thus, to follow up initial QTL mapping by the traditional approach, the QTL of interest must first be isolated from other unlinked loci before undertaking a lengthy breeding program to create a congenic strain. In contrast, CSSs permit a move immediately to fine-structure mapping by crossing any CSS of interest to the host strain. Relatively few offspring for good resolution are required from such crosses, and the progeny can also be used to rapidly produce congenic strains carrying a small interval around the QTL. Finally, molecular identification of QTLs is aided by the availability of both genome sequences for the A/J and B6 strains to facilitate gene discovery.[52]

On the other hand, the CSS approach does require a CSS panel for the strain combination of interest. At present, the CSS approach is limited to the A/J and B6 strains that are available as a research resource at the Jackson Laboratory.[18]

Commentary

It thus seems clear that QTL analysis can increase the understanding of the underlying process or pathogenesis of traits under polygenic control and can contribute to the dissection of allele-specific interactions involved. Just how successful searches of homologous regions of the human genome will be in identifying genes for corresponding human syndromes is less certain. There is no reason, for example, to think that the human homologues of the morphine preference loci of mice[46] will play a similar role in human morphine addiction or substance abuse. Adapting strategies for the identification of loci in model systems to maximize the chances of identifying loci of human relevance is still a major hurdle.[53]

Because of difficulties that may be encountered, only a few of approximately 1000 QTLs have been identified at the molecular level. Probably, the combination of multiple perspectives on genome sequence, variation, and function will be required to reveal molecular mechanisms of phenotypic variation.[5] It is reasonable to expect that QTL gene identification will be advanced if genetic mapping can be combined with genomic sequence, gene expression array, and proteomic data. The conception and design of QTL experiments may be assisted if blocks of ancestral identity among mouse strains can be identified by high-density SNP maps and correlated with phenotypes. And testing of candidate genes will be facilitated through the construction of transgenic mice.[54] The availability of the complete genomic sequences of mice[5] and rats[41] should further enhance prospects for success.

MODELING WITH SIMPLE EUKARYOTIC ORGANISMS

Human and mouse genomes have dominated the literature of genome science, but the annotation of the sequences of several nonmammalian eukaryotic organisms (yeast, fruit fly, nematode, zebrafish) provides additional opportunities to use comparative genomics for pharmacogenomic analysis and therapeutics.[55]

Successful use of simpler organisms in medical research implies that important biologic processes have remained essentially unchanged throughout evolution and that these processes are easier to dissect in simpler models. Additional advantages of these models for genetic studies are their short generation time and the fact that mutants responsible for specific phenotypes can be generated efficiently. Apart from the conservation of genomic sequences across species, the usefulness of a particular model is dictated primarily by its suitability for the study of specific cellular pathways. For example, yeast cells are particularly advantageous as a model for studies of cell cycle events and the effects of mutations on cell division, fly embryos for understanding genes that regulate the organization of tissues and differentiation of cells, and nematodes for investigating the developmental fate of individual cells and for apoptosis.[55] The zebrafish may greatly facilitate the study of genotype–phenotype relationships because the zebrafish genome is thought to contain a counterpart for almost every disease-causing gene in humans, and because the study of the consequences of aberrant gene expression can be readily studied at the level of the whole organism.[56]

Clues to several human genetic defects of pharmacogenomic interest have now been identified in simple eukaryotic models by genetic screening. Thus, germline mutations in the human ortholog of the fly gene, *patched,* have been found as somatic mutations in most cases of sporadic basal cell cancer.[57,58] The human ortholog of the zebrafish gene, *ferroportin1,* was found to be mutated in certain cases of autosomal-dominant hemochromatosis.[59,60] These models can also provide a means of defining cellular pathways by placing genes within a functional pathway—so-called modifier genes. Modifier genes often function in the same pathway as a gene of interest. Modifier screening in flies and nematodes has shown that abnormal expansion of glutamines is causative of various inherited diseases of neurodegeneration such as Huntington's disease and spinocerebellar atrophy.[61] In flies, overexpression of the gene for α -synuclein causes degenerative changes in dopaminergic neurons and abnormalities in movement that may prove to be of interest in connection with Parkinson's disease.[62]

Genetic screening in yeast, flies, and nematodes might also provide powerful optional approaches to the discovery of therapeutic agents. Although genetic screening in these models has not led to any drugs in current use, two agents with therapeutic potential have been identified.[55] One, cyclopamine, is beneficial in the treatment of basal cell cancer,[63] and the other, sirolimus, may be beneficial in the treatment of tuberous sclerosis. Cyclopamine causes prosencephaly in sheep, and a similar abnormality occurs in mice and humans lacking a hedgehog gene. In flies, cyclopamine interacts with *patched* and its partner (*Smoothened*) to suppress the hedgehog signaling cascade. But *patched* is known to be a target of mutations in the basal cell cancer syndrome raising the possibility that cyclopamine could be useful in treating this cancer. The other example of genetic screening in flies concerns the discovery of the potential therapeutic effect of sirolimus, also known as rapamycin, in the treatment of the congenital anomaly tuberous sclerosis. Rapamycin, an immunosuppressive antibiotic, was found to antagonize the function of TOR (target of rapamycin) kinase, a signaling molecule activated by several growth-promoting stimuli.[64] Tuberous sclerosis genes, TSC1 and TSC2, restrict cell growth, while mutations in TSC1 and TSC2 cause excessive TOR kinase and augment cell growth. These observations provide a rationale for the possible use of rapamycin in the treatment of tuberous sclerosis.[65]

SUMMARY

Pharmacogenetic studies are undertaken with the primary goal of detecting hereditary peculiarities in the human drug response and to elucidate these traits in accordance with the basic principles of pharmacology and genetics, but this goal can often be very difficult to attain solely through studies in human subjects. A convincing animal model can provide insights into the potential origin of the human condition and reveal features that are exceptionally difficult or impossible to demonstrate because of ethical or methodological limitations that apply to human studies. The ability to construct knockout and transgenic "humanized" experimental models through gene targeting and the capacity to conduct comparative genomic studies across many organisms were monumental advances toward the functional analysis of almost any gene. By exploiting a combination of these techniques and recombinant and congenic strains for analysis of monogenic traits, QTL mapping of gene loci for the analysis of polygenic traits, and simple eukaryotic organisms (yeast, flies, worms, zebra fish) for rapid, accessible ways of genetic screening, model systems provide powerful, wide-ranging toolsets to discern the molecular basis of hereditary peculiarities in individual responses to therapeutic agents and other exogenous substances in the human environment.

REFERENCES

1. Staats J. Standardized nomenclature for inbred strains of mice: Seventh listing for the International Committee on Standardized Genetic Nomenclature for Mice. Cancer Res 1980; 40(7):2083–2128.
2. Bedell MA, Jenkins Na, Copeland NG. Mouse models of human disease. Part I: Techniques and resources for genetic analysis in mice. Genes Dev 1997; 11(1): 1–10.
3. Bedell MA, Largaespada DA, Jenkins Na, Copeland NG. Mouse models of human disease. Part II: Recent progress and future directions. Genes Dev 1997; 11(1): 11–43.
4. Beck JA, Lloyd S, Hafezparast M, Lennon-Pierce M, Eppig JT, Festing MF, et al. Genealogies of mouse inbred strains. Nat Genet 2000; 24(1):23–25.
5. Waterston RH, Lindblad-Toh K, Birney E, Rogers J, Abril JF, Agarwal P, et al. Initial sequencing and comparative analysis of the mouse genome. Nature 2002; 420(6915):520–562.
6. Evans MJ. The cultural mouse. Nat Med 2001; 7(10):1081–1083.
7. Gregory SG, Sekhon M, Schein J, Zhao S, Osoegawa K, Scott CE, et al. A physical map of the mouse genome. Nature 2002; 418(6899):743–750.
8. Austin CP, Battey JF, Bradley A, Bucan M, Capecchi M, Collins FS, et al. The knockout mouse project. Nat Genet 2004; 36(9):921–924.
9. Wade CM, Kulbokas EJ III, Kirby AW, Zody MC, Mullikin JC, Lander ES, et al. The mosaic structure of variation in the laboratory mouse genome. Nature 2002; 420(6915):574–578.
10. Frankel WN. Taking stock of complex trait genetics in mice. Trends Genet 1995; 11(12):471–477.
11. Snell GD. Congenic resistant strains of mice. In: Morse HC III, editor. Origins of Inbred Mice. New York: Academic Press, 1978: 119–156.
12. Flaherty L. Congenic strains. In: Foster HL, Small JD, Fox JG, editors. The Mouse in Biomedical Research. History, Genetics and Wild Mice. New York: Academic Press, 1981: 215–222.
13. Lander ES, Schork NJ. Genetic dissection of complex traits. Science 1994; 265(5181):2037–2048.
14. Yui MA, Muralidharan K, Moreno-Altamirano B, Perrin G, Chestnut K, Wakeland EK. Production of congenic mouse strains carrying NOD-derived diabetogenic

genetic intervals: An approach for the genetic dissection of complex traits. Mamm Genome 1996; 7(5):331–334.

15. Morel L, Yu Y, Blenman KR, Caldwell RA, Wakeland EK. Production of congenic mouse strains carrying genomic intervals containing SLE-susceptibility genes derived from the SLE-prone NZM2410 strain. Mamm Genome 1996; 7(5):335–339.

16. Jeffs B, Negrin CD, Graham D, Clark JS, Anderson NH, Gauguier D, et al. Applicability of a "speed" congenic strategy to dissect blood pressure quantitative trait loci on rat chromosome 2. Hypertension 2000; 35(1 Pt 2):179–187.

17. Nadeau JH, Singer JB, Matin A, Lander ES. Analysing complex genetic traits with chromosome substitution strains. Nat Genet 2000; 24(3):221–225.

18. Consomic Mice. Bar Harbor, ME: Jackson Laboratory, 2006.

19. Nebert DW, Goujon FM, Gielen JE. Aryl hydrocarbon hydroxylase induction by polycyclic hydrocarbons: Simple autosomal dominant trait in the mouse. Nat New Biol 1972; 236(65):107–110.

20. Thomas PE, Kouri RE, Hutton JJ. The genetics of aryl hydrocarbon hydroxylase induction in mice: A single gene difference between C57BL-6J and DBA-2J. Biochem Genet 1972; 6(2):157–168.

21. Poland A, Glover E, Taylor BA. The murine Ah locus: A new allele and mapping to chromosome 12. Mol Pharmacol 1987; 32(4):471–478.

22. Poland A, Palen D, Glover E. Analysis of the four alleles of the murine aryl hydrocarbon receptor. Mol Pharmacol 1994; 46(5):915–921.

23. Swanson HI, Bradfield CA. The AH-receptor: Genetics, structure and function. Pharmacogenetics 1993; 3(5):213–230.

24. Birnbaum LS, McDonald MM, Blair PC, Clark AM, Harris MW. Differential toxicity of 2,3,7,8-tetrachlorodibenzo-p-dioxin (TCDD) in C57BL/6J mice congenic at the Ah locus. Fundam Appl Toxicol 1990; 15(1):186–200.

25. Hahn ME, Gasiewicz TA, Linko P, Goldstein JA. The role of the Ah locus in hexachlorobenzene-induced porphyria. Studies in congenic C57BL/6J mice. Biochem J 1988; 254(1):245–254.

26. Paigen B, Holmes PA, Morrow A, Mitchell D. Effect of 3-methylcholanthrene on atherosclerosis in two congenic strains of mice with different susceptibilities to methylcholanthrene-induced tumors. Cancer Res 1986; 46(7):3321–3324.

27. Lahvis GP, Pyzalski RW, Glover E, Pitot HC, McElwee MK, Bradfield CA. The aryl hydrocarbon receptor is required for developmental closure of the ductus venosus in the neonatal mouse. Mol Pharmacol 2005; 67(3):714–720.

28. Mouse Phenome Database. Bar Harbor, ME: Jackson Laboratory, 2006.

29. Levy GN, Martell KJ, DeLeon JH, Weber WW. Metabolic, molecular genetic and toxicological aspects of the acetylation polymorphism in inbred mice. Pharmacogenetics 1992; 2(5):197–206.

30. DeLeon JH, Martell KJ, Vatsis KP, Weber WW. Slow acetylation in mice is caused by a labile and catalytically impaired mutant N-acetyltransferase (NAT2 9). Drug Metab Dispos 1995; 23(12):1354–1361.

31. Nerurkar PV, Schut HA, Anderson LM, Riggs CW, Fornwald LW, Davis CD, et al. Ahr locus phenotype in congenic mice influences hepatic and pulmonary DNA adduct levels of 2-amino-3-methylimidazo[4,5-f]quinoline in the absence of cytochrome P450 induction. Mol Pharmacol 1996; 49(5):874–881.

32. Nerurkar PV, Schut HA, Anderson LM, Riggs CW, Snyderwine EG, Thorgeirsson SS, et al. DNA adducts of 2-amino-3-methylimidazo[4,5-f]quinoline (IQ) in colon, bladder, and kidney of congenic mice differing in Ah responsiveness and N-acetyltransferase genotype. Cancer Res 1995; 55(14):3043–3049.

33. Goldstein JL. Laskers for 2001: Knockout mice and test-tube babies. Nat Med 2001; 7(10):1079–1080.
34. Smithies O. Forty years with homologous recombination. Nat Med 2001; 7(10): 1083–1086.
35. Capecchi MR. Generating mice with targeted mutations. Nat Med 2001; 7(10):1086–1090.
36. Kuhn R, Schwenk F, Aguet M, Rajewsky K. Inducible gene targeting in mice. Science 1995; 269(5229):1427–1429.
37. Furth PA, St Onge L, Boger H, Gruss P, Gossen M, Kistner A, et al. Temporal control of gene expression in transgenic mice by a tetracycline-responsive promoter. Proc Natl Acad Sci USA 1994; 91(20):9302–9306.
38. Peltonen L, McKusick VA. Genomics and medicine. Dissecting human disease in the postgenomic era. Science 2001; 291(5507):1224–1229.
39. Paterson AH, Lander ES, Hewitt JD, Peterson S, Lincoln SE, Tanksley SD. Resolution of quantitative traits into Mendelian factors by using a complete linkage map of restriction fragment length polymorphisms. Nature 1988; 335(6192):721–726.
40. Doerge RW. Mapping and analysis of quantitative trait loci in experimental populations. Nat Rev Genet 2002; 3(1):43–52.
41. Gibbs RA, Weinstock GM, Metzker ML, Muzny DM, Sodergren EJ, Scherer S, et al. Genome sequence of the Brown Norway rat yields insights into mammalian evolution. Nature 2004; 428(6982):493–521.
42. Lander ES, Botstein D. Mapping mendelian factors underlying quantitative traits using RFLP linkage maps. Genetics 1989; 121(1):185–199.
43. Lander ES, Green P, Abrahamson J, Barlow A, Daly MJ, Lincoln SE, et al. MAPMAKER: An interactive computer package for constructing primary genetic linkage maps of experimental and natural populations. Genomics 1987; 1(2):174–181.
44. Jacob HJ, Lindpainter K, Lincoln SE, Kusumi K, Bunker RK, Mao P, et al. Genetic mapping of a gene causing hypertension in the stroke-prone spontaneously hypertensive rat. Cell 1991; 67:213–224.
45. Butler MA, Iwasaki M, Guengerich FP, Kadlubar FF. Human cytochrome P-450PA (P-450IA2), the phenacetin O-deethylase, is primarily responsible for the hepatic 3-demethylation of caffeine and the N-oxidation of carcinogenic arylamines. Proc Natl Acad Sci USA 1989: 86(20):7696–7700.
46. Berrettini WH, Ferraor TN, Alexander RC, Buchberg AM, Vogel WH. Quantitative trait loci mapping of three loci controlling morphine preference using inbred mouse strains. Nat Genet 1994; 7:54–58.
47. De Sanctis GT, Singer JB, Jiao A, Yandava CN, Lee YH, Haynes TC, et al. Quantative trait locus mapping of airway responsiveness to chromosomes 6 and 7 in inbred mice. Am J Physiol 1999; 277(6 Pt 1):L1118–L1123.
48. Hain HS, Belknap JK. Pharmacogenetic evidence for the involvement of 5-hydroxytryptamine (serotonin)-1B receptors in the mediation of morphine antinociceptive sensitivity. JPET 1999; 291(2):444–449.
49. Malkinson AM, Radcliffe RA, Bauer AK. Quantitative trait locus mapping of susceptibilities to butylated hydroxytoluene-induced lung tumor promotion and pulmonary inflammation in CXB mice. Carcinogenesis 2002; 23(3):411–417.
50. Belknap JK. Chromosome substitution strains: Some quantitative considerations for genome scans and fine mapping. Mamm Genome 2003; 14(11):723–732.
51. Singer JB, Hill AE, Burrage LC, Olszens KR, Song J, Justice M, et al. Genetic dissection of complex traits with chromosome substitution strains of mice. Science 2004; 304(5669):445–448.

52. CHORI-27 Mus musculus A/J BAC library. 2006.

53. Avner P. Quantity and quality: Polygenic analysis in the mouse. Nat Genet 1994; 7(1):3–4.

54. Cormier RT, Hong KH, Halberg RB, Hawkins TL, Richardson P, Mulherkar R, et al. Secretory phospholipase Pla2g2a confers resistance to intestinal tumorigenesis. Nat Genet 1997; 17(1):88–91.

55. Hariharan IK, Haber DA. Yeast, flies, worms, and fish in the study of human disease. N Engl J Med 2003; 348(24):2457–2463.

56. Renier C, Faraco JH, Bourgin P, Motley T, Bonaventure P, Rosa F, et al. Genomic and functional conservation of sedative-hypnotic targets in the zebrafish. Pharmacogenet Genomics 2007; 17(4):237–253.

57. Hahn H, Wicking C, Zaphiropolous PG, Gailani MR, Shanley S, Chidabaram A, et al. Mutations of the human homolog of *Drosophila* patched in the nevoid basal cell carcinoma syndrome. Cell 1996; 85(6):841–851.

58. Johnson RL, Rothman AL, Xie J, Goodrich LV, Bare JW, Boniface JM, et al. Human homolog of patched, a candidate gene for the basal cell nevus syndrome. Science 1996; 272(Jun 14):1668–1671.

59. Montosi G, Donovan A, Totaro A, Garuti C, Pignatti E, Cassanelli S, et al. Autosomal-dominant hemochromatosis is associated with a mutation in the ferroportin (SLC11A3) gene. J Clin Invest 2001; (1084):619–623.

60. Njajou OT, Vaessen N, Joose M, Berghis B, van Dongen JWF, Beurning MH, et al. A mutation in SLC11A3 is associated with autosomal dominant hemochromatosis. Nat Genet 2001; 28(Jul):213–214.

61. Gusella JF, MacDonald ME. Molecular genetics: Unmasking polyglutamine triggers in neurodegenerative disease. Nat Rev Neurosci 2000; 1(2):109–115.

62. Feany MB, Bender WW. A *Drosophila* model of Parkinson's disease. Nature 2000; 404(Mar 23):394–398.

63. Taipale J, Chen JK, Cooper MK, Wang B, Mann RK, Milenkovic L, et al. Effects of oncogenic mutations in Smoothened and Patched can be reversed by cyclopamine. Nature 2000; 406(Aug 31):944–945.

64. Schmelzle T, Hall MN. TOR, a central controller of cell growth. Cell 2000; 103(2): 253–262.

65. Kwiatkowski DJ, Zhang H, Bandura JL, Heiberger KM, Glogauer M, el-Hashemite N, et al. A mouse model of TSC1 reveals sex-dependent lethality from liver hemagiomas, and up-regulation of p70S6 kinase activity in Tsc1 null cells. Hum Mol Genet 2002; 11(5):525–534.

III

FUTURES

10
Drug Discovery

This chapter describes how genomics is involved in the discovery of new drugs for medical therapy. For at least a decade after numerous molecular benchmarks in enzyme and receptor pharmacogenetics had been established, the pharmaceutical industry did not vigorously pursue a gene-based approach to drug discovery.[1] Such an approach was initially viewed with skepticism, but in the 1990s genomics created a whole new direction for drug development,[2] and the elucidation of genetic diversity came to be regarded as an essential component of new drug discovery. By providing a better drug at the outset, genomics could improve safety and efficacy, and diminish costly drug failures.

Since 1995,[3–5] the number of new drugs in the drug discovery pipeline has fallen well short of Big Pharma's goals. An average of 31 new drugs had been approved each year with a downward trend more recently, including only a surprisingly small number of innovative targets, typically two to three a year.[6] In contrast, academic researchers, often in collaboration with new biotechnology companies, effectively applied genomics principles to new drug discoveries. By 2003, the proportion of new therapeutic agents that originated in biotech firms through gene-based approaches had reached 20–25%.

CHANGING PHARMACEUTICAL PERSPECTIVES

From the earliest of times, humanity has relied on natural sources for its medical needs.[7] But this picture began to change in 1805 when the medicinal value of opium was identified with its content of morphine. The isolation of caffeine and quinine in 1819, of codeine in 1832, and of papaverine in 1848 led medicinal and physiological chemists to purify, modify, and synthesize the biologically active components of natural products. Subsequently these substances provided a rich source of new drugs.

At the beginning of the twentieth century, epinephrine was one of the first of these naturally occurring substances to be obtained in pure form, and during the

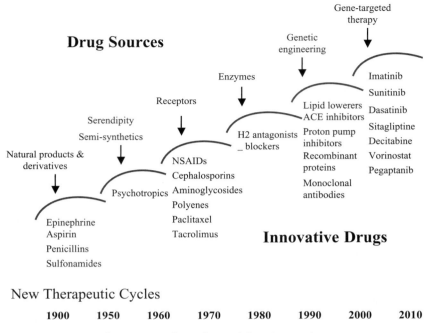

Figure 10.1 Chronology of drug innovation.

next 30 years a number of related drugs, such as phenylephrine and isoprenaline, were introduced as therapeutic agents (Figure 10.1). The identification of α- and β-adrenergic receptor subtypes by Ahlquist in 1948 opened further therapeutic opportunities, first realized in the development of antagonists for the α-adrenergic receptor, such as phentolamine, tolazoline, and prazosin, and for the β-adrenergic receptor, propranolol. When β-adrenergic receptors were divided into β_1, β_2, and β_3 subtypes, salbutamol emerged in 1967 as the first agonist with selectivity for the β_2 receptor, while metoprolol and atenolol were introduced later as selective antagonists for the β_1 receptor. Many drugs that were used therapeutically throughout the twentieth century, and currently, were discovered through the same or similar approaches.

Following these discoveries, additional medicines were obtained by modification of native forms of natural products. The initial success of the antibiotic penicillin as an antiinfective was followed quickly by the emergence of resistance, which in turn led medicinal chemists to modify the molecule to produce new, semisynthetic drugs with improved resistance profiles. During the 1960s and 1970s, the pharmaceutical industry focused major efforts on screening natural products both as extracts and in pure form, and through these efforts cephalosporins such as cefuroxime, aminoglycosides such as streptomycin, and polyenes such as amphotericin B were obtained. The discoveries of the anticancer agent, paclitaxel, of 3-hydroxy-3-methylglutaryl coenzyme A (HMG-CoA) reductase antilipid inhibitors such as atorvastatin derived from 3-hydroxycompactin, and of the immunosuppressant, FK506/tacrolimus, were additional triumphs of these efforts. In each of these instances, synthetic chemistry was used to improve the therapeutic efficacy and safety of the original, naturally occurring molecule.

In recent years, however, interest in natural products has waned and libraries of synthetic molecules have tended to replace them as the primary resource of chemical screens for new drugs.[8] Between 1981 and 2003 only 5% of 1031 new chemical entities approved by the Food and Drug Administration (FDA) were natural products while another 23% were derived from natural product molecules. However, these newer sources supplied fewer good leads than expected, and today there is a resurgence of interest in natural products obtained from marine organisms, rain forests, and soil as the search intensifies for targets identified via genetic technologies. Certainly, natural products are still major sources of innovative therapeutics and have proven useful as drugs or as leads as shown by vancomycin in the treatment of Gram-positive bacterial infections, by staurosporine as a lead structure for the inhibition of protein kinases at the ATP-binding site, by rapamycin as a lead for immunosuppression, and by Taxol for cancer chemotherapy. Even though the complexity of many natural products is a barrier to optimize their therapeutic use, the increasing efficiency of synthetic bioorganic chemistry is reducing this barrier, even for substances with very complex structures.[9]

HUMAN DRUG EFFICACY TARGETS

Following completion of the first phase of the Human Genome Project, Craig Venter and colleagues[10] observed that about 18% of the putative proteins represented in the human genome belonged to chemically defined families nominally regarded as major drug targets. The analysis by these investigators also identified sequences for receptors and select regulatory molecules, for transferase and oxidoreductase enzymes, kinases, ion channels, and transporters. On further analysis of these data, Jurgen Drews concluded that there were 5000–10,000 potential drug targets in the human genome, and that approved medicines exploited fewer than 500 of these as validated targets.[11]

Assignment of Drug Efficacy Targets

Hopkins and Groom[12] challenged Drews's estimate and suggested that rule-of-five* compliant drugs acted primarily through only 120 targets. In a subsequent

---

*Rule-of-five: Poor absorption or permeation of a compound is more likely when there are more than five hydrogen bond donors, the molecular mass is greater than 500, the calculated octanol/water partition coefficient ($c \log P$) is greater than 5, and the sum of nitrogen and oxygen atoms in a molecule is greater than 10. Many drugs are exceptions to this rule and often these are substrates for biological transporters.

report, Hopkins and colleagues reconciled these and other earlier reports through analysis of more than 21,000 drug products and reached a consensus of 324 molecular drug targets for all classes of approved therapeutic agents.[13] When products with duplicate active ingredients, supplements, vitamins, imaging agents, and so on were removed, only 1357 unique drugs remained, of which 1204 were "small molecule drugs" and 166 were "biological drugs." Among all small molecule drugs, 885 (74%) passed the rule-of-five test and at least 192 (16%) of them were prodrugs.

Protein molecular targets could be assigned to 1065 (78%) of the 1357 unique drugs via a comprehensive analysis of the literature. When possible, the particular binding domain of the protein as well as the binding residues was also assigned. Among the 324 molecular targets, 266 were found to be human genome-derived proteins; the remainder comprised nonhuman (bacterial, viral, fungal, or other pathogenic organism) targets. Small molecule drugs were found to modulate 248 proteins, of which 207 were targets encoded by the human genome. Oral, small molecule drugs targeted 227 molecular targets, of which 186 were human targets. Biological drugs, on the other hand, targeted 76 proteins with monoclonal antibody therapeutics acting on 15 distinct human targets. Only nine targets were found to modulate both small molecule and biological drugs. For example, the biological drugs cetuximab and panitumumab target the extracellular domain of the receptor tyrosine kinase epidermal growth factor receptor (EGFR) (ERBB1), whereas the small molecule drugs gefinitib and erlotinib target the adenine portion of the ATP-binding site of the cytosolic catalytic kinase domain of the same receptor.

Many drugs are capable of interacting with more than one valid target and exhibit clinically relevant, multitarget effects. Members of the class of protein kinase inhibitors encoded by the BCR/ABL fusion gene, such as the small molecule drug imatinib mesylate (Gleevec®), provide excellent examples of such "clinical polypharmacology." Following the introduction of imatinib for the treatment of chronic myeloid leukemia, studies revealed that it targets kinases other than BCR/ABL such as c-Kit, expanding its clinical relevance in myeloid disorders to gastrointestinal stromal tumors and glioblastomas. The clinical polypharmacology of imatinib and newer protein kinase inhibitors such as sorafenib and sunitinib with target footprints similar to imatinib can be rationalized by similarities of key pharmacophores.[†] Recent research on such polypharmacological interactions reveals the extent of clinically relevant drug promiscuity.[14] Taking account of polypharmacological interactions and putting them on a sound footing represent other major challenges to the discovery of safe and effective clinical therapies.

[†]Pharmacophore: An ensemble of steric and electronic features that is required to ensure optimal interactions with a specific target structure and to trigger (or block) its biological response.

Gene Families as Drug Targets

A large number of receptor superfamilies encompassing both membrane receptors [e.g., G-protein-coupled receptors (GPCRs), tyrosine kinase receptors, ligand- and voltage-gated ion channels, and integrins] and intracellular nuclear receptors have evolved to accommodate the selective recognition of a large and diverse number of endogenous and exogenous ligands. Analysis of the gene-family distribution of drug targets for both small molecule and biological drugs by Overington and colleagues revealed that more than 50% of drugs targeted only four key gene families: Class I GPCRs, nuclear receptors, ligand-gated ions channels, and voltage-gated ion channels (Figure 10.2). Several additional features of gene-family targets for current drugs are brought out by the analysis of Overington et al. (1) Approximately 130 "druggable" domains cover all current drug targets, a number that contrasts markedly with the number of protein families (>16,000) and protein folds (~10,000). (2) Approximately 60% of current drug targets are located at the cell surface, compared with only ~22% of all proteins in the human genome. (3) Only 1620 distinct human protein sequences are linked directly to a genetic disease. Of these, 105 are drug targets, corresponding to 47% of human drug targets that are directly linked with a disease. (4) The determination of the potency distribution of marketed small molecule drugs shows that the median affinity for all current small molecule drugs is around 20 nM. (5) Analysis of the protein domains shows that new domains join the drugged domain set relatively infrequently. For example, of 361 new molecular entities (NMEs) approved by the FDA between 1999 and 2000, 76% targeted a previously drugged domain and only 6% targeted a previously undrugged

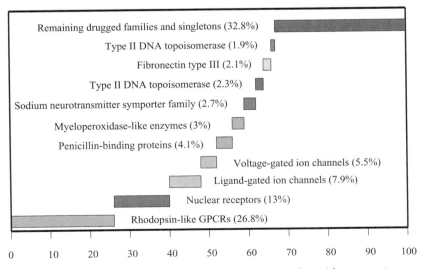

Figure 10.2 Gene family distribution (percentage drugs/drug target).

domain; the remainder had either unknown targets (4%) or were believed not to act at distinct molecular targets (17%). (6) The rate of target innovation averaged 5.3 new drugged targets per year but was quite variable year by year.

APPLYING GENOMICS TO DRUG DISCOVERY

Typically, new drug discovery begins with the selection of promising candidate chemical entities having biological activities that correlate with relevant treatment targets. Following the identification of the better candidates as leads, the process proceeds through preclinical and clinical phases to validate the safety and efficacy of the better leads.[3] Candidates should consistently lead to phenotypic changes that are in harmony with the desired therapeutic effects, effects should be dose dependent, the desired phenotypic change should be inducible or mimicked in one or more relevant animal or experimental models, and the mechanism by which the target molecule brings about a particular phenotype should be known or determined. Until recently, studying functional changes of single genes in appropriate animals and in human cells were the primary approaches to validate the target. Though such approaches are powerful and time tested, they are also slow, labor intensive, and expensive.

By knowing the full complement of human genes, however, scientists have at their disposal a much broader range of targets at which to aim potential therapeutic interventions. They may also take advantage of high-throughput technologies, global gene expression analysis, and genome-wide functional analyses. With the aid of gene expression profiling, investigators can readily analyze the effects of hundreds or thousands of genes on toxicity and the efficacy of drug candidates, conducting thousands of tests in parallel instead of sequentially, thus streamlining the drug discovery process while enhancing prospects for better therapies.[15] Thus, the real challenge of gene-based approaches to drug discovery is to define a consistently effective process, or processes, to translate gene-sequence data into drugs that provide defined physiological and clinical endpoints, or, to put it more simply, to find efficient ways to move from gene sequence data (or the protein the sequence encodes) to drug entity.

Some incremental advances have already been achieved in this endeavor as shown by the following descriptions of several successful or promising applications of genomics/proteomics to the discovery or improvement of small molecule drugs, recombinant DNA products, and monoclonal antibodies suitable for human therapy.

SMALL MOLECULE DRUG DISCOVERY

Targeting Enzymatic Drug Inactivation Mechanisms

Once an enzyme has been identified as an attractive target, drug designers have tended to frame their approach in terms of designing enzyme inhibitors that bind to the active conformation of the enzyme. For tyrosine kinases, work by Schindler and colleagues[16] on the antileukemic drug STI-571 suggested that the inactive conformation of the enzyme might make a better drug target than the active conformation. STI-571, the most potent of a series of 2-phenylaminopyridines, had been exceptionally successful as a therapeutic agent in clinical trials on patients with chronic myeloid leukemia. It blocked the oncogenic form of ABL, a tyrosine kinase whose activation by the acquisition of a phosphate group is linked to the proliferation of leukemic cells in affected patients, but it did not alter the activity of some 50 other closely related kinases. Studies of the crystallographic structure of the ABL–drug complex that were undertaken to explain the specificity of STI-571 for the ABL kinase revealed that the drug bound to the inactive conformation of ABL, locking the enzyme in an inactive conformation and preventing the acquisition of the activating phosphate by the drug–enzyme complex. While the active kinases looked very similar structurally to each other, the inactive kinases looked very different, which explained why STI-571 was selective for ABL, and why this drug did not exhibit selectivity for other kinases.

The discovery and clinical development of STI-571, now called imatinib (Gleevec®), is an excellent example of how knowledge of a specific enzyme inactivation mechanism was used to design a therapeutic agent. Imatinib mesylate has specific indications for treating chronic myelogenous leukemia, a clonal hematological disorder that is characterized by a reciprocal translocation between chromosomes 9 and 22. As a consequence of the creation of the BCR-ABL fusion gene, proliferation of leukemic cells occurs in affected patients. Binding of imatinib to the inactive conformation of ABL prevents proliferation of the cancer cells. The first patient was treated with imatinib in 1998, and within 3 years three large clinical trials showed the drug to be a safe and effective treatment for all stages of chronic myelogenous leukemia. In 2001, imatinib received FDA approval for treating this disorder, and in 2002, it received approval for the treatment of gastrointestinal stromal tumors.[17]

Imatinib mesylate (Gleevec®) is a highly effective treatment for chronic myelogenous leukemia and causes remarkably few side effects. Unfortunately, some patients relapse and die because of Gleevec resistance.[18] However, additional inhibitors of BCR-ABL appear to be active against several kinase mutations found in patients who develop Gleevec resistance.[19] Recently, investigators have tested such a compound as a prototype of a new generation of anti-BCR-ABL compounds that appears to be more effective than Gleevec.[20] In 2006, two second-generation tyrosine kinase inhibitors, Sutent (Sunitinib malate, Pfizer) and Sprycel (Dasatinib, Bristol-Myers Squibb), both received FDA approval for the treatment of chronic myelogenous leukemia.[4]

The success of imatinib suggests that strategies that target distinctive inactivation mechanisms can provide a compelling approach to rational drug discovery.

Targeting Inhibitor Chemical Switches

The development of small molecule inhibitors of tyrosine kinases such as imatinib was an important advance in drug design, but the study of individual kinases has also presented a formidable problem because they are so numerous—more then 500 have been identified in the human genome[21]—and because they have such similar active sites. A new method of small molecule target identification, termed "chemical genetics," has recently been reported.[22] The chemical genetic approach devised by Shokat and colleagues[23] provides a strategy, among a number of other strategies that have been proposed,[24] to engineer proteins with specificity and sensitivity to small molecule, cell-permeable protein kinase inhibitors. Submitting this method to the kinase family of enzymes provides a rigorous test of this strategy because protein kinase signaling pathways are highly conserved, central mediators of many different cell signaling events, and because highly selective kinase inhibitors for dissection of these pathways have proven difficult to obtain.

In Schokat's approach, a functionally silent mutation is inserted into a kinase (e.g., v-src protein kinase) by replacing a bulky amino acid in the active site (such as threonine) by glycine (or alanine). This modification has little effect on the ability of the src kinase to transfer the activating phosphate efficiently in cells and animals, and the modified kinase retains its ability to confer unrestrained growth on cells in culture equivalent to that of the unmodified gene. However, the modified kinase can be distinguished from all other cellular kinases by an inhibitor especially synthesized for this purpose. And when the gene that encodes the modified enzyme is inserted into cells and/or living animals, its activity can be switched off by administering (feeding) them the inhibitor.

The generality of the strategy was demonstrated by repeating the procedure in several protein kinases from five distinct families, again by substituting a bulky amino acid with a glycine.[23]

The researchers say that the chemical genetic strategy has key advantages over strategies to study the function of closely related proteins that involve mutating or knocking out the genes that encode them, or by studying temperature-sensitive mutants.[23] They point out that mutations or knockouts may disrupt embryonic development, or be lethal, and that studies of temperature-sensitive mutants can be hard to interpret because the temperature change may affect cellular processes of direct interest as well as processes other than those directly altered by the target protein.

Targeting G-Protein-Coupled Receptors

Analysis of the human genome reveals the existence of 735–802 GPCR open reading frames, of which ~375 are neither olfactory nor taste receptors.[25,26] Based on sequence homology and pharmacological similarities, human GPCRs are divisible into five families: A (rhodopsin), B (secretin), C (glutamate), and adhesion and Frizzled/Smoothened/Taste2.[26] Family A is the largest and its members recognize ligands including odorants, biogenic amines, neuropeptides and peptidic hormones, lipids, nucleotides, proteases, and photons. Family B recognizes hormones and peptides and family C recognizes amino acids, ions, and tastants. Adhesion receptors are believed to interact with extracellular matrix or membrane-bound proteins, while Frizzled and Taste2 receptors are activated by Wnt proteins and tastants, respectively.

The GPCR family represents one of the most attractive therapeutic targets in the human genome. According to Drews,[11] cell membrane receptors constitute the largest subgroup with 45% of all therapeutic targets. In 2001, 50–60% of all therapeutics in use targeted GPCRs. The GPCR family, represented by more than 600 genes, is one of the largest gene families in the genome.[10] These receptors conduct, or participate in, a wide variety of disorders associated with dysfunctional central and peripheral neurotransmission, as well as with impaired autocrine, hormonal, and paracrine systems. Traditionally, therapeutic agents intended to modulate GPCR function act as agonists or antagonists. GPCRs consist of membrane-bound molecules that are usually classified according to the drug ligand they bind; the major GPCR classes are those that bind bioaminergic, peptide, opioid, protease, chemokine, or fMLP (chemotactic) ligands or substrates. GPCRs that have been extensively studied, or are currently of considerable interest, include the β_2-adrenoceptor, the dopamine receptor, the V2 vasopressin receptor, the chemokine receptor, and the protease receptor.

A significant degree of individual variability is associated with therapeutic responses to GPCR agonists and antagonists. But pharmacogenomic studies on GPCRs are relatively scarce, and the therapeutic relevance of GPCRs is often not well defined.[27] Attempts to assess the relevance of specific and variant forms of GPCR alleles are often thwarted by a variety of factors including the cross reaction of a single drug with multiple receptors, poorly defined ligand-binding receptor pockets that can accommodate drugs in different orientations and at alternative domains, the possibility of multiple receptor conformations with distinct functions, and multiple signaling pathways engaged by a single receptor.

Nevertheless, insights into the nature and significance of GPCR variability that are of interest to drug discovery are advancing. Characterization of GPCR genetic variability reveals that as much as 60% of this variability is attributed to genetic causes, and functional polymorphisms occur in multiple, potentially critical, genomic regions of GPCR genes. Studies of the β_2-adrenoceptor, for example, suggest that such variability might have evolved through expression, ligand binding, G-protein coupling, or regulation, but the data indicate that variability developed most commonly in the transmembrane-spanning domains that are typical of ligand binding.[28] It was suggested that there is a need to be cognizant of ligand-binding single-nucleotide polymorphisms (SNPs) and to seek to delineate such variability early in the discovery process. Also, false nonsynonymous polymorphisms of GPCR genes are frequently reported (68%), and caution is advised against exclusive reliance on databases for the selection of candidate GPCR polymorphisms for pharmacogenetic studies or disease associations.[29]

Targeting RGS Proteins and GPCR Regulation

The regulator of G-protein signaling (RGS) family is a recently identified protein family that plays a major role in regulating GPCR signaling pathways by modulating the activity of G-proteins.[30,31] Despite advances in the understanding of GPCR signaling pathways, none of the known regulatory mechanisms satisfactorily explained the rapid turnoff of G-protein signaling. Generally speaking,

G Protein Cycle

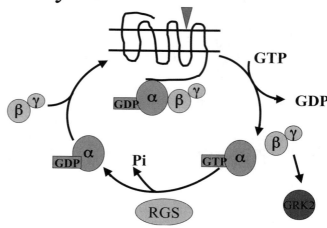

Figure 10.3 Regulator of G-protein signaling (RGS) proteins.

G-proteins are fairly stable and the levels of G-protein expression do not vary significantly under different physiological conditions. In contrast, several RGS mRNAs do vary under these circumstances, suggesting that RGS proteins might provide an important mechanism for regulating G-protein signaling (Figure 10.3).

Such a rapid turnoff mechanism generally applicable to G-proteins emerged only a few years ago with the discovery of the RGS protein family.[30,31] This highly diverse protein family was discovered when a conserved sequence of 120 amino acids was observed across yeast and worm proteins. Shortly thereafter, several investigators showed that RGS proteins were GTPase accelerating proteins. The GTPase activating activity of the RGS domain of the RGS proteins accounts for the rapid suppression of G-protein signaling by accelerating GTP hydrolysis of the GTP bound to the α-subunit of the G-protein. The RGS family of proteins exerts a number of additional effects on cell signaling, but their GTPase activity explains the paradox that some signals, visual responses, and cardiac potassium channels turn off much faster than expected given the slow hydrolysis of GTP by purified α-subunits.

RGS proteins are believed to act selectively by localizing to specific cell types and distinct intracellular sites, by the timing of their expression, and by the presence of domains other than the RGS domain that link these proteins to diverse signaling pathways. The gene structure, tissue-specific expression, chromosomal location, and regulation of RGS proteins in mammalian systems are as yet at an early stage of investigation, and the evidence for the physiological roles of RGS proteins as they are currently perceived comes mainly from model studies in *Saccharomyces cerevisiae* and *Caenorhabditis elegans*. However, multiple RGS mRNAs have been found in every mammalian tissue and cell type examined so far. Alternatively spliced RGS mRNAs may explain the multiplicity of RGS proteins, but many of these isoforms are incompletely characterized. Further characterization of the molecular characteristics and transcriptional regulation should be helpful in elucidating the potential involvement of RGS proteins in disorders of phamacogenetic interest.

As regulators of GPCRs, RGS proteins present numerous opportunities for new drug development. The fact that levels of RGS proteins have an important effect on GPCR signaling pathways suggests that RGS dysregulation might lead to pathological states. Because of a defect in transcriptional regulation such that RGS proteins are not expressed, or are mistargeted, G-protein signaling would be prolonged. On the other hand, should such a defect lead to RGS overexpression, they might represent potential targets for drug discovery. In their recent review of RGS proteins as novel multifunctional drug targets, Neubig and Siderovski speculate on ways that RGS inhibitors could be used, either alone or in combination with other drugs, for a variety of clinical indications.[32] For example, an inhibitor that targeted RGS proteins in brain regions involved in pain control might serve as an analgesic or an analgesic potentiator. As another example, an RGS inhibitor might serve to modify and/or increase the specificity of an administered agonist. Thus a drug that decreased RhoGEF activity, an oncogene that has a role in stimulating leukemic cell proliferation and possesses an RGS homology region, could be useful as an anticancer agent. Additional possibilities for RGS proteins as attractive drug targets are also discussed.[32]

The structural and biochemical properties of the RGS proteins enable them to interact with a growing list of proteins with diverse cellular functions. Their ability to suppress or silence GPCR signaling pathways provides a compelling reason to investigate their role in human variations in response to drugs and other exogenous chemicals. Information gained will not only make possible a broader understanding of the physiological roles of RGS proteins, but may also open new avenues to the discovery of more effective drugs and individualized drug therapy.

RNA Aptamers as Therapeutic Agents

Finding that cells contain a bevy of RNA snippets was another genomics discovery with surprising therapeutic implications.[33] These short segments of RNA, called aptamers, can bind to ligands with high affinity and specificity. This property, plus their low molecular weight, stability, and ease and low cost of preparation, suggests therapeutic aptamers may ultimately be superior to small molecule-based and monoclonal antibody therapeutics.[34]

Aptamers typically bind to their targets with dissociation constants in the high picomolar to low nanomolar range. They achieve their tight binding and specificity by adapting precise three-dimensional structures on binding and becoming encapsulated by the ligand. This property distinguishes them from antisense oligonucleotides and ribozymes that are linear and act to disrupt protein expression at the mRNA level via traditional hydrogen bond interactions. Studies in cell culture and of animals have shown that functionally, aptamers can be potent biological antagonists.

In addition to their high affinity and specificity, RNA aptamers can be modified relatively easily to improve their stability and bioavailability. They are nontoxic and are of low immunogenicity or are nonimmunogenic. While the first generation of aptamers was limited by nuclease sensitivity, poor availability, fast renal clearance, and limited uptake, these limitations have been largely overcome. Another significant advance in aptamer technology has shown that "antidotes," which are short complementary sequences (antisense) to the aptamers, can reverse the inhibitory properties of aptamers.

At the present time, Macugen® (Pegaptanib sodium) is the only FDA-approved aptamer drug. It improves vision in some patients afflicted with age-related wet macular degeneration, the leading cause of blindness in the elderly.[35] Age-related wet macular degeneration is characterized by blood vessel growth in the back of the eye or leakage of blood vessels that results in total loss of vision. The PEGylated, nuclease-stabilized aptamer is a selective antagonist of the vascular endothelial growth factor (VEGF) that plays a crucial role in angiogenesis. Macugen retards loss of vision and is currently in trial for diabetic macular edema and retinal vein occlusion.

Several additional RNA aptamers are currently in clinical development. Included among these are aptamers that target transcription factor decoys (for E2F, which plays a role in cardiovascular disease, and for nuclear factor NF-κβ), thrombin, several coagulation factors including Factors IXa, VIIa, and XII, and nucleolin.[34] Aptamers designed to target extracellular as well as intracellular sites present additional prospects for antiviral therapy, including HIV therapy. The anti-HIV aptamer, RNA aptamer B4, targets the extracellular, envelop protein gp120, which controls viral entry through its interaction with chemokine receptors. This aptamer was found to be highly effective in neutralizing HIV infectivity in human blood mononuclear cells by more than 1000-fold. Other viral infections being targeted for aptamer intervention include hepatitis C virus (HCV), Rous sarcoma virus, and cytomegalovirus.

PROTEIN THERAPEUTICS

Recombinant Proteins

The synthesis of recombinant therapeutic proteins traces back to two studies performed in the early 1970s. In 1972, Paul Berg and colleagues first described the biochemical technique for joining two DNA molecules from different sources to produce a "recombinant plasmid."[36] Following this lead, Stanley Cohen and Herbert Boyer used such a construct to transform *Escherichia coli* cells and replicate the recombinant protein encoded in the DNA of the construct. The perfection and commercialization of this technology by the 1980s, complemented by the polymerase chain reaction invented in 1986, provided a rapid, reliable means for producing unique recombinant proteins in quantities sufficient for therapeutic purposes.

This technology was used initially to produce recombinant versions of biological proteins heretofore available only from extracts derived from natural sources such as insulin from pigs and cows and growth hormone and antihemophilia factor from human tissues. The first human recombinant protein, recombinant insulin (Humulin), was approved for marketing in 1982, the second recombinate product in 1985 was the human growth hormone, somatotropin, while the third, antihemophilia factor, was not produced until 1992 (Table 10.1). From 1982 through 2002, 54 rDNA products (Table 10.1) received FDA approval for therapeutic use. During this 20-year period, the number of approved products expanded rapidly with 6 approved between 1985 and 1989, 11 between 1990 and 1994, 19 between 1995 and 1999, and 17 between 2000 and 2002. Approximately half of these were approved between 1997 and 2002. Recombinant DNA technology permits the synthesis of rDNA products that are slightly altered, or completely different from naturally occurring proteins, and hence may have superior safety and efficacy profiles. Today, the rDNA product industry numbers more than 100 companies, over 70 marketed products, and more than 100 new products in clinical development.

To be efficacious and safe, a successful recombinant protein must satisfy several criteria. Optimally, its efficacy should closely match that of the native protein, and it should have high affinity and specificity, and good stability. It must also have properties favorable to expression in cell culture, fold and secrete correctly, be subject to the appropriate posttranslational modifications, and be soluble at concentrations apropos of those used under therapeutic conditions. Delivery of protein drugs presents another problem. As oral administration results in their denaturation by the acid in the stomach, protein drugs must be delivered parenterally. Still further, as the half-life of protein products in the body is usually very short, it is advantageous if its clearance can be slowed. Drug formulation relies on a strategy known as PEGylation for this purpose.[37]

As genetic engineering technology improved, different cell lines were employed for production of rDNA products. Between 1980 and 1983, most (86%) therapeutic products were produced in *E. coli* while only one (14%) was produced in a mammalian cell line, whereas between 1984 and 1987 the percentage produced in *E. coli* dropped to 58% with 25% produced in mammalian cell lines and 17% in yeast. Between 1988 and 1991, the preferred cell line for production was mammalian (60%, Chinese hamster ovary and baby hamster kidney cells). But bacterial, mammalian, and yeast cell lines differ in the abilities regarding protein glycosylation, glycosylation pattern, and posttranslational modification, and mammalian cell lines were not necessarily better and did not supplant older cell lines. In 2002, 46% of approved products were produced in *E. coli,* with 38% produced in mammalian cell lines and 15% produced in yeast.[38]

Some interesting trends are revealed by the time intervals required for completion of the clinical development and FDA-approval phases of rDNA therapeutics.[38] When the data were stratified according to the therapeutic indication (Table 10.2A), it is apparent that the mean clinical phase varied greatly and depended on the indication. Products with immunological and antiinfective

Table 10.1 Charting the Growth of Drug Discovery

| FDA approval | Recombinant proteins | | Monoclonal antibodies (mAbs) | | | Breakthrough targets | | FDA approval |
	Trade name (generic name)	Protein type	Generic name	Description	Application	Drug	Target	
1982	Humulin (insulin)	Insulin						1982
1985	Prototropin (somatotropin)	Human growth hormone (HGH)						1985
1986	Intron A (interferon-α-2b)	Interferon	Muromonab-CD3	Murine, IgG2α, anti-CD33	Immunological			1986
	Roferon (interferon-α-2a)	Interferon						
1987	Humatropin (somatotropin)	HGH						1987
	Activase (alteplase)	tPA						
1989	Epogen (epoetin α)	Growth factor						1989
1990	Actimmune (interferon-γ1b)	Interferon						1990
1991	Neupogen (filgrastim)	Interferon						1991
	Leukine (sargramostim)	Growth factor						
	Novolin (insulin)	Insulin						

Year		Type					Year
1992	Proleukin (aldesleukin)	Interleukin					1992
	Recombinate (antihemophilic factor)	Coagulation factor					
1993	Kogenate (antihemophilic factor)	Coagulation factor					1993
	Betaseron (interferon-β-1b)	Interferon					
	Nutropin	HGH					
	Pulmozyme (dornase α)	Enzyme					
1994	Cerezyme (imiglucerase)	Enzyme	ReoPro (Abciximab)	Hemostasis — Chimeric, IgG$_1$, anti-GPIIb/IIIa	Glucophage	Perhaps acetyl-CoA carboxylase	1994
1995	Norditropin (somatotropin)	HGH			Precose	α-Glucosidase	1995
	Bio-Tropin (somatotropin)	HGH			Cozaar	Angiotensin receptor AT$_1$	
	Genotropin (somatotropin)	HGH			Cell Cept	Inosine monophosphate dehydrogenase	
					Fosamax	Perhaps farnesyl diphosphate synthase	
1996	Avonex (interferon-β-1a)	Interferon			Accolate	Leukotriene receptor	1996
	Humalog (insulin lispro)	Insulin					
	Serostim (somatotropin)	HGH					
	Retavase (eteplase)	TPA					

(continued)

311

Table 10.1 (*continued*)

	Recombinant proteins		Monoclonal antibodies (mAbs)			Breakthrough targets		
FDA approval	Trade name (generic name)	Protein type	Generic name	Description	Application	Drug	Target	FDA approval
1997	BeneFIX (Factor IX)	Coagulation factor	Rituxan (rituximab)	Chimeric, IgG$_{1\kappa}$, anti-CD20	Antineoplastic	Plavix	Platelet P2Y$_{12}$ receptor	1997
	Follistim (rFSH)	Fertility hormone	Zenapax (daclizumab)	Humanized, IgG$_{1\kappa}$, anti-CD25	Immunological	Rezulin	Peroxisome proliferator activated receptor	
	Gonal-F (follitropin α)	Fertility hormone						
	Infergen (interferon alfacon-1)	Interferon						
	Neumega (oprelvekin)	Interleukin						
	Regranex (becaplermin)	Growth factor						
1998	Refludan (lepirudin)	Protein inhibitor	Simulect (basiliximab)	Chimeric, IgG$_{1\kappa}$, anti-CD25	Immunological	Celebrex	Cycloxygenase 2	1998
	Glucagen (glucagons)	Glucagon	Synagis (palivizumab)	Humanized, IgG$_{1\kappa}$, antirespiratory syncytial virus	Antiinfective	Aggrastat integrilin	Platelet glycoprotein IIb/IIIa receptor	
	Glucagon (glucagons)	Glucagon	Remicade (infliximab)	Chimeric, IgG$_{1\kappa}$, antitumor necrosis factor (TNF-α)	Immunological	Viagra	Phosphodiesterase 5	

Year	Product	Class	Molecular description	Application	Trade name	Target	Year
	Enbrel (etanercept)	Protein inhibitor			Enbrel remicade	Recombinant receptor or antibody to bind TNF-α	
1999	Ontak (denileukin)	Interleukin					
	Herceptin (trastuzumab)		Humanized, IgG$_{1\kappa}$, anti-HER2	Antineoplastic	Herceptin	ERBB2 (or HER/neu)	1999
					Rapamune	FK-binding protein 12 and target of rapamycin (TOR kinase)	
	Novoseven (Factor VIIa)	Coagulation factor			Xenical	Gastrointestinal lipase	
					Targretin	Retinoid X receptors	
2000	ReoFacto (Factor VIII)	Coagulation factor					
	Mylotarg (gemtuzumab ozogamicin)		Humanized, IgG$_{4\kappa}$, anti-CD33, immunotoxin	Antineoplastic	Mylotarg	Antibody to CD33	2000
	Lantus (insulin glargine)	Insulin					
	TNKase (tenectplase)	tPA					
	Novolog (insulin aspart)	Insulin					
	Ovidrel (choriogonadotrophin α)	Fertility hormone					

(continued)

Table 10.1 (*continued*)

	Recombinant proteins		Monoclonal antibodies (mAbs)			Breakthrough targets		
FDA approval	Trade name (generic name)	Protein type	Generic name	Description	Application	Drug	Target	FDA approval
2001	PEG-intron (PEG-interferon-α-2b)	Interferon	Campath-1H (alemtuzumab)	Humanized, IgG$_{1\kappa}$, anti-CD52	Antineoplastic	Gleevec	BCR-ABL	2001
	Natrecor (neseritide)	Protein inhibitor				Natrecor	Recombinant B-type naturetic peptide	
	Aranesp (darbepoietin α)	Growth factor				Tracleer	Endothelin receptor	
	OP-1 implant (osteogenic protein 1)	Growth factor						
	Kineret (anakinra)	Interleukin				Kineret	Recombinant interleukin 1 receptor antagonist	
	Xigris (drotrecogin α)	Coagulation				Xigris	Recombinant activated protein C	
2002	Neulasta (pegfilgrastim)	Growth factor	Zevalin (ibritumomomab tiuxetan)	Murine, IgG$_{1\kappa}$, anti-CD20, radiolabeled (yttrium-90)	Antineoplastic			2002
	Rebif (interferon-β-1a)	Interferon	Humira (adalimumab)	Humanized, IgG$_{1\kappa}$, anti-TNF-α	Immunological			

	InFuse Bone Graft/L0CAGE (dibotermin α)	Growth factor				
	Elitek (rasburicase)	Enzyme				
	Pegasys (perinterferon-α-2a)	Interferon				
	Forteo (teriparatide)	Hormone				
2003			Xolair (omalizumab)	Humanized, $IgG_{1\kappa}$, anti-IgE	Immunological	2003
			Bexxar (tositomomab)	Murine, $IgG_{2a\lambda}$, anti-CD20, radiolabeled (iodine-131)	Antineoplastic	
			Raptiva (efalizumab)	Humanized, $IgG_{1\kappa}$, antiCD11a	Immunological	
2004	Apidra (insulin glusiline)	Insulin	Erbitux (cetuximab)	Chimeric, $IgG_{1\kappa}$, antiepidermal growth factor receptor	Immunological	2004
	Luveris (lupotropin alfa)	Hormone	Avastin (bevacizumab)	Humanized, $IgG_{1\kappa}$, antivascular endothelial growth factor	Antineoplastic	
	Kepivance (palifermin)	Growth factor	Tysabri (natalizumab)	Humanized, $IgG_{4\kappa}$, antiα_4-integrin	Multiple sclerosis	

(continued)

Table 10.1 (*continued*)

	Recombinant proteins		Monoclonal antibodies (mAbs)			Breakthrough targets		
FDA approval	Trade name (generic name)	Protein type	Generic name	Description	Application	Drug	Target	FDA approval
2005	Naglazyme (galsulfase)	Enzyme						2005
	Levemir (insulin determir)	Insulin						
	Fortical (calcitonin)	Hormone						
	Increlex (mecasermin)	Growth factor						
	Hylenex (hyaluronidase)	Enzyme						
	Iplex (mecasermin rinfabate)	Growth factor						
	Orencia (abatacept)	Protein inhibitor						
2006			Lucentis (ranibizumab)	Humanized, IgG$_1$, anti-VEGF, Fab fragment	Macular degeneration			
			Vectibix (panitumumab)	Human IgG$_{2\kappa}$, anti-EGFR antibody	Antineoplastic			

Source: Compiled from Owens,[4] Zambrowicz and Sands,[6] Reichert,[7] Brown,[8] and Reichert and Paquette.[38]

Table 10.2 Mean Clinical and FDA Approval Phases for Therapeutic Recombinant Proteins

A. For Various Therapeutic Indications

Therapeutic indication	Number of proteins	Interval	
		Clinical phase (months)	Approval phase (months)
Immunological	4	92.1	13.3
Antiinfective	4	91.4	17.9
Hemostatic	7	58.0	23.2
Cardiovascular	4	55.6	21.1
Endocrine	13	48.6	17.5
Antineoplastic	4	46.6	27.6
Blood cell deficiency	6	39.8	14.7

B. For Various Types of Recombinant Proteins

Protein type	Number of proteins	Interval	
		Clinical phase (months)	Approval phase (months)
Protein inhibitor	3	79.8	19.8
Interferon	8	75.4	18.8
Interleukin	4	72.2	22.5
Fertility hormone	3	66.5	26.3
Growth factor	8	56.1	18.7
Coagulation factor	6	51.2	24.7
TPA	3	49.1	14.9
Insulin	5	45.4	15.3
Enzyme	3	34.8	17.3

Source: Modified from Reichert and Paquette.[38]

indications (92.1 and 91.4 months) had the longest mean clinical phases while products that increased the production of blood cells were in clinical development for less than half the time (39.8 months). Compared to new chemical entities approved between 1993 and 2001 (data not shown), rDNAs for cardiovascular, endocrine, and antineoplastic indications had shorter clinical phases, but longer phases for antiinfective indications. It is also apparent from Table 10.2A that the mean approval phases were much shorter than the corresponding clinical phases, but they also varied with the indication, with the immunological products reviewed in less than half the time of the antineoplastic products. When the data were stratified according to the type of protein studied (Table 10.2B), the protein type affects but is less likely to be a major factor in determining the length of the clinical phase. And protein type was unlikely to be a major determinant of the length of the mean approval phase.

Recombinant proteins add another option to the physician's therapeutic armamentarium by being complementary to treatment with small molecule drugs. For example, when disease is caused by the absence of a specific protein in the

FUTURES

affected person, such as in Type 1 diabetes or hemophilia, then replacement with insulin or hemophilia factor is an obvious choice. However, because proteins do not readily enter cells, the drug target must be extracellular and usually involves cell surface receptors. Cell surface receptors account for the actions of the majority of biological responses because of their capacity to bind such a wide variety of biologically active substances including biogenic amines, protein and polypeptide hormones, autocoids, neurotransmitters, and environmental chemicals. Therapeutic proteins may be the preferred option for treatment requiring a natural agonist (or antagonist), particularly if a suitable small molecule replacement is not available or is difficult to obtain. Inspection of recombinant proteins (Table 10.1) reveals that the majority of approved recombinant proteins do, in fact, act as cell surface receptor agonists or antagonists.

Monoclonal Antibodies

The discovery of hybridoma technology in 1975 by Kohler and Milstein, who demonstrated that fusion of myeloma cells with antibody cells from mouse spleen was capable of producing an unlimited supply of monoclonal antibodies (mAbs), initiated a new era in antibody research and clinical development.[39] Transfer of this technology to therapeutic trials in human patients with leukemia and lymphoma enabled clinical investigators to show that antibodies directed against normal lymphoid antigens administered to such patients achieved important antitumor effects. In one early case report, Miller and colleagues[40] showed that hybridomas resulting from non-immunoglobulin-secreting human malignant B cells fused to myeloma cells secreted substantial quantities of the malignant B cell surface immunoglobulin, which they used in mice to generate monoclonal anti-idiotype antibodies. Administration of these monoclonal antibodies to a 67-year-old man with B cell lymphoma produced a dramatic response that persisted several years, well beyond the period of passive therapy.

When mAbs were first generated it was expected that therapeutic products would soon follow because of their specificity and unlimited supply. But the first wave of reliable FDA-approved immunotherapeutic reagents was of unmodified murine origin and repeated administrations of these agents often provoked severe antimouse antibody responses that limited or prevented multiple applications.[41] In 1986, for example, the therapeutic mAb approved for human use, muromonab-CD3 (also called OKT3), failed as a treatment for transplantation rejection, primarily for this reason. In many of the early trials, exceedingly small quantities of material were administered, which were insufficient to produce a therapeutic response, and because of their murine origin, had a very short half-life in humans, further reducing the effective dose. The failure of muromonab-33 was so influential that more than 8 years elapsed before the introduction of the chimeric mAb, abciximab (ReoPro) in 1994, the second mAb approved for human therapy. Three years later another chimeric mAb, rituximab (Rituxan), received FDA approval, after which there was a surge of approved therapeutic mAbs. Currently, chimeric and humanized mAbs make up the bulk of mAbs approved for human use (Table 10.1).

Engineering Monoclonal Antibodies

By the early 1990s, emerging recombinant DNA technologies enhanced the clinical efficacy of mouse antibodies including the construction of chimerized, humanized, and fully human antibodies. Chimeric mAbs are 65–90% human. In their most basic form, chimeric mAbs are composed of murine variable regions for antigen recognition and constant regions derived from the equivalent human genes, most often the κ light chain and the immunoglobulin G (IgG_1) heavy chain. The IgG_1 subclass was preferred because it was among the most active in the immune system, capable of engaging Fcγ receptors (FcγRs) situated on cytotoxic cascade cells and activating complement that efficiently destroys target cells.[42] In a refinement of this strategy, humanized antibodies, which are 95% human, were constructed. In humanized mAbs the constant regions and most of the structural elements of the variable regions are replaced by human sequences leaving only the complementary determining regions (CDRs) of murine origin. Human mAbs are fully human sequences, usually derived from transgenic animals that have had their antibody genes replaced by the human equivalent sequences, or by the generation of synthetic antibody libraries.[43]

Figure 10.4 shows schematically the entire IgG molecule and different fragments that have been engineered.[44] Because antibodies are multidomain proteins with highly organized, differentiated structures, they can be altered by a variety of strategies to enhance their therapeutic relevance. Innovative structural designs have improved the pharmacokinetics, expanded the immune repertoires, and permitted screening against refractory targets and complex proteome arrays. New

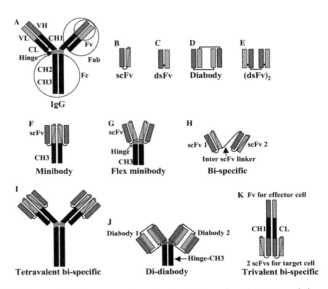

Figure 10.4 Schematic diagram of a whole IgG molecule (A) and fragments that have been engineered (B–K). With permission from Elsevier Limited.

molecular strategies have enhanced the affinity, stability, and expression efficiency, while primary structures have been manipulated to incorporate chemical and posttranslational modifications and the construction of fusion partners for unique clinical applications.[41,45] Several examples that illustrate the application of these strategies to construct specific therapeutic antibodies for unique clinical applications are described below.

To simplify the following discussion, therapeutic antibodies are divided into those that are unconjugated and those that are conjugated, because these two groups exert their effects in different ways. Unconjugated antibodies act via recruitment and activation of effector cells by antibody-dependent cellular cytotoxicity (ADCC), by blocking receptor interactions, or by induction of an intracellular signal such as apoptosis. Conjugated antibodies are used to deliver agents such as radioisotopes, toxins, or drugs that have additional cytotoxic effects. Radioisotope (such a iodine-131 or yttrium-90) conjugates can deliver ionizing radiation to the site of the disease whereas toxins such as *Pseudomonas* toxin attached to mAbs can disrupt protein synthesis, while drugs such as calicheamicin can damage DNA and initiate apoptosis.

The therapeutic efficacy of an antibody is largely dependent on its pharmacokinetics and biodistribution. An intact immunoglobulin (Figure 10.4A) of 150 kDa mass diffuses slowly and is cleared slowly from the body; for IgG_1s, the half-life is about 3 weeks. Both clearance and tissue/tumor penetration of the antibody can be increased by removing the constant region, or the Fc portion; these maneuvers generate fragments such as Fvs and Fabs, or diabodies and minibodies. The Fv region is the smallest antibody fragment that retains antigen-binding specificity characteristic of the whole IgG. Further engineering can be performed to covalently connect the two V-domains of Fv (by introducing two cysteine residues in the framework region of VH and VL resulting in a disulfide stabilized Fv) thereby preventing intramolecular unfolding and intermolecular aggregation. Additionally, Fvs, diabodies, $(dsFv)_2$, and minibodies are excellent vehicles to target radionuclides for tumor imaging or to target toxins to specific cells to produce cytotoxicity because of their small size and rapid clearance.

While rapid clearance is desirable for certain therapeutic indications, prolonged clearance may be preferred for other indications. PEGylation, a process whereby polyethyleneglycol chains are conjugated to the antibody, or antibody fragments, is one strategy that is commonly employed for this purpose. PEGylation not only prolongs the half-life of the protein but also offers a means of reducing its immunogenicity, increasing its solubility, and protecting it from protease attack.[37] PEGylation results in some loss of antigen binding, but this effect can be minimized by PEGylation of the antibody at a site distant from the antigen-binding site, or by introducing a free cysteine at the end of the hinge region of the antibody. Altering the ionization properties (pI) of the antibody offers another strategy that can improve therapeutic efficiency. For example, by lowering the pI of immunotoxin, hepatotoxicities can be reduced. Additionally, a high scFv pI value favors its reabsorption in the kidney leading to renal accumulation and toxicity while reducing the pI opposes these effects without significant loss of antigen-binding activity.

Other engineering strategies can also be used to improve mAb effector function or to introduce a new effector function into the mAb. Effector functions include ADCC, or complement-dependent cytotoxicity (CDC). In ADCC, the antigen–antibody complex binds to FcγRs and attracts effector cells, such as natural killer (NK) cells, that lead to lysis or opsonization of the target cells. In CDC, the antigen–antibody complex activates the complement system that leads to lysis or opsonization of the target cells. Thus, engineering an mAb to improve binding to FcγRs, or to complement factors, may lead to improvement in its therapeutic efficacy. Several approaches that involve mapping and mutating the residues in the hinge IgG region that contribute to FcγR binding, or that involve glycoengineering of the IgG component of the antibody, have succeeded in improving ADCC and CDC activity.[44]

To engineer a new effector function into a mAb, the mAb (or its antigen-binding domain) can be conjugated with molecules such as toxins, enzymes, cytokines, or radioisotopes. Mylotarg (gemtuzumab ozogamicin), for example, is a humanized anti-CD33 IgG$_4$ that has been conjugated with the cytotoxic drug calicheamycin. (Table 10.1). Mylotarg is used for the treatment of patients who have acute myeloid leukemia and who are not eligible for, or are resistant to chemotherapy. Another example with antineoplastic indications is designated as "antibody-directed enzyme prodrug therapy" (also called ADEPT). In this case, the therapeutic antibody is conjugated with an enzyme that introduces a new effector function. ADEPT therapy is administered in two phases. First, the antibody–enzyme conjugate is administered systemically and allowed to home in on tumor sites and to be cleared from normal tissues. In the second phase, a nontoxic prodrug is administered and converted by the enzyme conjugated to the antibody into a highly cytotoxic drug within the tumor. The most widely studied ADEPT drugs are conjugates between anti-CEA antibodies, A5B7 and MFE-23, and the bacterial carboxyl peptidase, CPG2. In this instance, the conjugate was synthesized in yeast to introduce high mannose glycans into the N-linked glycosylation sites of CPG2. This step was very helpful in overcoming the slow clearance of the conjugate from normal tissues by way of the mannose receptors.[44]

Selected Protein Therapeutics Currently Marketed

Several protein therapeutics have been engineered to improve their therapeutic relevance. Table 10.3 presents a selected list of protein therapeutics, including both recombinant DNA products and monoclonal antibodies, that are currently marketed.[45,46]

Vaccines

An upsurge of new, life-threatening infectious disorders and the resurgence of old infectious diseases of long-standing during the past 25 years, combined with the more recent global threat of infectious disease, have intensified interest in the development of prophylactic vaccines.[47] Analysis indicates that a total of 15 vaccines received FDA approval between 1996 and 2005,[7] only 25% of which

Table 10.3 Engineered Therapeutic Recombinant Proteins and Monoclonal Antibodies Marketed[45,46]

Recombinant protein® (generic name)	Family	Medical indication	Modification	Property
Betaseron (interferon-β-1b)	IFN-β	Multiple sclerosis	Mutated free cysteine	Decreased aggregation
Lantus (glargine)	Insulin	Diabetes	Precipitates in derms	Sustained release
Enbrel (etanercept)	TNF receptor	Rheumatoid arthritis	Fc fusion	Longer plasma half-life, increased avidity
Neulast (pegfilgrastim)	Granulocyte colony-stimulating factor	Leukemia	PEGylation	Increased plasma half-life
Aranesp (darbepoietin alfa)	Erythropoietin	Anemia	Additional glycosylation sites	Increased plasma half-life, weaker receptor binding

Monoclonal antibody (generic)	Target	Medical indication	Mode of action	Type
Rituxan (rituximab)	CD20	B cell non-Hodgkin's lymphoma	Complement-dependent cytotoxicity	Chimeric
Mylotarg (gemtuzumab ozogamicin)	CD33	Relapsed acute myeloid leukemia	Toxin-mediated killing	Humanized
Campath-1H (alemtuzumab)	CD52	Chronic lymphocytic leukemia	Complement-dependent cytotoxicity	Humanized
Zevalin (ibritumomab tiuxetan)	CD20	Rituximab-failed non-Hodgkin's lymphoma	Targeted radiolysis (yttrium-90)	Murine radiolabeled
Bexxar, Corixa (tositumomab)	CD20	Chemotherapy-refractory B cell non-Hodgkin's lymphoma	Targeted radiolysis (iodine-131)	Murine, radiolabeled
Erbitux (cetuximab)	EGF	Colon and certain other solid cancers	Antiepidermal growth factor receptor	Chimeric
Herceptin (trastuzumab)	HER2	HER2-positive breast cancer	Antibody cell-mediated cytotoxicity	Humanized
Avastin (bevacizumab)	VEGF	Colorectal cancer	Inhibition angiogenesis	Humanized

were products for a previously unmet medical need. Four products (for rotavirus, Lyme disease, and pneumococcal and meningiococcal vaccines) were considered innovative, and two of these are no longer on the market.

In the oncology area, 2006 also saw the first vaccine, Gardasil® (Merck), explicitly designed to prevent cancer induced by a virus.[4,48] Finding that infection with the human papilloma virus (HPV) is a critical factor in the majority of cases of cervical cancer allowed the development of strategies to prevent this form of cancer. It is important to note that in addition to cervical cancer, several other cancers including head and neck cancers are associated with HPV infection.[48]

The mean clinical developmental and approval phases for vaccines were 80.0 and 13.9 months, respectively, with the developmental phases for follow-on products tending to be shorter than the average for the innovative vaccines. The approval phases for the follow-on vaccines, however, were quite variable (3.2–97.4 months). Priority-reviewed vaccines had the shortest approval phases, whereas follow-on vaccines had lengthier approval phases (>2 years).

GENETIC PATHWAYS TO IMPROVED DRUG THERAPY

More recent drug discovery literature considers additional potentially productive pathways for discovering or improving drug therapy. One approach, inspired by the long successful history of combination therapy where a combination of drugs has become the standard of care for many diseases, considers the potential of a systems biology framework to drug discovery. Another approach makes use of large-scale mouse knockout programs combined with phenotypic screens to identify targets that are therapeutically relevant. A third possibility considers the advantages that simple model organisms such as yeast, flies, worms, and zebrafish might bring to drug discovery, and a fourth possibility addresses potential therapeutic options for epigenetic disorders.

Systems Biology Applied to Combination Drug Therapy

Combination drug therapy originated through happenstance by the deliberate mixing of drugs in a clinical setting. The practice of combining two or more drugs has had a successful history in various areas of medicine including cancer, infectious diseases, and cardiovascular and central nervous system (CNS) disorders. In many instances, such testing has been conducted when the rationale for the combination is evident, or with agents known to be effective in a therapeutic area of specific interest as exemplified by the synergistic combination of a diuretic and an angiotensin-converting enzyme inhibitor for treatment of hypertension and heart failure. As a small number of compounds would provide a very large number of combinations, such an empirical approach would sample only a small fraction of combination space and would not be likely to result in the selection of optimal combinations. A collection of 1000 compounds, for example, would yield almost 500,000 pairwise combinations (i.e., $[n(n-1)/2]$). Combinations of three or more drugs could lead to many additional possibilities because variations in the molar ratio and in the time of compound administration could be relevant.

Since human cells and tissues are composed of complex networks comprising redundant, convergent, and divergent signaling pathways, a systems biology framework that entails identification of combinations of small molecules that perturb signaling pathways in desirable ways would appear to offer a reasonable approach to drug discovery. Borisy and colleagues have brought these issues into sharper focus by devising a high-throughput screening method for identifying effective combinations of therapeutic compounds.[49] Borisy's method incorporates both an experimental strategy and analytical methods to determine whether a beneficial interaction occurs between compounds. The application of this method to screen approximately 120,000 different two-component combinations of drugs for unexpected synergist interactions attributable to signaling networks within and between cells has yielded some promising results. Among these, they identified (1) a fungistatic (fluconazole) and a urinary analgesic agent (phenazopyridine) that together generated fungicidal activity in drug-resistant *Candida albicans,* (2) a glucocorticoid (dexamethasone) and an antiplatelet agent (dipyridamole) that together suppressed the production of tumor necrosis factor (TNF)-α in human primary peripheral blood mononuclear cells, and (3) an antipsychotic (chlorpromazine) and an antiprotozoal agent (pentamidine) that together prevented the growth of tumors in mice.

Because the molecular mechanisms and targets of the drugs subjected to testing were well studied, the investigators believed that the information obtained might aid in understanding the underlying biological pathways that are perturbed by combination treatment. The combination of fluconazole and phenazopyridine was more effective in inhibiting fluconazole-resistant *C. albicans* than that of either compound alone, and the combination did not significantly affect the proliferation of another human cell, primary lung fibroblasts. To explain its effectiveness, a dye efflux experiment was performed to test the possibility that this combination inhibited the ability of the fungal cell to eliminate fluconazole through multidrug resistance pumps. Finding that neither agent alone had any effect on dye efflux while the combination of fluconazole and phenazopyridine efficiently inhibited dye efflux probably explains in part the effectiveness of the combination.

Another interesting example that emerged from the screen was the combination of the antipsychotic drug, chlorpromazine, and the antiprotozoal drug, pentamidine. This combination selectively prevented tumor cell growth of A549 lung carcinoma cells *in vitro* and *in vivo.* Each of these compounds exhibited moderate antiproliferative activities *in vitro* against A549 lung carcinoma cells, but not at clinically relevant concentrations. The combination, however, prevented the growth of these cells *in vitro* and in a human tumor xenograft assay in mice, suggesting that the combination might possess therapeutically useful antitumor-selective activity. In a further series of studies on the basis for its effectiveness, the investigators found that the antiproliferative effect of the combination of chlorpromazine and pentamidine was highly complex and likely to involve several components including calmodulin inhibition, DNA binding, modulation of poly-amine levels, and possibly other mechanisms.

Borisy and co-workers noted that screening such small molecule combinations may also help define the interactions among human genes and proteins, and the reagents that act on them. They also point out that their procedure for improving drug therapy by screening small molecule drug combinations could be adapted to other methods of cell signal perturbation such as cDNA overexpression or RNA interference-based messenger RNA knockdown. In practical terms, this meth-odology might be promising for the rapid production of effective medicines and could be useful for the systematic discovery of new therapeutics.

Finding Targets by Reverse Genetics in Knockout Mice

Mouse knockout (KO) technology provides a powerful means of elucidating the physiological functions of mammalian genes (see Chapter 9) and recent studies have demonstrated the utility of KO mice in the identification of drug targets.

Predicting Drug Efficacy of Pipeline Drugs

In 2003, Zambrowicz and Sands systematically analyzed the potential of KO mice to predict drug efficacy. In the first part of the study, they evaluated the extent to which KO mice predicted drug efficacy for drugs then currently in the pipeline of the pharmaceutical industry.[50] They focused on new targets for which there were published mouse KOs. While they found a few targets for which KOs did not exist, the published KOs represented the majority of the pipeline targets of the top 10 pharmaceutical companies for drugs in Phase 2 clinical trials and be-yond. The KO phenotypes included 24 targets distributed among five neurolog-ical, three metabolic, six cardiac, six immunological, three oncological, and one osteological agent (Table 10.4).

This part of the study showed that KO mouse phenotypes provided useful criteria for predicting drug efficacy phenotypes for at least 85% of the drug targets in the pipeline. Only two targets, NHE1 and PDE4, did not reveal a convincing therapeutic strategy. NHE1 KO mice demonstrated multiple developmental de-fects, making interpretation of the phenotype and pursuit of the medical indi-cation (ischemic heart disease) difficult, whereas PDE4 KO mice demonstrated an antiinflammatory phenotype that was related only indirectly to the multifac-torial disease pursued (chronic obstructive pulmonary disease).

Prospects for Discovering Future Targets
of Likely Pharmaceutical Value

In the second part of the study, Zambrowicz and colleagues assessed the pros-pects of KO mice to discover future drug targets by retrospective evaluation of mouse KOs.[6] They compared the phenotypes of intact mice administered a given drug with those of KO mice that had the putative drug target of the drug knocked out. Drugs taken from the 100 best selling drugs were tested. To achieve their ultimate goal, the technology employed for target identification had to fulfill two

Table 10.4 Drug Targets for Pipeline Pharmaceutics[50]

Indication	Target	Drug	Drug type
Obesity and nicotine addiction	Central cannabinoid CB1 receptor	Rimonabant (Sanofi-Syntheabo)	Antagonist
Obesity	Serotonin 5-HT$_{2C}$ receptor	BVT-933 (GSK)	Agonist
Gallstones, obesity	Cholicystokinin (CCK$_1$) receptor	GI-181771 (GSK)	Agonist
Depression, nausea, pain	NK$_1$ receptor	TAK-637 (Abbott with Takeda), Emend (Merck)	Antagonist
Pain	Adenosine A$_1$ receptor	GW-493838 (GSK)	Agonist
Diabetes	Glp-1 receptor	Exenatide, GLP-1 (Lilly)	Protein ligand agonist
Diabetes	Dipeptidyl peptidase V	LAF-237 (Novartis) P32/98 (Merck)	Antagonist
Diabetic peripheral neuropathy	PKC-β	Unnamed (Lilly)	Antagonist
Atherosclerosis	ACAT2	Avasimibe (Parke-Davis, Pfizer)	Antagonist
Thrombosis	Thromboxane–A2 receptor	Ifetroban (BMS)	Antagonist
Renovascular hypertension	Vasopeptidase	Gemomoaptrilat omapatrilat (Vanlev, BMS), fasidotril (Lilly), reacecadotril (GSK)	Dual ACE + NEP inhibitor
Hypertension, cardiac failure	Aldosterone receptor	Epierenone (Novartis–Pfizer, Pharmacia)	Antagonist
Antidiuretic hormone (ADH) syndrome, glaucoma	Vasopressin AVPR2	SR-121463 (Sanofi-Syntheabo)	Antagonist
Ischemic heart disease	Na$^+$/H$^+$ exchanger (NHE1)	Zoniporide (CP-597396, Pfizer)	Antagonist
Multiple sclerosis and other autoimmune diseases	CTLA4	BMS-188667, BMS-224818 (Bristol-Myers Squibb Co.)	Protein therapeutic
Allergic rhinitis	IgE	Omalizumab (Genentech), TNX-901 (Roche with Novartis and Tanox)	Monoclonal antibody
COPD, asthma, allergic rhinitis, rheumatoid arthritis	Phosphodiesterase 4	Roflumilast (Pfizer), AWD-12291 = GW-842470), cilomilast GSK, PDE4 inhibitor (Merck)	Antagonist
Inflammatory bowel disease, rheumatoid arthritis	TACE	BMS-561392 (BMS)	Antagonist
Allergic rhinitis, asthma	A$_4$/β$_1$ integrin	GW-559090 (GSK), R-411 (Roche)	Antagonists and monoclonal antibodies
Organ transplantation, autoimmune disease	EDG receptors	FTY-720 (Novartis)	Agonist

Table 10.4 (*continued*)

Indication	Target	Drug	Drug type
Age-related macular degeneration, diabetic retinopathy, cancer	VEGF receptor	Pegaptanib, SU-6668 (Pfizer), vatalanib midostaurine (mixed; Novartis), ZD-6474 (Astrazeneca), ranbizumab, bevacizumab (Roche opt-in right from Genentech)	Antagonists and monoclonal antibodies
Solid tumor, cancer, myeloproliferative disorder	EGF receptor	GS-572016 (GSK), Cl-1033, CP-547632 (Pfizer), erlotinib (Tarceva; Pfizer/Roche), gefitinib, cetuximab (Iressa, Astrazeneca)	Antagonists and monoclonal antibody
Nervous system injury, mucositis, inflammatory bowel disease, ulcerative colitis, wound healing, skin ulcer, Crohn's disease	Keratinocyte growth factor-2	Repifermin (GSK with HGS)	Secreted protein therapeutic
Osteoporosis	Cathepsin K	AAE-581 (Novartis)	Antagonist

requirements: first, it had to provide a large number of potential drug target candidates, and second, it had to filter out less promising targets. More than 750 gene KOs that were created and the number of biologically validated, therapeutically relevant drug targets that offered a realistic possibility of drug discovery in the human genome were predicted from these KOs (Table 10.5).

Fourteen of the drugs tested were antiinfective and hence did not have human targets, while the remaining 86 drugs modulated approximately 46 targets. This compilation shows how large-scale, reverse genetics could be used to discover those genes among thousands of sequences that encode new targets likely to be of value for pharmaceutical development.

Several points of interest flow from this analysis. (1) About 75%[34] of the targets were knocked out, and the majority of those[29] were informative for illuminating gene function and of pharmaceutical interest. (2) The targets that produced a physiological change in the individual to alter a disease process are mainly key biochemical switches. This observation suggests that such switches are more likely to be efficacious drug targets and that drug discovery strategies should be directed toward the identification of members of this class of targets instead of disease genes. (3) Concerns about physiological differences between mice and humans were not a major issue for most of the important targets, nor were mutations that operate throughout development, gene compensation, and embryonic lethality. (4) In this study[50] complete KO and phenotypic analysis of 1250 genes were completed, suggesting that after completing a total of 5000 "druggable" genes, 100–150 new targets may be identified.

Table 10.5 Medical Indications and Human Genomic Targets of 100 Top Selling Drugs of 2002

Indication	Target	Drug	Mouse phenotype
Acne	Retinoic acid receptor	Accutane	Gross developmental defects and early lethality
Allergy	Histamine H_1 receptor	Claritin, Allegra, Zyrtec	Decreased T and B cell response, decreased alertness and altered activity level
Anemia	Erythropoietin	Procrit, Epogen	Failure to produce blood cells, embryonic lethal
Arthritis	COX2	Vioxx, Celebrex	Reduced inflammation, reduction in collagen-induced arthritis, reduced febrile response, decreased polyp formation
Arthritis	COX1 and COX2	Voltaren	COX1: decreased acute inflammation, decreased pain, decreased clotting, increased sensitivity to GI damage, decreased polyp formation; see COX2
Arthritis	TNF-α	Enbrel, Remicade	Decreased contact hypersensitivity and decreased IgG and IgE
Asthma	β-Adrenergic receptor	Serevent	Complicated by multiple targets, but target implicated for CV disease and KOs have defined the targets for β-blockers, impaired relaxation of heart, no data on bronchodilation
Asthma	Glucocorticoid receptor	Floven, Advair, Pulmicort, Flonase	Null mutations result in early lethality; point mutations used to demonstrate role in inflammation
Asthma	Leukotriene receptor	Singulair	Decreased extravasation in ip zymosan challenge; 5-lipoxygenase KOs have decreased airway responsiveness in the ovalbumin challenge and reduced pulmonary fibrosis
Atherosclerosis	$P2Y_{12}$	Plavix	Decreased platelet aggregation
Breast cancer	Estrogen receptor	Noladex	Reproductive defects, reduced bone mineral density
Breast cancer	β-Tubulin	Taxotere	Not available

Table 10.5 (*continued*)

Indication	Target	Drug	Mouse phenotype
Cholesterol	HMG-CoA reductase	Zocor, Lipitor, Pravachol, Mevalotin	Not available
Colorectal cancer	Topoisomerases	Camptosar	Premature senescence
Depression	Dopamine and noradrenaline transporters	Wellbrutin	Multiple targets; however, increased activity levels (dopamine transporter), increased struggle in tail suspension
Depression	Serotonin transporter	Paxil, Zoloft, Prozac, Effexor, Celexa	Altered open-field behavior
Diabetes	Insulin	Humulin/insulin, Humalog	No phenotype for KO of *insulin I* and *insulin II*, insulin-receptor KO mice display hyperglycemia, ketoacidosis, increased triglyceride levels, and fatty liver; 10% of heterozygotes develop diabetes
Diabetes	Peroxisome proliferator activated receptor (PPAR-γ)	Avandia	Increased insulin sensitivity in heterozygotes; embryonic lethal homozygotes
Diabetes	Unknown, probably ACAC2	Glucophage	Antidiabetic effects seen in *Acac2* KOs
Epilepsy	Unknown	Depakote, Neurontin	Not available
Erectile dysfunction	Phosphodiesterase 5 (PDE5)	Viagra	Not available
Gastrointestinal reflux disease	H^+/K^+-ATPase	Prilosec, Prevacid, Takepron, Pantozol	A polypeptide KO: pH of gastric contents is close to neutral rather than 3.14; β polypeptide KO stomachs are achlorhydric
Gastrointestinal reflux disease	Histamine H_2 receptor	Gaster, Zantac	Induction of gastric acid secretion by histamine or gastrin is completely abolished
Glaucoma	Prostanoid receptors	Xalatan	Intraocular pressure not tested in Prostanoid receptor KOs
Hypercalcemia	Farensyl diphosphate synthase, probably	Aredia	Embryonic lethal; heterozygous males have increased bone mineral density
Hypertension	β-Adrenergic receptor	Toprol	Complicated by multiple targets, but targets implicated for CV disease and KOs have defined the targets for β-blockers, impaired relaxation of heart, no data on bronchodilation

(*continued*)

Table 10.5 (*continued*)

Indication	Target	Drug	Mouse phenotype
Hypertension	Angiotensin-converting enzyme	Vasotec, Prinivil, Zestril, Lotensin, Tritace, Accupril	Low blood pressure
Hypertension	Angiotensin receptor	Cozaar	Low blood pressure
Hypertension	AT1	Diovan	Low blood pressure
Hypertension	Cardiac L-type Ca^{2+} channel α_{1C}	Norvasc, Adalat	Not available
Insomnia	GABA receptor	Ambien, Stilnox	Hyperactive, hyperresponsive
Lymphoma, non-Hodgkin's disease	CD20	Rituxan	Depletion of a subpopulation of B cells
Menopause/ osteoporosis	Estrogen receptor	Premarin, Evista, Noladex (breast)	Reproductive defects, reduced bone mineral density
Migraine	Serotonin 5-HT$_{1D}$ receptor	Imitrex	Not available
Multiple sclerosis	INF-β-1a	Avonex	Not available
Multiple sclerosis	INF-β-1b	Betaseron	Not available
Nausea/vomiting	Serotonin 5-HT$_1$ receptor	Zofran	Not available
Neutropenia	Granulocyte colony-stimulating factor	Neupogen	Deficiency in the total bone marrow cells, granulocytes and monocyte precursors in the bone marrow
Obesity	Lipases	Xenical	PLRP2, decreased fat absorption, carboxyl ester lipase reduced dietary cholesterol ester absorption
Osteoporosis	Farensyl diphosphate synthase, probably	Fosamax	Embryonic lethal; heterozygous males have increased bone mineral density
Ovarian, breast, and lung cancer	β-Tubulin	Taxol	Not available
Overactive bladder	Muscarinic M$_3$ receptor	Detrol	Increased urine retention in males
Pain	μ-Opioid receptor	Duragesic, Ultram	Increased sensitivity to pain
Prostate	Luteinizing hormone	Lupron, Leuplin, Zoladex	Luteinizing hormone receptor: releasing hormone hypogonadism and reduced steroidogenesis
Psychosis	Dopamine, serotonin, and histamine receptors	Zyprexa, Risperidal, Seroquel	Multiple targets; related KOs display behavioral phenotypes (movement, activity, and anxiety)
Thrombosis	Factor X	Lovenux/Heparin	Neonatal death due to massive bleeding

Table 10.5 *(continued)*

Indication	Target	Drug	Mouse phenotype
Transplant rejection	Calcineurin, thymocytes, defective leukocytes	Sandimmun	KO of calcineurin Aβ exhibits reduced T cells in periphery, reduced activation, and impaired allograft rejection
Transplant rejection	Inosine monophosphate dehydrogenase	CellCept	Embryonic lethal; heterozygotes show significant impairment of T cell activation and function

Source: Modified from Zambrowicz and Sands[6] (Table 8).

These two studies indicate that KO mice can be highly informative in the discovery of efficacious drug targets. They suggest that the prospective application of "reverse genetics" to KO mice is likely to afford a productive source of new targets for future drug discovery.

Simple Eukayotic Organisms in Drug Discovery

The use of simple eukaryotic organisms as models for the study of human disease (see p. 292) can be extended to the discovery of better therapeutics.[51–53] For instance, Giaever and colleagues[53] have recently explored the possibility of the genomic profiling of yeast *S. cerevisiae* for drug sensitivities via induced haploinsufficiency. This approach is based on the idea that lowering the dosage of a single gene from two copies to one in diploid yeast yields a heterozygote that is sensitized to any drug that acts on the product of this gene. The "haploinsufficient" phenotype serves to identify the gene product of the heterozygous locus as the drug target.

This observation was exploited in a genomic approach to drug-target identification as follows. First, a set of heterozygous yeast strains was constructed carrying deletions in genes encoding drug targets. Next, each strain was grown in the presence of sublethal concentrations of the drug that directly targets the protein encoded by the heterozygous locus and was analyzed for drug sensitivity (e.g., a reduced growth rate in the presence of the drug) on high-density oligonucleotide microarrays. A feasibility study on individual heterozygous strains verified six known targets. In each case, the result was highly specific as no sensitivity was exhibited when these strains were tested with other drugs. Additionally, parallel analysis of a mixed culture of 233 strains in the presence of the drug tunicamycin (a well-characterized glycosylation inhibitor) identified the known target and two unknown hypersensitive loci.

Today, drug discovery is driven, in part, by combinatorial chemistry followed by high-throughput screening of agents against a preselected target. Giaever's method does not require any prior knowledge of the target, and will identify only those targets that affect the fitness of the organism. The discovery that both drug target and hypersensitive loci exhibit drug-induced haploinsufficiency may help elucidate mechanisms underlying heterozygous disease phenotypes as well as variable drug toxicities.

Yeast, Flies, Worms, and Zebrafish in Drug Discovery

In the search for the genetic basis of a disease, it is not uncommon to discover a new protein whose normal function is unknown. Information about a new protein may be obtained by studying its distribution in normal tissues and subcellular compartments, or alternatively by examining the consequences of overexpression of the protein in cultured cells, or inactivation of the corresponding gene in knockout mice, as noted above.

In their article on yeast, flies, worms, and zebrafish, Hariharan and Haber[54] discuss the usefulness of these simple model organisms for the identification of genes with direct relevance to human disease, a topic of great interest to new drug discoveries, noting that the use of simple organisms in medical research is based on two premises. The first is that most of the important biological processes that occur in simple organisms have remained unchanged throughout evolution and are conserved in humans. The second is that these processes are easier to dissect in simple organisms than in humans. Their short generation times accelerate genetic studies of these organisms, mutant strains can be generated efficiently, and the effects of gene inactivation or overexpression on phenotype can be identified rapidly. Finally, the genetic approaches used to study each of these organisms have been extensively described.

Apart from the study of disease-causing genes, the potential usefulness of yeast, flies, worms, and zebrafish to pharmacological and toxicological studies has recently gained momentum. Their usefulness is dictated in part by their suitability for investigating particular cellular pathways. Yeast cells are particularly suited for studying the effects of mutations on cell division while fly embryos are well suited for studying mutations that disturb tissue organization and cell differentiation, Genetic studies in worms, in which the developmental fate of individual cells can be tracked, are especially suited for understanding programmed cell death (apoptosis). Vertebrate zebrafish, which have a counterpart for almost every disease-causing gene in humans, have been used mainly in the fields of molecular genetics and developmental biology of vertebrates. But since their amenability to large-scale forward genetic screens, a technique previously limited to yeast, flies, and worms, was demonstrated in 1996, zebrafish have been explored as a model to accelerate drug discovery.[55,56] They are amenable to high-throughput chemical screens because of their small size, and are more permeable than invertebrates because of the absence of a cuticle. The genes of zebrafish show an overall identity of about 70% with human orthologs at the amino acid level, but the similarity is much higher in functional domains. In substrate-binding regions, for instance, identity approaches 100%, which explains why many drugs elicit responses in this organism comparable to those in humans, and why zebrafish are suitable for modeling human pharmacological, toxicological, and behavioral research.[57] Because zebrafish combine a way to study the physiological complexity in the whole organism with high-throughput scale of *in vitro* screens, useful in drug target identification, lead discovery, and toxicology, this model offers an alternative opportunity to decrease the time and cost, simplify the performance, and enhance the prospects for new drug discovery.

A Perspective on Epigenetic Therapy

Methylation of CpG islands and conformational changes in chromatin involving histone acetylation are reversible, interacting processes that are associated with transcriptional silencing of gene expression (Figure 6.6). Disruption of either or both of these processes can lead to inappropriate gene expression, resulting in epigenetic disease including cancer (Table 6.2). Encouraged by the possibility that reversal of these processes and upregulation of genes could be important in preventing or reversing the disease phenotype, these processes have become therapeutic targets in the treatment of cancer and other epigenetic disorders.

Numerous preclinical and clinical trials have resorted to the treatment of various hemoglobinopathies (β-thalessemia, sickle cell anemia), myelodysplastic and leukemic syndromes, and the fragile-X syndrome with demethylating agents, histone deacetylase (HDAC) inhibitors, or the combined manipulation of cytosine methylation and histone acetylation, as described earlier (see p. 172). Agents used in these trials included older (5-azacytidine, 2-deoxy-5-azacytidine, or decitabine) and newer (MG98, an antisense DNMT1 inhibitor) demethylating agents, older (sodium butyrate, sodium phenyl butyrate), and newer (trichostatin, suberoylanilide hydroxamic acid, and depsipeptide) HDAC inhibitors. The results of most of these trials, though limited in scope, were encouraging, but the risks of such therapy at present would appear to be largely unknown. First, it is clear that hypomethylation is observed in malignant cells *in vivo* at doses of demethylating agents such as decitabine that overlap with clinical responses. Second, it should be noted that multiple genes may be methylated, or undergo histone modification in epigenetic diseases, and there is the possibility of hitting many targets with one drug. The evidence for decitabine, for example, favors DNMT inhibition as the critical event in demethylation, but other possible events might include reactivation of hypermethylated tumor suppressor genes and activation of retroposons through hypomethylation. Furthermore, the extent to which other downstream events such as apoptosis and differentiation might occur is unclear. And finally, because methylation increases with age, demethylation might contribute to senescence and the development of age-related chronic diseases, including cancer, in the elderly.[58–60]

In 2004, 5-azacytidine was the first agent to receive FDA approval for the treatment of several myelodysplastic syndromes. In 2006, one demethylating agent, Decitabine® (5-aza-2′-deoxycytidine), received FDA approval for the treatment of the myelodysplastic syndrome, and one HDAC inhibitor, Zolinza® (vorinostat), received FDA approval for the treatment of cutaneous T cell lymphoma.[4] Several other epigenetic drugs are capable of altering DNA methylation patterns or of the modification of histones. Those targeting methylation include

FCDR (5-fluoro-2′-deoxycytidine), EGCG (epigalocatechin-3-gallate), zebular-ine, procainamide, SAHA (suberoylanilide hydroxamic acid, vorinostat, Zolinza), Psammaplin A, and antisense oligomers. Those targeting HDACs include phe-nylbutyric acid, SAHA, depsipeptide, and valproic acid. Several of these agents are in clinical trial.[59,61]

We are just beginning to understand the contributions of epigenetics to human disease, and how to optimize its management. As we learn more about the proteins that are targeted by therapeutic agents, and the molecular interactions that they perturb, rationally designed drugs and individualized therapy may be-come reasonable goals.[58–60] Various HDAC inhibitors seem to enhance the tumor response to ionizing radiation and thereby may protect normal tissues from ra-diation damage, and combinations of demethylating agents with HDAC inhibi-tors are also being studied with great interest.[61]

SUMMARY

The completion of the human genome sequence coupled with advances in ge-nomic and proteomic technologies has ushered in a new era in drug target dis-covery and in the development of new drugs. Genomics is helping the pharma-ceutical industry move toward these goals, but the translation of gene sequence information into new drug entities has not kept pace with the demands for con-tinued innovation. The application of genomic principles to drug design com-bined with the miniaturization, automation, and parallelization of genomic technologies has led to the engineering of increasing numbers of therapeutic monoclonal antibodies, the production of therapeutic recombinant proteins such as human insulin, growth factor, and erythropoietin, and the development of new prophylactic vaccines for the prevention of infectious diseases, but the yield of new small molecule drugs is much smaller than anticipated. Several useful strategies have emerged for enhancing the understanding of biological function and chemicobiological interactions and the efficiency of new drug discovery through systems biology, reverse genetics in knockout mice, and the use of simple model organisms.

REFERENCES

1. Marshall A. Getting the right drug into the right patient. Nat Biotechnol 1997; 15(12):1249–1252.
2. Drews J, Ryser S. The role of innovation in drug development. Nat Biotechnol 1997; 15(13):1318–1319.
3. Drews J. Strategic trends in the drug industry. Drug Discov Today 2003; 8(9):411–420.
4. Owens J. 2006 drug approvals: Finding the niche. Nat Rev Drug Discov 2007; 6(2):99–101.
5. Cutler DM. The demise of the blockbuster? N Engl J Med 2007; 356(13):1292–1293.

6. Zambrowicz BP, Sands AT. Knockouts model the 100 best-selling drugs—will they model the next 100? Nat Rev Drug Discov 2003; 2(1):38–51.

7. Reichert JM. Trends in US approvals: New biopharmaceuticals and vaccines. Trends Biotechnol 2006; 24(7):293–298.

8. Brown D. Overview of sources of new drugs. In: Kennewell PD, editor. Global Perspective. Amsterdam: Elsevier, 2007: 321–353.

9. Clardy J, Walsh C. Lessons from natural molecules. Nature 2004; 432(7019): 829–837.

10. Venter JC, Adams MD, Myers EW, Li PW, Mural RJ, Sutton GG, et al. The sequence of the human genome. Science 2001; 291(5507):1304–1351.

11. Drews J. Drug discovery: A historical perspective. Science 2000; 287(5460):1960–1964.

12. Hopkins AL, Groom CR. The drugable genome. Nat Rev Drug Discov 2002; 1(9):727–730.

13. Overington JP, Al Lazikani B, Hopkins AL. How many drug targets are there? Nat Rev Drug Discov 2006; 5(12):993–996.

14. Paolini GV, Shapland RH, van Hoorn WP, Mason JS, Hopkins AL. Global mapping of pharmacological space. Nat Biotechnol 2006; 24(7):805–815.

15. Chanda SK, Caldwell JS. Fulfilling the promise: Drug discovery in the post-genomic era. Drug Discov Today 2003; 8(4):168–174.

16. Schindler T, Bornmann W, Pellicena P, Miller WT, Clarkson B, Kuriyan J. Structural mechanism for STI-571 inhibition of abelson tyrosine kinase. Science 2000; 289(5486):1938–1942.

17. Capdeville R, Buchdunger E, Zimmermann J, Matter A. Glivec (STI571, imatinib), a rationally developed, targeted anticancer drug. Nat Rev Drug Discov 2002; 1(7): 493–502.

18. Gorre ME, Sawyers CL. Molecular mechanisms of resistance to STI571 in chronic myeloid leukemia. Curr Opin Hematol 2002; 9(4):303–307.

19. La Rosee P, Corbin AS, Stoffregen EP, Deininger MW, Druker BJ. Activity of the Bcr-Abl kinase inhibitor PD180970 against clinically relevant Bcr-Abl isoforms that cause resistance to imatinib mesylate (Gleevec, STI571). Cancer Res 2002; 62(24): 7149–7153.

20. Huron DR, Gorre ME, Kraker AJ, Sawyers CL, Rosen N, Moasser MM. A novel pyridopyrimidine inhibitor of abl kinase is a picomolar inhibitor of Bcr-abl-driven K562 cells and is effective against STI571-resistant Bcr-abl mutants. Clin Cancer Res 2003; 9(4):1267–1273.

21. Manning G, Whyte DB, Martinez R, Hunter T, Sudarsanam S. The protein kinase complement of the human genome. Science 2002; 298(5600):1912–1934.

22. Zhu H, Bilgin M, Bangham R, Hall D, Casamayor A, Bertone P, et al. Global analysis of protein activities using proteome chips. Science 2001; 293(5537):2101–2105.

23. Bishop AC, Ubersax JA, Petsch DT, Matheos DP, Gray NS, Blethrow J, et al. A chemical switch for inhibitor-sensitive alleles of any protein kinase. Nature 2000; 407(6802):395–401.

24. Gura T. A chemistry set for life. Nature 2000; 407(6802):282–284.

25. Kroeze WK, Sheffler DJ, Roth BL. G-protein-coupled receptors at a glance. J Cell Sci 2003; 116(Pt 24):4867–4869.

26. Fredriksson R, Lagerstrom MC, Lundin LG, Schioth HB. The G-protein-coupled receptors in the human genome form five main families. Phylogenetic analysis, para-logon groups, and fingerprints. Mol Pharmacol 2003; 63(6):1256–1272.

27. Sadee W, Hoeg E, Lucas J, Wang D. Genetic variations in human G protein-coupled receptors: Implications for drug therapy. AAPS PharmSci 2001; 3(3):E22.

28. Small KM, Tanguay DA, Nandabalan K, Zhan P, Stephens JC, Liggett SB. Gene and protein domain-specific patterns of genetic variability within the G-protein coupled receptor superfamily. Am J Pharmacogenom 2003; 3(1):65–71.

29. Small KM, Seman CA, Castator A, Brown KM, Liggett SB. False positive non-synonymous polymorphisms of G-protein coupled receptor genes. FEBS Lett 2002; 516:253–256.

30. Hepler JR. Emerging roles for RGS proteins in cell signalling. TIPS 1999; 20(Sep): 376–382.

31. De Vries L, Zheng B, Fischer T, Elenko E, Farquhar MG. The regulator of G protein signaling family. Ann Rev Pharmacol Toxicol 2000; 40:235–271.

32. Neubig RR, Siderovski DP. Regulators of G-protein signalling as new central nervous system drug targets. Nat Drug Discov 2002; 1(March):187–197.

33. Zaman GJR, Michiels PJA, van Boeckel CAA. Targeting RNA: New opportunities to address drugless targets. Drug Discov Today 2003; 8(7):297–306.

34. Que-Gewirth NS, Sullenger BA. Gene therapy progress and prospects: RNA aptamers. Gene Ther 2007; 14(4):283–291.

35. Pollack A. RNA trades bit part for starring role in the cell. New York Times 2003; D1–D4.

36. Jackson DA, Symons RH, Berg P. Biochemical method for inserting new genetic information into DNA of simian virus 40: Circular SV40 DNA molecules containing lambda phage genes and the galactose operon of *Escherichia coli*. Proc Natl Acad Sci USA 1972; 69(10):2904–2909.

37. Whelan J. Beyond PEGylation. Drug Discov Today 2005; 10(5):301.

38. Reichert JM, Paquette C. Therapeutic recombinant proteins: Trends in US approvals 1982 to 2002. Curr Opin Mol Ther 2003; 5(2):139–147.

39. Kohler G, Milstein C. Continuous cultures of fused cells secreting antibody of pre-defined specificity. Nature 1975; 256(5517):495–497.

40. Miller RA, Maloney DG, Warnke R, Levy R. Treatment of B-cell lymphoma with monoclonal anti-idiotype antibody. N Engl J Med 1982; 306(9):517–522.

41. Hudson PJ, Souriau C. Engineered antibodies. Nat Med 2003; 9(Jan):129–134.

42. Deo YM, Graziano RF, Repp R, van de Winkel JG. Clinical significance of IgG Fc receptors and Fc gamma R-directed immunotherapies. Immunol Today 1997; 18(3): 127–135.

43. Glennie MJ, Van de Winkel JGJ. Renaissance of cancer therapeutic antibodies. Drug Discov Today 2003; 8(11 June):503–510.

44. Chowdhury PS, Wu H. Tailor-made antibody therapeutics. Methods 2005; 36(1):11–24.

45. Marshall SA, Lazar GA, Chirino AJ, Desjarlais JR. Rational design and engineering of therapeutic proteins. Drug Discov Today 2003; 8(5):212–221.

46. O'Mahony D, Bishop MR. Monoclonal antibody therapy. Front Biosci 2006; 11: 1620–1635.

47. Snell NJ. Examining unmet needs in infectious disease. Drug Discov Today 2003; 8(1):22–30.

48. Baden LR, Curfman GD, Morrissey S, Drazen JM. Human papillomavirus vaccine—opportunity and challenge. N Engl J Med 2007; 356(19):1990–1991.

49. Borisy AA, Elliott PJ, Hurst NW, Lee MS, Lehar J, Price ER, et al. Systematic discovery of multicomponent therapeutics. Proc Natl Acad Sci USA 2003; 100(13): 7977–7982.

50. Zambrowicz BP, Turner CA, Sands AT. Predicting drug efficacy: Knockouts model pipeline drugs of the pharmaceutical industry. Curr Opin Pharmacol 2003; 3(5): 563–570.

51. Marton ML, DeRisi JL, Bennett HA, Iyer VR, Meyer MR, Roberts CJ, et al. Drug target validation and identification of secondary drug target effects using DNA microarrays. Nat Med 1998; 4(11):1293–1301.

52. Hughes TR, et al. Functional discovery via a compendium of expression profiles. Cell 2000; 102(Jul 7):109–126.

53. Giaever G, Shoemaker DD, Jones TW, Liang H, Winzeler EA, Astromoff A, et al. Genomic profiling of drug sensitivities via induced haploinsufficiency. Nat Genet 1999; 21(3):278–283.

54. Hariharan IK, Haber DA. Yeast, flies, worms, and fish in the study of human disease. N Engl J Med 2003; 348(24):2457–2463.

55. Zon LI, Peterson RT. In vivo drug discovery in the zebrafish. Nat Rev Drug Discov 2005; 4(1):35–44.

56. Langheinrich U. Zebrafish: A new model on the pharmaceutical catwalk. BioEssays 2003; 25(9):904–912.

57. Renier C, Faraco JH, Bourgin P, Motley T, Bonaventure P, Rosa F, et al. Genomic and functional conservation of sedative-hypnotic targets in the zebrafish. Pharmacogenet Genomics 2007; 17(4):237–253.

58. Issa JP, Garcia-Manero G, Giles FJ, Mannari R, Thomas D, Faderl S, et al. Phase 1 study of low-dose prolonged exposure schedules of the hypomethylating agent 5-aza-2'-deoxycytidine (decitabine) in hematopoietic malignancies. Blood 2004; 103(5): 1635–1640.

59. Egger G, Liang G, Aparicio A, Jones PA. Epigenetics in human disease and prospects for epigenetic therapy. Nature 2004; 429(6990):457–463.

60. Oki Y, Aoki E, Issa JP. Decitabine—bedside to bench. Crit Rev Oncol Hematol 2007; 61(2):140–152.

61. Conley BA, Wright JJ, Kummar S. Targeting epigenetic abnormalities with histone deacetylase inhibitors. Cancer 2006; 107(4):832–840.

11
Predictive Biology

After its emergence as a discipline akin to both pharmacology and genetics, pharmacogenetics focused on determining the relationships between variations in single genes and variations in the response of individuals to drugs and other exogenous substances. The intent of pioneer investigators was firmly rooted in learning how human responsiveness to these agents was linked to the molecular processes of cells and tissues. After biologists deciphered the mechanisms by which cells read information encoded in the human genome and invented genomics technologies, the switch from pharmacogenetics to pharmacogenomics began, bringing about dramatic changes in the pace and scope of pharmacogenetics from the mid-1980s to the present time.

Going from genetics to genomics resulted in a flood of new gene discoveries and new approaches to the identification of drug susceptibility loci; applications of genomics principles led to the discovery of many gene-based drug targets and to incremental advances in the development of new therapeutic agents. Today, the composition and function of hundreds or thousands of human genes spanning large fractions of the genome in many individuals and populations can be examined efficiently as a result ot advances in high-throughput genomic technologies combined with new methods to store, access, and analyze genomic data. A plethora of conferences, workshops, and educational programs focusing on a wide variety of themes helped everyone keep pace, while academic and industrial scientists, including many whose skills and immediate interests lay outside biology, lent their expertise to pharmacogenomic initiatives.

The traits that we use to illustrate the principles and consequences of pharmacogenetics throughout this book typically fall into three groups: those associated with the altered transport, distribution, and elimination of therapeutic agents, those resulting from the adverse effects of such agents, and those associated with genetic variations of the targets for these agents. These traits are representative of dozens of other genetic markers of human drug responses not specifically mentioned. Although the means of detecting and characterizing any specific trait are likely to change in the future, the vital characteristics of the trait—that is, its genetics (inheritance, allelic frequencies, and population variation), molecular basis (genes responsible and their mutation spectrum), and medical or biological significance—are not.

By the year 2000, as the Human Genome Project approached maturation, a strong case could be made for the structural and functional analyses of genomic diversity aimed at producing a complete catalog of human pharmacogenomic diversity [single-nucleotide polymorphisms (SNPs), copy number variation, deletions, insertions, repeats, rearrangements, and mobile elements]. By establishing associations between the unique genetic makeup of individuals and their responsiveness to specific drugs, foods, and other exogenous substances, the discovery of better therapies and improved prospects for individualized medicine were anticipated.

As a consequence of decades of detailed studies on the biochemical and molecular basis of physiological and pharmacological cell functions in humans and model systems and the development of analytical and computational technologies, pharmacogenetics has been transformed from a descriptive to a predictive science. The field has reached a point at which many of the complexities of the human drug response are understood and some can be predicted. It is also evident that we are just beginning to appreciate the extreme complexity of biological systems and that the biological landscape will continue to change rapidly, delivering new insights that must be considered as the genetics and genomics of human drug responses advance. As in most other biological fields, pharmacogenetics is primarily a data-driven science without which attempts at prediction are likely to fail. This chapter considers a number of areas and topics, derived mainly from the recent literature, that are likely to aid prediction and to be important to the future of pharmacogenetics and pharmacogenomics.

INDEXING PHARMACOGENETIC KNOWLEDGE

Modern biological research, training, and education rely largely on databases to store, analyze, and disseminate information. Most of the widely used biomedical databases are of limited scope: GenBank contains DNA sequences, the Protein Data Bank contains three-dimensional coordinates of macromolecules, Online Mendelian Inheritance in Man (OMIM) and Gene Cards contain a record of human genetic disease, and PubMed contains the biomedical literature. Pharmacogenetics, on the other hand, requires a much broader kind of database that is flexible enough to accommodate phenotypes whose characteristics are undefined and at the same time provides a repository from which biologists can construct new analyses and new hypotheses. If we accept as a general principle that *variation in a gene is related to variation in the phenotype associated with a drug,* and subgroup (index) phenotypes according to the four types of information commonly reported, the following classification described by Altman et al.[1] would appear to represent pharmacogenetic datasets in a way suitable for retrieval and analysis.

In 1998, The National Institute of General Medical Sciences (NIGMS), recognizing the challenges and obstacles facing pharmacogenetics, convened a

Phenotypic Variation	Variation in clinical outcomes
	Pharmacodynamic (drug response) variation
	Pharmacokinetic variation
	Molecular and cellular variation
Genotype Variation	

working group of biological and medical scientists charged with the purpose of identifying ways to facilitate research that would advance the science of pharmacogenetics and pharmacogenomics.[2] Based upon their deliberations and recommendations, the Pharmacogenetics Research Network (PGRN) was established in 2000 to generate knowledge concerning the relationships among genes, drug responses, and disease, to establish an interactive network of investigators appropriately schooled in the knowledge, tools, and resources of pharmacogenetics, and to create a publicly available knowledge base to store and curate pharmacogenetic and pharmacogenomic knowledge linking phenotypes to genotypes. The PGRN knowledge base is available at www.pharmgkb.org.

The PGRN is funded as a trans-National Institutes of Health (NIH) effort with the NIGMS leading the initiative, and at present is in its second 5-year renewal period. As originally organized, the PGRN was intended as a research tool that cut a wide swath across drugs and diseases. It currently is composed of 12 independently funded research groups and includes about 200 investigators at some 40 different sites in the United States and Canada.[2–4] It encompasses seven major topics including informatics, cardiovascular, pulmonary, addiction, cancer, transport, and metabolism. Another major component focuses on specific proteins, transporters, and drug-metabolizing enzymes that participate in drug disposition and elimination. Table 11.1 summarizes the current goals, findings, and future directions of each research group. The long-term goal for all research groups is to translate pharmacogenetic and pharmacogenomic knowledge into safe and effective drug therapies designed for individual patients.

EDGING TOWARD PERSONALIZED MEDICINE

The pharmaceutical industry has traditionally relied on population averages to develop new drugs, and despite its capacity to produce a variety of therapeutics, made little or no attempt to differentiate patients according to differences in their response to these agents. Physicians were thus forced to decide on treatment and dosage empirically from information gathered on population averages instead of individual profiles.[5,6]

Table 11.1 Goals, Findings, and Future Directions of Current Pharmacogenomics Research Network (PGRN) Projects [2–4]

Research project	Goals	Findings	Future directions
Informatics	Goals of PharmGKB are to identify interactions between genetic variability and drug response from (1) genotyping data, (2) phenotypic measures, (3) published literature, (4) drug response pathways, and (5) very important pharmacogenes	The Informatics knowledge base includes data on more than 200 genes and their variants, 300 diseases, and 400 drugs	Studies are underway to develop an enhanced system for annotating pharmacogenomic information and to understand applications and requirements of site users
Cardiovascular	Antihypertensive pharmacogenomics: to identify genetic determinants of individual variability of (1) diazide diuretics and (2) β-adrenergic receptor blockers	Analyses include genes that are involved in response variability to hydrochloro-thiazide and to β-blockers	Studies are continuing to define therapeutic and ADR response profiles (1) of hydrochlorothiazide and (2) of atenolol and hydrochlorothiazide in mild to moderate hypertensives
	Statin pharmacogenomics: to identify genetic determinants of phenotypic variability in response to statins	Up to 30% of patients do not respond to lipid lowering by statins	Studies are continuing to improve the understanding of ethnicity (Caucasian vs. Afro-American) response and age- and gender-related LDL responsiveness in smokers vs. nonsmokers
	Pharmacogenomics of antiarrhythmia therapy: to fine-tune drug selection in LQT-induced arrhythmias and to better define genetic determinants of arrhythmias in high-risk patients	Drugs and loss-of-function mutations in SCN5A that predispose to ventricular fibrillation were identified	Studies are continuing to identify new genetic determinants for ventricular and atrial fibrillation
		Variants of KCNA5 that predispose to atrial fibrillation were described	

(continued)

Table 11.1 (*continued*)

Research project	Goals	Findings	Future directions
	Pharmacogenomics of antiplatelet therapy: to identify specific gene variants and the mechanistic basis of individual variability to antiplatelet therapy and distinguish responsive from nonresponsive patients to antiplatelet therapy	Platelet aggregation and thrombosis are major factors leading to vascular occlusive and thrombotic events	Studies are continuing to identify genes that determine the response to clopidogrel and clopidogrel plus aspirin via candidate gene and genome-wide association studies in a closed founder population of Amish families
Pulmonary	Pharmacogenomics of asthma therapy: to identify genetic determinants of the response to drug therapy to β-adrenergic agonists, corticosteroids, and leukotriene antagonists	Responses to asthma therapy are characterized by marked inter- and intraindividual variability; current studies are evaluating 2013 SNPs in 220 candidate genes for responses to inhaled corticosteroids and β-agonists	Studies are continuing to develop predictive models of treatment response to β-adrenergic agonists, corticosteroids, and leukotriene antagonists for pharmacogenetic asthmatic phenotypes
Nicotine addiction	Pharmacogenomics of nicotine addiction: to design individualized smoking cessation treatment programs	Rapid metabolizers of nicotine smoke more, take in more smoke, and have altered responses to antismoking therapy; CYP2A6 variability only partially explains the variability metabolism of nicotine	Studies are continuing to better understand the role of genotype (CYP2A6, CYP2B4) in nicotine metabolism and smoking cessation treatment with bupropion
Cancer	Pharmacogenetics of anticancer research: to identify genetic polymorphisms in pharmacokinetic (PK) and pharmacodynamic (PD) drug target pathways that are important for safe and efficacious anticancer chemotherapy	Drug targets of primary interest in PK pathways: variability in CYP3A enzyme family, the UGT enzyme family, and the efflux transporter P-glycoprotein (P-gp)\n\nDrug targets of primary interest in PD pathways: genes associated with sensitivity and resistance to cisplatin and EGFR overexpression, and enzymes (and genes) involved in the metabolism of antileukemic agents	Studies are continuing to identify specific genetic variants responsible for variations in CYP3A enzymes, MDR1, and UGT relevant to safe and efficacious anticancer chemotherapy\n\nStudies will be initiated to determine genetic profiles responsible for cisplatin cytotoxicity, for variability in responses to EGFR inhibitors, and for fine-tuning therapy in leukemic patients

	Pharmacogenomics of breast cancer: to evaluate the role of genes in estrogen metabolism that control the activation, distribution, and elimination of antiestrogen drugs in breast cancer therapy	Three classes of drugs (anti-ER modulators, aromatization inhibitors, and ER down regulators) represent the cornerstones of breast cancer chemotherapy; as the genes (and proteins they encode) serve as targets of these agents, and modulators of their biological effects, they are rich areas for individualization of breast cancer therapy; PK studies have shown that CYP2D6 catalyzes the conversion of tamoxifen to the active metabolite, endoxifen, and that treatment with SSRIs for depression and hot flashes results in lower concentrations of endoxifen	Studies are continuing (1) to compare women of several phenotypes (hot flashes, quality of life, bone mineral density, weight gain, etc.) and multiple genotypes (CYP2D6, sulfatases, ER, coactivators, and repressors) who are initiating tamoxifen therapy to determine the importance of the PK observation, (2) to evaluate whether there is any association between CYP2D6 status and tamoxifen against breast cancer, and (3) to compare the pharmacogenomics of different aromatase inhibitors in postmenopausal women and identify biomarkers of response to individual agents
Transport	Pharmacogenomics of membrane transporters: to understand how genetic variation in membrane transporters contributes to variation in drug response by identifying sequence variants in transporters in ethnically diverse populations and characterizing them in cellular systems	Many new variants were identified in ethnically diverse populations; functional analyses of 88 variants reveal that 22 exhibited more than a 40% decrease in transport with 14 showing almost complete loss of function; since substrate-specific effects were also observed for several variants, these findings may be of interest in clinical association studies	Resequencing and cellular phenotyping effects are continuing with the aim of understanding the extent and significance of variations in noncoding regions, particularly in promoter regions of transporter genes

(continued)

Table 11.1 (*continued*)

Research project	Goals	Findings	Future directions
		Special interest attaches to therapeutic and adverse responses to selective serotonin reuptake inhibitor (SSRI) antidepressants and genetic variations in monoamine membrane transporters, focusing on serotonin transporter-linked promoter region variants (5-HTTLPR) of the serotonin transporter (SLC6A4)	Studies are continuing to search for functional variants in SLC6A4 that may be associated with a greater likelihood of a sustained response to fluoxetine and paroxetine, two common SSRI medications
Metabolism	Pharmacogenetics of Phase II drug-metabolizing enzymes: the major focus of this research is to characterize the functional implications and mechanisms responsible for the effects of nonsynonymous coding region SNPs	Many polymorphisms have been identified and functionally characterized, most notably the family of thiopurine methyl-ltransferases (TPMTs) that metabolizes 6MP, 6TG, and 8-azathiopurine; most often, the altered function of the variant TPMT enzymes is due to an alteration in protein quantity resulting from various mechanisms involving aberrant folding and accelerated degradation	Studies are continuing on the use of a yeast genetic system to identify a series of genes involved in trafficking and targeting TPMT*3A for degradation and aggregation Additionally, two major collaborative translational studies have been initiated that have evolved from gene sequencing efforts; they are focused on anastrazole, an aromatase inhibitor used to treat breast cancer, and escitalopram, an SSRI.

Recently, the enormity of pharmacoeconomic problems associated with population averages as the approach to drug therapy has been clarified.[7] Epidemiological studies reveal many approved drugs work as intended in only a fraction of patients, and may be accompanied by serious adverse reactions. Efficacious responses for many drugs range from about 40% to 75%; the highest percentage, 80%, responds to Cox-2 inhibitors, and the lowest, 25%, responds to cancer chemotherapy.[8] Adverse drug reactions rank as a leading cause of hospitalizations and death,[9] and are estimated to cost more than 177 billion U.S. dollars annually.[10] Cost-effectiveness studies of the potential benefits of pharmacogenomics suggest that some types of disease and drugs are more suited to individualized therapy than others.[7,11] In their evaluation of these issues, Veenstra et al.[12] have identified five criteria governing the cost-effectiveness of genotyping in conjunction with drug use: (1) the avoidance of severe outcomes when genotype information is available, (2) the existing methods for measuring drug responses are inadequate, (3) established genotype–phenotype associations exist, (4) the availability of a rapid, accurate genetic test, and (5) a relatively common occurrence of the variant genotype. The authors conclude that these criteria are likely to result in clinically useful and economically viable improvements in the care of patients.

Genetic Markers of Human Drug Response

Drug-metabolizing enzyme polymorphisms are valuable genetic markers predictive of adverse drug reactions. These proteins are implicated in the disposition and elimination of the majority of drugs, occur at high frequencies in human subjects, have been characterized in many human populations, and have been used extensively to characterize the genetics and molecular basis of normal and genetically altered drug responses and to document the diversity in different raciogeographic populations. Those listed in Table 11.2 with their relevant characteristics are representative of many additional enzymes, receptors, and other proteins that might be utilized for predicting drug responsiveness (see also Appendix A).

CYP2D6 Polymorphism and Codeine

CYP2D6 polymorphisms define four phenotypes (poor, intermediate, extensive, and ultrarapid metabolizers) that control the elimination of at least 25% of all prescribed drugs and a higher proportion of drugs that are most commonly prescribed.[28–30] At least 80 CYP2D6 polymorphisms have been identified, although the most common six CYP2D6 alleles appear to account for 95–99% of the detected phenotypes worldwide. CYP2D6 poor metabolizers are at increased risk of toxicity from drugs and interactions between them when they are administered at the usual dosages, while ultrarapid metabolizers may not reach therapeutic levels because duplicated genes (2- to 12-fold) produce increased amounts of enzyme that are responsible for increased elimination. Ethnogeographic differences in the frequencies of all four are pronounced.

The susceptibility to altered responses to the widely used analgesic drug, codeine, attributable to the CYP2D6 polymorphism is an important example of

Table 11.2 Genetic Markers Predictive of Adverse Drug Reactions

Genetic marker	Drug	Subjects studied	Adverse reaction	Comment	Reference
CYP2C9	Warfarin	561 subjects	Bleeding	Reduced dose associated with variant CYP2C9 alleles	13
	Acenocoumarol	35 subjects	Bleeding	Low dose requirement of acenocoumarol associated with a *3 allele	14
	Phenytoin	60 epileptic subjects	Phenytoin toxicity	Raised drug levels associated with *2 and *3 alleles	15
		31-year-old (y/o) woman	Phenytoin toxicity	Associated with *3 homozygosity and CYP2C19*2 heterozygosity	16
		45-y/o woman	Phenytoin toxicity	Association of fluoxamine with CYP2C9 and CYP2C19 wild-type alleles attributed to drug interaction	17
CYP2C19	Triple therapy for *H. pylori* GI infection (omeprazole or lansopromazole plus amoxicillin or clathromycin)	261 patients	*H. pylori* eradication rate reduced in 2C19 extensive metabolizers	Reduced eradication rate attributed to homozygous (72.7%) and heterozygous (92.1%) extensive metabolizers compared to poor metabolizers (97.8%)	18
CYP2D6	Prozac® (fluoxetine)	9-y/o boy	Seizures, cardiac arrest, and death	Toxicity and death associated with CYP2D6 poor metabolizer genotype	19

Enzyme/Gene	Drug	Patient	Clinical Effect	Comments	Ref.
	Codeine	33-y/o woman	Morphine toxicity	Toxicity attributed to an ultrarapid CYP2D6 genotype	20–21
VKORC1	Warfarin		Varying degrees of warfarin response	Warfarin patients segregate into low-dose (mean ~3 mg/day) and high-dose (~7 mg/day) phenotypes	22
Dihydropyrimidine dehydrogenase	5-Fluorouracil	44-y/o woman	Stomatitis, diarrhea, and pancytopenia	Toxicity attributed to a nonfunctional enzyme due to a point mutation in the splice site	23, 24
Glucuronosyltransferase (UDPGT-1A1)	Irinotecan	49-y/o woman and 63-y/o man	Neutropenia and diarrhea	Severe toxicity attributed to a mutant promoter UDPGT1A1*28	25
Thiopurine methyltransferase	6-Mercaptopurine, 6-thioguanine, azathioprine	Several case histories	Severe neutropenia	Neutropenia and CNS leukemia associated with TPMT deficiency; leukemic relapse associated with elevated TPMT activities	26
	Azathioprine	65-y/o man with heart transplant	Severe neutropenia, sepsis	Death due to sepsis acquired after neutropenia	27

347

clinical interest. CYP2D6 catalyzes the conversion of the prodrug codeine to morphine. Poor metabolizers, who typically carry null alleles of CYP2D6, found in as many as 6% of Caucasians,[29] do not obtain pain relief from ingestion of codeine.[31] CYP2D6 ultrarapid metabolizers have an enhanced capacity to metabolize codeine to morphine and hence may exhibit an exaggerated response such as abdominal cramping, fuzzy vision, and disorientation.[20,21,32]

CYP2C19 Polymorphism and Proton Pump Inhibitors (PPIs)

CYP2C19 is the major route of metabolism for numerous frontline drugs of several classes including the antimalarial agent proguanil, many antidepressants, hypnotic barbiturates, and most proton pump inhibitors.[33] More than 10 different alleles of CYP2C19 have been identified, most of which are defective. There are also marked ethnic differences in the frequency of the poor metabolizer phenotype, which comprises 2–5% of Caucasian subjects but 13–23% of Orientals; extreme frequencies reported in small ethnic populations can be as low as 0% in Cuna Indians and as high as 79% in Pacific Islanders.[34] By genotyping for the CYP2C19*2 and *3 alleles, 84% of poor metabolizers would be identified among white subjects, greater than 90% among blacks, and approximately 100% among Asians.

Many good examples of in vivo correlations between the CYP2C19 genotype and phenotype have been reported for probe drugs,[34] but overlap occurs between heterozygous and homozygous extensive metabolizers. A considerable proportion of the variation in the metabolism of PPIs can be attributed to variability in CYP2C19.[33] The plasma concentrations of racemic omeprazole, of lansoprazole, or of pantoprazole in poor metabolizers is 5–12 times higher than in extensive metabolizers.[34] There is a clear correlation between mephenytoin S/R status and the metabolizer status of these three drugs, so that any of them can be used for phenotyping. However, the S-omeprazole enantiomer is less dependent on CYP2C19 and it is not suitable for phenotyping.

CYP2C9 Polymorphism and Warfarin

The CYP2C family metabolizes approximately 20% of clinically important drugs,[35] including the anticoagulant warfarin.[36] While the drug is customarily administered as the racemate, the active enantiomer is S-warfarin. Six SNPs affecting three amino acids have been characterized in this gene.[37] Between 5% and 40% of humans depending on ethnicity carry at least one copy of either of two genetic variants with reduced enzymatic activity for S-warfarin and many other CYP2C9 substrates.[13,38–40]

Warfarin has a narrow therapeutic window and is used to prevent and treat thromboembolic disease. Inappropriate dosing leads to excessive and occasionally life-threatening bleeding in 2–12% of patients per year.[41] The risk is greatest during initiation of therapy.[42,43] Carriers of common variants metabolize warfarin more slowly, requiring lower daily doses of the drug. A recent retrospective analysis[40] established that the CYP2C9 genotype affected the maintenance dose, the time to stable dosing, the level of anticoagulation, and the risk of bleeding events.[13,38,39] CYP2C9 genotyping prior to warfarin treatment could benefit patients, particularly during the high-risk period of warfarin therapy initiation, by reducing risk and decreasing monitoring requirements.[37,40,44] The CYP2C9 genotype predicts approximately 10% of the variability in the warfarin dose.[22]

VKORC1 Polymorphisms and Warfarin

Warfarin exerts its pharmacological effect by inhibiting the vitamin K epoxide reductase complex 1 (VKORC1). VKORC1 is the vitamin K cycle enzyme controlling the regeneration of reduced vitamin K, an essential cofactor that drives the formation of blood clotting factors II, VII, IX, X, and protein C/S. Patients with varying degrees of warfarin resistance carry genetic variants of one copy of VKORC1, although the severity of phenotypes is based on small numbers of patients and should be viewed as tentative. Five haplotypes typified by noncoding polymorphisms that associate with the variability in warfarin dose requirements have been identified. Haplotypes H1 and H2 (group A) confer the low-dose warfarin phenotype (mean $\sim$3 mg/day) and haplotypes H7–H9 (group B) confer the high-dose phenotype (mean $\sim$7 mg/day). An SNP at the allelic site 1173T/C in intron 1 assigns European-American subjects to either groups A or B 95% of the time. This polymorphism is associated with the optimal warfarin dose in both European and Asian patients, and the reduced average maintenance dose required for Asians is largely a result of the low frequency of the high-dose 1173T allele. In Caucasian and Asian populations, the VKORC1 genotype predicts approximately 25% of the variability in the warfarin dose.[22]

By combining the clinical characteristics with knowledge of the genotypes of CYP2C9 and VKORC1, as much as 60% of the variability in the warfarin dose can be explained.

ALDH2 Polymorphism and Alcohol

Variant forms of aldehyde dehydrogenase (ALDH2) are important markers of altered alcohol metabolism. ALDH2 deficiency occurs in 8–45% of Mongoloid populations (defined as inclusive of some 14 subpopulations divided among Orientals, South American Indians, North American Indians, and Mexican Indians), resulting in facial flushing and acute vasomotor dilation in response to ethanol. Nearly 86% of Japanese subjects who always experienced flushing have inactive ALDH2, while infrequent flushing is associated with active ALDH2.[45] As a consequence of this aversive effect of alcohol, Japanese men and women with inactive ALDH2 drink significantly less alcohol and are highly protected from alcoholism compared to those with active ALDH2.[45]

Dihydropyrimidine Dehydrogenase (DPD) Polymorphism and 5-Fluorouracil

DPD deficiency is estimated to occur in 1–3% of an unselected group of cancer patients.[46] A homozygous DPD-deficient person given the chemotherapeutic nucleoside 5-fluorouracil exhibits an altered pattern of drug metabolites, resulting in prolonged exposure to the parent drug and severe drug-related toxicity. As 5-fluorouracil occupies a pivotal role in the treatment of cancers of the gastrointestinal tract, breast, and head and neck, DPD deficiency is an important genetic marker. To date, at least 19 mutations of DPD have been identified. Recently, it has been shown that a G → A point mutation is an invariant slice site that is by far the most common one (52%) among patients with complete DPD deficiency.[23,24] This mutation leads to skipping of exon 14 and yields a completely nonfunctional form of DPD. It occurs in the normal (Dutch) population at a sufficiently high frequency (1.8% heterozygotes) that these investigators suggest genetic screening for its presence is warranted in cancer patients before the administration of 5-fluorouracil.

Glucuronosyltransferase Polymorphism and Irinotecan

A polymorphism resulting from a mutated promoter of UGT1A1, termed UGT1A1*28, is responsible for the impaired glucuronosyltransferase activity of UGT1A1. This polymorphism is associated with Gilbert's syndrome, a relatively mild, nonpathogenic, hyperbilirubinemic, often undiagnosed disorder that occurs in up to 19% of individuals. Biotransformation of irinotecan, an anticancer prodrug, involves its sequential conversion by carboxylesterase to SN-38, and subsequently detoxification to the pharmacologically inactive SN-38 glucuronide. SN-38 is a potent topoisomerase inhibitor, but SN-38 glucuronide formation is impaired by the polymorphism of UGT1A1*28. This polymorphism is due to an additional TA repeat in the TATA sequence of the UGT1A1 promoter [(TA)$_7$TAA, instead of (TA)$_6$TAA]. The frequency of the 7/7 polymorphism in Caucasians is 20%. Persons with this polymorphism are predisposed to severe grades of diarrhea and leukopenia. The UGT1A1*28 polymorphism may serve as a marker predictive of patients with lower SN-38 glucuronidation rates and greater susceptibility to irinotecan-induced gastrointestinal and bone marrow toxicity.[25]

Thiopurine Methyltransferase (TPMT) Deficiency and Immunosuppressive/Antileukemic Drugs

TPMT deficiency is ascribed to a series of SNPs that result in low TPMT activity. TPMT deficiency is associated with serious acute and delayed intolerance to immunosuppressive and antileukemic drugs (6-mercaptopurine, 6-thioguanine, azathioprine). At least eight alleles that confer low levels of TPMT have been reported, but only two of these appear to account for the majority of subjects with low TPMT activity.[26,47] TPMT deficient persons administered these agents are predisposed to several forms of toxicity. They may suffer bone marrow toxicity that is potentially fatal. TPMT-deficient or heterozygous patients treated with mercaptopurine while receiving cranial radiotherapy for CNS leukemia are at risk of developing secondary brain tumors. However, in the latter group, patients received more intensive systemic antimetabolite therapy before and during radiotherapy. Studies have also suggested that the TPMT genotype may influence the risk of secondary malignancies such as acute myelogenous leukemia.[26] Clinically significant interactions may also occur when agents that are potent TPMT inhibitors (e.g., olsalazine) are coadministered with standard doses of thiopurine drugs to produce phenocopies of subjects with genetically low TPMT activity.[48] It is also known that thiopurine efficacy is low in persons with high TPMT activity,[49] which may require higher thiopurine doses. However, a dose increase of thiopurines for such patients may cause adverse effects. For instance, a patient with high TPMT who receives 6-mercaptopurine generates methylmercaptopurine, a cytotoxic by-product that can cause serious side effects such as hepatotoxicity.[50]

It has been shown that an average of 78% of adverse drug reactions from thiopurine drugs is not associated with TPMT polymorphisms.[51] Nevertheless, a strong argument can be made for pharmacogenetic testing prior to thiopurine treatment and is being practiced clinically.[52]

Developing Prospective Pharmacogenetic Profiles

Drug therapy tailored to the individual and rational discovery of better therapies are exciting prospects that have universal appeal. Science and technology have provided the framework and tools for genetic analysis of the human drug response, but whether these advances will improve patient care in a cost-effective manner remains to be established. It is the hope of personalized medicine that patient treatment guided by profiles individualized for specific drugs can provide an approach that will meet these objectives. It is reasonable to expect that risk profiles for drug susceptibility based on predictive genetic markers would provide the means to translate the molecular foundations of pharmacogenetics into these objectives.

The construction of risk profiles necessitates the collection of genomic data on a large scale. Pharmacogenetics is well positioned to construct such profiles suitable for medical practice from the extensive knowledge accumulated on monogenic pharmacogenetic traits. At present, the number of pharmacogenetic markers that have been characterized exceeds by a considerable margin the estimate of several dozen made almost two decades ago. Furthermore, recent molecular studies indicate that such traits are often associated with a limited number of functionally important variants, raising the prospect that the responsible genes may be cataloged in the near future.[53,54] With the Human Genome Project completed, with genomics technologies for identifying and scoring polymorphisms, and with bioinformatics tools for handling large data sets well in hand, important parts of this task are already in place.

Despite the documented functional relevance of many drug-metabolizing genes, prospective gene-based drug prescribing has not yet been translated into clinical practice.[13,34,55–59] Although scientifically sound, the pharmacogenetic evidence linking single-gene polymorphisms to functional outcome has often been incomplete or difficult to access, complicating its translation into clinical practice. The reasons for this are numerous and complex:

1. *Pharmacogenetic studies often have not assessed clinically relevant endpoints.* Many early investigations were performed to test proof of concept, i.e., to examine the relevance of genetic diversity to variations in human drug response. The pharmacogenetic studies performed during the 1960s and into the 1980s were not usually conceived or designed to assess clinical endpoints in a clinical setting. Only with ample evidence that genetic diversity was an important contributor to human drug response were the aims of research altered to assess clinically relevant endpoints.

2. *Objective criteria appropriate for assessing clinically relevant outcomes were lacking.* Most investigators in the earlier studies used one or more unfamiliar variables (genotypes, drug metabolite ratios, urinary drug/metabolite patterns, drug plasma concentrations, etc.) to express the outcome, and the clinical implications of such variations may not have been clearly or sufficiently defined.

3. *The statistical power of studies was low.* Many of the early studies were limited to a small number of individuals or small populations, so their statistical power was low.

4. *Many studies failed to evaluate the effects of modifying genes.* The evidence suggests that most pharmacogenetic markers are monogenic in origin (i.e., in any particular family, only one responsible locus is thought to be defective). As these traits are examined in greater depth, we find that analyses at a single locus will reliably predict few phenotypic outcomes. Principal among the problems encountered in dissecting the molecular basis of even the simplest disorders attributed to mutations of a single gene, as Peltonen and McKusick[60] observed recently, are the modifying effects of other genes. Existing information about monogenic disorders demonstrates that modifier genes can bring about substantial variations in the clinical phenotype for diseases such as cystic fibrosis and Hirschsprung's disease. Arguably, the metabolism of certain drugs is governed by a single rate-limiting step, and for them a close genotype–phenotype correlation might be expected. Admittedly, however, among all of the pharmacogenetic traits that have been characterized, none to our knowledge has tested the hypothesis that the modifying effects of other genes have no effect on the expression of the trait. Hence, establishing the relationship of genotype to phenotype for the human drug response represents a major challenge to the construction of genetic susceptibility profiles.

5. *Drug susceptibility profiling implies a causal relationship between genotype and phenotype.* Somehow, the belief that knowledge of the genotype is sufficient to determine the phenotype and predict the response of susceptible individuals has gained a credible audience. However, this notion ignores our ignorance of biology and defies expert opinion. First, the potential effects of modifying genes on the expression of a trait for a specific drug must be taken into account, as noted previously. Second, the functional consequences of genetic diversity must be precisely defined for each drug specified and for each of the separable phenotypes that characterize a given trait. This means that the drug susceptibility phenotype that is expressed in response to a specific drug must be causally related to the genotype (or haplotype) of a specific individual as precisely as data will allow.

6. *Adequate methodology for high-throughput phenotyping is not available.* As was noted in points 4 and 5 above, knowledge of genotype alone is usually insufficient to predict drug-specific phenotypes. Progress toward partial resolution of this problem has been made by technical means. Genotyping complemented by phenotyping with probe substrates has been used to determine the activity of specific drug-metabolizing enzymes.[61–64]

For example, Frye et al.[61] showed that a cocktail of noninteracting probe drugs (caffeine, chloroxazone, dapsone, debrisoquin, and mephenytoin) can be administered simultaneously to estimate *in vivo* activities of several CYP450 and *N*-acetyltransferase enzymes. Subsequently, Dierks and co-workers[62] developed a method for simultaneously evaluating the activities of seven major human drug-metabolizing P450s (CYP1A2, 2A6, 2C8, 2C9, 3A4, 2D6, and 2C19) using midazolam, bufuralol, diclofenac, ethoxyresorufin, *S*-mephenytoin, coumarin, and paclitaxel as probe substrates to monitor activity, and ketoconazole, quinidine, sulfaphenazole, tranylcypromine, quercetin, furafylline, and 8-methoxypsoralen as inhibitors to monitor inhibition in human liver microsomes. These techniques have been employed mainly in a research setting, but there is a pressing need for phenotyping methodology applicable to large-scale, high-throughput analyses of therapeutic drugs. The method of Frye et al. appears to be directly applicable to this end, and perhaps the other methods could be adapted to this purpose.

7. *Knowledge of physiological or pathological factors that affect the regulation of genetic markers is lacking.* Infections or inflammatory stimuli, or cytokines and interferons employed as therapeutic agents, as well as hormones and nutritional status can cause changes in the activities or expression of various forms of human drug-metabolizing enzymes.[65–67] These factors have the potential to alter, adversely or beneficially, the therapeutic or toxic effects of drugs, and these effects are particularly crucial for drugs with a low therapeutic index. For certain drugs, the effects of these factors on the drug level have been known for many years (see Table 1 in Morgan[65]), but systematic investigation of their effects on the expression of Phase 1 and Phase 2 drug-metabolizing enzymes has only recently begun.

Factors Affecting the Clinical Practice of Gene-Based Therapy

In addition to the incompleteness and inaccessibility of scientific evidence, socioeconomic factors have probably hindered translation of the science into clinical practice.[59] While clinical data increasingly suggest that characterization of genetic variability in drug disposition and response, particularly for drugs with low safety margins, would improve patient care, the cost of genotyping large populations at risk as well as the practice efficiency, education of physicians and patients, and data security remain undetermined and need to be assessed if gene-based drug prescribing is to succeed.

At present, two main factors appear to affect the clinical realization of gene-based drug prescribing: compelling scientific evidence, a force tending to advance this process, and unproven economic benefits, a force tending to retard the process. Wilke et al. explored some of the issues relevant to prospective gene-based therapy in the context of three drug classes that are widely used in medical practice, PPIs antiulcer therapy, anticoagulation by coumarin drugs, and statin hypolipidemic therapy.[59]

On the Economics of Gene-Based PPI Therapy

Most PPIs are subject to metabolism by CYP2C19 polymorphism, and the CYP2C19 metabolizer status of the majority of whites (~84%), blacks (>90%), and Asians (~100%) can be determined by genotyping only two variant alleles, CYP2C19*2 and CYP2C19*3, as described above.

Desta and colleagues have explored the economic utility of CYP2C19 genotyping for the treatment of peptic ulcer disease with PPIs.[33] Assuming treatments of 3 months for extensive metabolizers, 2 months for intermediate metabolizers, and 1 month for poor metabolizers, and a conservative genotyping cost saving of U.S. $10 per allele, they estimated a cost saving of equal or greater than U.S. $5000 per 100 Asian patients genotyped. Because of differences in the frequencies of CYP2C19 alleles, the cost:benefit ratio for prospective gene-based prescribing might be quite different in white and black populations. Despite lower minor allele frequencies in non-Asian populations, CYP2C19 might still lead to improved, cost-effective care. Since *Helicobactor pylori* eradication rates in homozygous (~80%) and heterozygous (~98%) extensive metabolizers and poor metabolizers (~100%) differ significantly,[68,69] and since extensive metabolizers have lower eradication rates, Lehmann et al. postulated that gene-based therapy would be cost effective if extensive metabolizers were given a regimen containing anti-*H. pylori* treatment and an H2-histamine receptor blocker (ranitidine) instead of a PPI.[70] Lehmann et al. predicted a breakeven cost of approximately U.S. $90–119 per genotype on implementing CYP2C19-based testing for non-Asian patients within the United States. For Pacific Rim (Asian) patients, they found the cost savings of CYP2C19 genotyping was greater (U.S. $495–2195).

Savings are relatively modest in this example, but it should be recognized that the PPIs as a class have a wide therapeutic index. Hence, the potential savings might be amplified for drugs with a narrower safety margin, particularly for drugs with clinically severe toxicity. Warfarin is such an example and is considered below.

On the Convergence of Safety and Economics of Gene-Based Warfarin Anticoagulation

Therapy with warfarin and other coumarin anticoagulant drugs is challenging because of the wide variability in patient response due to many factors including drug-, dietary-, and disease-related factors and genetic factors.[71] It is clear that genetic polymorphisms in genes affecting metabolism (CYP2C9) and response (VKORC1) are associated with warfarin response. A strong case can be made for prospective genotyping of patients who receive warfarin because optimal dosing determines safe and efficacious anticoagulant responses to this agent.[22,40]

Several attempts have been made to estimate cost savings that attach to prospective gene-based therapy with warfarin. Higashi et al.[40] estimated the CYP2C9 genotyping cost at U.S. $135 per patient, and subsequently predicted that 13 patients would need to be treated for the cost of genotyping to offset the cost of each adverse event avoided. The study population consisted of 526 patients of European (91%), Asian (4%), African (3%), and Hispanic (2%) origin. You and colleagues tested a decision tree designed to simulate clinical outcomes of warfarin therapy in a series of Caucasian populations with and without the benefit of CYP2C9 genotype.[72] Their model projected 9.58 versus 10.48 adverse events per 100 patient years in the genotyped group compared to those in the nongenotyped group. The cost saved was estimated to be approximately U.S. $5778 per additional major bleeding event avoided.

These analyses were conducted on retrospective study populations of relatively homogeneous ethnicity adhering to standardized anticoagulant therapeutic protocols. The findings have been extended to measure the effect of the CYP2C9 genotype in a context of various clinical covariates. Wadelius et al.[73] demonstrated that 29% of the total variance in stable warfarin dosing could be explained by age, gender and CYP2C9 genotype. Hillman et al.[74] found that 34% of the total variance could be explained by a model that included age, gender, body size, CYP2C9 genotype, comorbidity, and concomitant medication, and Gage explained 39% of the variance by developing a model that considered ethnicity, genotype, and the clinical covariates noted above.[75]

Prospective studies have been designed to characterize the clinical utility and economic impact of CYP2C9 gene-based warfarin dosing, and pilot trials have been performed by Russell Wilke and colleagues as part of the Marshfield Clinic Personalized Medicine Project.[76] In one study, the influence of several clinical covariates (age, gender, body composition, comorbidity, and concomitant medication) on the rate of rise for prothrombin time during the first 30 days of warfarin therapy was assessed in the context of the CYP2C9 genotype in a large retrospective patient cohort followed regularly in an outpatient anticoagulation clinic.[71] This study showed that age and concomitant sulfonylurea therapy altered the rate of anticoagulation during the first 30 days of therapy. The influence of the CYP2C9 genotype was marginally significant. A second study performed by Wilke and co-workers evaluated the feasibility of applying a CYP2C9 gene-based warfarin dosing model in clinical practice.[77] Candidates were recruited from clinic patients eligible for warfarin for inclusion in this prospective, randomized single-blinded pilot trial. Results suggested that CYP2C9 gene-based multivariate warfarin dosing is technically feasible and acceptable to patients and providers. Although the study involved only a few patients, the results suggested that those with variant CYP2C9 genotypes appeared to benefit from the use of gene-based models to dose warfarin.

Metabolic variations in all of the models mentioned above were based on genetic variations in CYP2C9, but improved models must still be developed that include variations in response due to polymorphisms in vitamin K epoxide reductase complex 1 (VKORC1), the enzyme known to mediate vitamin K-dependent clotting factors, and the vitamin K-dependent inhibitory factors. Shikata et al. have explained as much as 50% of the variance in warfarin maintenance dosing.[78]

These advances led to speculation that the Food and Drug Administration (FDA) might require labeling of warfarin to require pharmacogenetic testing, but this change probably awaits the results from prospective randomized clinical trials. Meanwhile, the search continues for new candidate genes and for genetic variations in CYP2C9 and VKORC1 among minority populations.[22]

A Broad Range of Genetic Diversity Impinges on Statin Hypolipidemic Therapy

Several large, multicenter trials have demonstrated that statin therapy reduces both primary and secondary coronary artery disease. Worldwide, the statins represent one of the most widely prescribed classes of drugs. Although they interact with a variety of cellular processes, the statins derive their primary therapeutic effect by attenuating lipoprotein synthesis and upregulating the expression of low-density lipoprotein cholesterol receptors. Currently, there are at least half a dozen statin drugs on the market, and despite their clinical efficacy, statin therapy can be complicated by differential properties of individual statins. Some are highly lipophilic while others are hydrophilic, and the resultant profiles differ from one statin to another.

Wilke et al.[59,79] have summarized the pharmacokinetics of several statins of particular interest. Each of three common Phase I enzymes, CYP2C9, 2D6, and 3A4/5, interacts differently with each of the currently available statins. Atorvastatin is oxidized primarily by the CYP3A family. This family of enzymes also contributes to the metabolism of simvastatin, while CYP2D6 contributes to the further metabolism of simvastatin metabolites. Unlike atorvastatin and simvastatin, fluvastatin is metabolized mainly by CYP2C9, and the CYP2C9 variants implicated in warfarin kinetics also appear to alter fluvastatin kinetics. Certain statins such as atorvastatin are extensively metabolized while others such as pravastatin are less extensively metabolized, and the primary enzyme often differs. Phase 1 (P450) metabolism of statins typically results in a variety of hydroxyl metabolites. Atorvastatin, for example, is converted mainly by CYP3A/5 to 2-hydroxy (OH) atorvastatin and 4-OH atorvastatin, while simvastatin is converted via CYP2D6 to 3-OH simvastatin and 6-OH simvastatin. Hydroxylated statin metabolites are often further metabolized through Phase II conjugation through the glucuronosyltransferase *UGT1*. Gemfibrizol, a drug that lowers triglycerides, is believed to alter the pharmacokinetics and clinical outcomes of a variety of statin drugs via a UGT-dependent interaction. Inhibition of glucuronidation of simvastatin hydroxyl acid by gemfibrizol attenuates the biliary excretion of simvastatin and increases the risk of statin-related toxicity.

Membrane transporters also modulate a variety of statin-related clinical outcomes. Polymorphisms in the organic anion transporter (OATP-C) have been associated with alterations in the hepatic uptake of pravastatin. Gemfibrizol attenuates the OATP-C-dependent uptake of rosuvastatin and cerivastatin. Whether gemfibrizol alters other statin-related outcomes through UGT-1 and OATP-C interactions is unclear, but Wilke and co-workers have recently demonstrated a hidden interaction between CYP3A/5 binding affinity and atorvastatin-induced myopathy.[80] However, statin binding affinity varies from statin to statin, and these investigators note that this relationship may differ for other statin drugs.

Thus, it is apparent that the metabolism and transport of statins differ so remarkably from statin to statin that gene-based models for each statin will need to be developed and refined before they can be implemented in the clinic.

Implementing Personalized Medicine

The completion of the Human Genome Project (HGP) brought with it the opportunity to explore the whole spectrum of human health and disease from the fresh perspective of genome science. The vision of genomics research as detailed in the blueprint for the genomic era[81] was formulated into three major themes—genomics and biology, genomics in health, and genomics to society—and six elements cross-cutting all three thematic areas. The six elements were resources, technology development, computational biology, training, ethical, legal, and social implications (ELSI), and education. Finally, a series of bold achievements was proposed that would have profound implications for genomics research and its applications to medicine.

As to the second of the major themes set forth in the blueprint, genomics in health, the original framers of the HGP were explicit in their expectation that it would lead to improvements in human health. With the completion of the HGP, the vision included the development and application of strategies to identify genes and pathways with roles in health and disease and how they interact with the environment; to develop, evaluate, and apply genome-based diagnostic methods for the prediction of susceptibility to disease, drug response, early detection, and accurate molecular classification of disease; and to develop methods that catalyze the translation of genomic knowledge into therapeutic advances.

Collins and colleagues[81] and Khoury[82] both argued for the organization of large, longitudinal population-based prospective cohort studies as resources to meet the goals outlined above. Projects such as the UK Biobank (www.ukbiobank.ac.uk), the Estonian Genome Project (www.geenivaramu.ee), and the Marshfield Clinic Personalized Medicine Research Project (www.mfldclin.edu/pmrp) were already seeking to provide such resources.

The Marshfield Personalized Medicine Research Project

The Marshfield Clinic's Personalized Medicine Research Project was conceived in 2000.[76,83] The project was designed to coordinate existing resources of the Clinic that were unique and robust in aggregate. These resources included (1) a 12-year-old epidemiological study area encompassing 80,000 patients who had received their health care at the Clinic for several decades, (2) a highly sophisticated electronic medical record that tracked and integrated the outpatient and inpatient health care events for the Clinic population consisting of over 1.2 million electronic records spanning over 20 years, (3) a data warehouse and provider-initiated lexicons that allowed data retrieval for specific clinical phenotypes, (4) extensive experience in human genotyping through the Center for Medical Genetics that developed the Marshfield Maps used globally for evaluating the genetic basis of disease, and (5) extensive infrastructure and experience in patient recruiting and consenting for over 700 clinical research projects on an annual basis.

Since the population of the Marshfield Epidemiological Study Area (MESA) was known to be representative of statewide disease distribution by several criteria, the goal of this project was to recruit all of the patients in the MESA over the age of 18 years, draw blood samples from these patients for DNA, plasma, and serum collection, and then create a database linking genetic information with phenotypic information extracted from the patient's medical record (see http://www.mfldclin.edu.prmp/).

The project confirmed through focus groups the sensitivity of patients to the maintenance of privacy for their genetic and health care information and their concerns regarding potential discrimination by employers and insurers based on genetic information. Consequently, a nationally expert Ethics and Security Advisory Board was formed to ensure the security and confidentiality of the database. The database was in a secure area and was free standing, that is, free of connections to the remainder of the Clinic's information system or the Internet. The data were one way encrypted. In addition, the project received a Certificate of Confidentiality from the National Institutes of Health that protected the data against forced release even under court order.

A Scientific Advisory Board was also organized composed of genetic epidemiologists, pharmacogeneticists, and computational geneticists to address the ability of the population to address the pertinent questions, to aid in prioritizing projects, and to help structure the project into a proper multiuser resource.

Patient recruitment began in late September 2002, with 3300 patients enrolled by mid-January 2003, and enrollment continuing at 60–70 patients daily. Funding for the project has come from grants through the Health Resources and Services Administration (HRSA) to address the ethical and scientific issues, through the State of Wisconsin to recruit the patients and collect the biological samples, and through the Marshfield Clinic to further support infrastructure development.

The project is directed toward delineating the predictability of the genetic markers of drug response, outcomes analysis of genetically based prescriptive practices, preventive medicine based on the genetic basis of disease, and answering important questions in population genetics. The hope of this project is that it will allow physicians to use genetic information to be proactive rather than reactive in freeing patients of disease.

The Personalized Medicine Coalition (PMC)

The concept of personalized medicine has repercussions well beyond those of the science that made it possible. Its adoption will without doubt require changes in numerous aspects of health care as in healthcare infrastructure, diagnostics and therapeutics business models, reimbursement policy from government and private payers, and a different approach to regulatory oversight. While the details surrounding these issues are beyond the scope of this presentation, they are being considered by a variety of groups and organizations such as the PMC.[84]

The PMC (URL: http//:www.personalizedmedicinecoalition.org/newsevents/news.php) was formed as a nonprofit umbrella organization of pharmaceutical, biotechnology, diagnostic, and information technology companies, healthcare providers and payers, patient advocacy groups, industry policy organizations, major academic institutions, and government agencies. The PMC provides a structure for achieving consensus on crucial public policy issues that will be vital to translating personalized medicine into clinical practice. In a recent article, the PMC outlines its goals and the strategies it will take to foster communication and debate and to achieve consensus on issues such as genetic discrimination, reimbursement for pharmacogenomic drugs, diagnostics, regulation, physician training, medical school criteria, and public discussion.[84]

DIGGING DEEPER INTO HUMAN GENETIC VARIATION

Synonymous Codons Are Not Always Silent

Each of several amino acids is represented by more than one codon (triplet of nucleotide bases) in accordance with the genetic code. Such codons are termed "synonymous" because they do not translate into a change in the amino acid composition of the protein; they have usually been categorized as "silent" because it has been assumed that they exert no discernible effect on gene function or phenotype. Nonsilent polymorphisms involve those variations in a gene that do lead to amino acid changes in the protein product. In the human genome roughly 99.8% of DNA sequence variations in coding regions are synonymous, and synonymous SNPs show a higher frequency than both missense SNPs and SNPs in noncoding regions. They are also the most polymorphic, suggesting they may be functionally neutral. This does not mean, however, that every synonymous site is nonfunctional or neutral.[85]

Recently, Michael Gottesman and colleagues described a synonymous polymorphism in the gene that codes for P-glycoprotein (P-gp), MDR1, which is not silent.[86,87] The MDR1 protein resides in cell membranes where it transports drug molecules out of cells and renders many human cancers resistant to a diversity of anticancer drugs. Gottesman's group discovered that combinations of three previously known SNPs for the *MDR1* gene (C1236T, G2677T, and C3435T) give rise to versions of MDR1 that are less effective at expelling drugs from cells than the wild-type protein. The C1236T polymorphism changes a GGC codon to GGT at codon 412 of the polypeptide (both encode glycine), while the C3435T polymorphism changes ATC to ATT at codon 1145 (both encode isoleucine). Both polymorphisms result in changes from frequent to infrequent codons. The investigators hypothesized that substitution of an infrequent codon for a more frequent codon would delay protein synthesis because there is less of the infrequent codon available, and because of the delay, the growing variant protein would have the opportunity to fold in a different final conformation. Limited proteolysis and the use of a conformation-sensitive monoclonal antibody revealed structural differences between the protein derived from wild-type MDR1 and the polymorphic haplotypes in support of this hypothesis. However, the mechanical details of the altered folding need to be worked out.

A study by Luda Diatchenko and colleagues sheds additional light on this issue by assessing the significance of synonymous variations for another protein, catechol-*O*-methyltransferase (COMT).[88] Diatchenko's group, like Gottesman's group, found that different synonymous codons in the gene for COMT led to changes in the properties of the expressed protein. Human COMT, an enzyme responsible for metabolic inactivation and elimination of catecholamines, has recently been implicated in the modulation of persistent pain. Three common haplotypes of the human *COMT* gene, divergent in two synonymous and one nonsynonymous position, code for differences in COMT enzymatic activity and are associated with differences in pain sensitivity and the likelihood of developing temporomandibular joint disorder (TMJD). The haplotypes divergent in synonymous changes exhibited by far the largest difference in COMT activity, due to a reduced amount of translated protein. The major *COMT* haplotypes varied with respect to messenger RNA local stem–loop structures, such that the most stable structure was associated with the highest pain sensitivity and with the lowest protein levels and enzymatic activity. Because total RNA abundance and RNA degradation rates did not parallel COMT protein levels, the investigators hypothesized that differences in protein translation efficiency likely resulted from differences in the local secondary structure of corresponding RNAs. Site-directed mutagenesis that eliminated the stable structure restored the amount of translated protein affirming this hypothesis. Finding that alterations in mRNA secondary structure resulting from synonymous changes have such a profound effect on protein expression suggests that the mRNA secondary structure, not the nucleotides in the synonymous positions, are subject to selective pressure.

These two studies demonstrate that haplotype variants of naturally occurring synonymous SNPs can have stronger effects on gene function than nonsynonymous variations. They also suggest that synonymous changes should be given more weight and are likely to be of greater biological and medical significance than is generally recognized. It is not unreasonable to think of targeting this mechanism in new drug discovery programs and personalized drug treatment.

Polymorphically Duplicated Genes Relevant to Pharmacogenetics

Initially, analysis of the human genome sequence suggested that SNPs, which occurred on average in 1 of 300 nucleotides, were believed to be the main source of genetic and phenotypic individual variation. However, the creation of genome-wide scanning technologies and comparative genomic-sequence analyses revealed the large extent of DNA variation involving DNA segments smaller than those recognizable microscopically, but larger that those detected by conventional sequence analysis. Estimates have suggested that as much as 5–7% of the human genome might be duplicated, but that may change as a more finished genomic sequence is obtained because identification of repeat-rich regions is technically challenging and their misidentification is likely to underestimate such architectural features.[89]

The concept of "genomic disorders" refers to disorders that result from DNA rearrangements of regional genomic architecture.[89] These rearrangements usually consist of blocks of DNA that span from about 400 kilobases up to 3 megabases of genomic DNA with at least 97% identity, and provide substrates for homologous recombination. They may comprise deletions, duplications, inversions, gene fragments, pseudogenes, endogenous retroviral sequences, intrachromosomal rearrangements, and large-scale copy number variants of entire genes or fragments of genes. In a broader sense they can be regarded as all genomic changes that are not single-base pair substitutions.[90] In some regions, such rearrangements have no apparent effect, but in other regions they may alter gene dosages to cause disease either alone or in combination with other genetic or environmental factors. Such variants are collectively referred to as copy number variants (CNVs) or copy number polymorphisms (CNPs).

Although a large number of Mendelian disorders have been shown to result from genomic rearrangements,[89,91,92] there has been no systematic search for the polymorphic duplication of genes. Several polymorphic duplications of pharmacogenetic interest have been found by chance as summarized in Table 11.3. Some of these duplications have been, or may be, associated with specific phenotypes. A few other duplications that may also express a functional phenotypic effect are also listed there.

Examples of Copy Number Variants

Butyrylcholinesterase (*BuCHE*) is responsible for the metabolic elimination of the muscle relaxant succinylcholine, an adjunct drug used during general anesthesia. Variant forms of this enzyme are responsible for prolonged apnea, an extension of its therapeutic effect that is sometimes fatal. BuCHE is specifically inhibited by agricultural organophosphate poisons such as parathion. Individuals expressing the "silent" phenotype of *BuCHE* produce a defective form of this enzyme, rendering them especially sensitive to parathion. In 1987, Prody et al.[93] found a 100-fold amplification in the *BuCHE* gene in two generations of a family under prolonged exposure to parathion.

Johansson and colleagues demonstrated that very rapid metabolism of several antidepressant and antipsychotic drugs could be explained by up to 12-fold amplification of CYP2D6.[95] Dalen and co-workers showed that the relationship between the CYP2D6 genotype and the oral clearance of the antidepressant drug nortriptyline in persons with 0, 1, 2, 3, and 13 functional CYP2D6 genes was 1:1:4:5:17.[96] The ethnic distribution of the ultrarapid metabolizer phenotype shows that Swedish and German populations carry 1–2% of the ultrarapid metabolizer phenotype, while the frequency of ultrarapid carriers in Ethiopia and Saudi Arabia approaches 29%. Subsequently, Ledesma et al. found CYP2D6 CNVs in approximately 12% (5.1% with deletion, CYP2D6*5), and 7.2% with duplication (CYP2D6x2), in a Spanish population.[109]

The study by McLellan and co-workers identified a duplicated functional *GSTM1* gene as the genetic basis for the ultrarapid phenotype observed in a small percentage of Saudi Arabian subjects.[98] The glutathione-*S*-transferases (GSTs) contribute to protection against a broad range of compounds including carcinogens, pesticides, antitumor agents, and environmental pollutants. *GSTM1* is polymorphic in humans, one allele of which, *GSTM1*O*, results from the deletion of the entire GSTM1 gene. Approximately 50% of the Caucasian population is homozygous deleted for this allele and fails to express the protein. Numerous studies suggest that GSTM1*O is associated with some types of lung cancer as well as cancers of the urinary bladder, stomach, colon, and pituitary gland. Although it seems likely that duplication of GSTM1 resulting in an ultrarapid phenotype may be protective against environmentally related disorders, this remains to be determined.

Patients with glucocorticoid-related aldosteronism (GRA) possess chimeric gene duplications fusing ACTH-responsive regulatory sequences of 11β-

Table 11.3 Polymorphic Duplication of Human Genes of Pharmacogenetic Interest

Gene (gene symbol)	Locus	Size of duplication	Frequency of duplication	Phenotype	Reference
Genes with phenotypes associated with duplication					
Butyryl cholinesterase (*BuCHE*)	3q26	100 copies of genomic BuCHE fragment	Undefined, identified in two members of a single family subjected to prolonged exposure to organo-phosphate insecticides	Not defined	93, 94
P450 CYP2D6 (*CYP2D6*)	22q13.1	2–13 copies of the entire CYP2D6 gene	1–29%; large ethnic variation	Ultrarapid phenotype: codeine toxicity; resistance to CYP2D6 substrates	95–97
Glutathione-*S*-transferase M1 (*GSTM1*)	1p13.3	3 copies of the entire GSTM1 gene	Undefined; identified in Saudi Arabian population	Ultrarapid phenotype: possibly protective against carcinogenic chemicals	98
P450 chimeric gene 11β-hydroxylase/aldosterone synthase (*CYP11B1/2*)	8q21	10 kb	True prevalence unknown; identified in a large kindred	Glucocorticoid remediable aldosteronism (GRA)	

Chemokine (CCL3-LI)	17q21.1	Entire gene	Average copy number varies from 2 to 7 among six ethnic populations tested	High copy numbers protect against susceptibility to and progression of HIV, whereas low copy numbers enhance both HIV susceptibility and progression	101, 102
Coagulation Factor VIII (Factor VIII)	Xq28	Intron 22 inversion and 9.5 kb duplication	0.57–0.59 in whites, Japanese, and Chinese	Accounts for at least half of hemophilia A cases	103
Genes with phenotypes that may be associated with duplication					
P450 CYP2A6*3 (CYP2A6*3)	19q13.2	Multiple CYP2A6/CYP2A7 gene conversions; >7 kb	0–1.7%	Potential effect on nicotine metabolism undefined	104, 105
Estrogen receptor	6q25	Exons 6 and 7 in breast cancer cell line (MCF-2A)	Undefined	May act to inhibit wild-type estrogen receptor	106, 107
Cytosine 5-methyltransferase (5-DNMT1)	19p13.3–13.2	1–4 copies of allele II entire gene	Undefined	Potential association with cancerogenesis not determined	108

hydroxylase to coding sequences of aldosterone synthase (see Appendix A). These chimeric species are specific for GRA and explain the biochemistry, physiology, and genetics of GRA and this form of hereditary hypertension.

In 2002, Townson et al.[101] found that copy number regulated the production of the human chemokine CCL3L1, a potent HIV-suppressive chemokine. They found that the *CCL3L1* copy number could vary from one to six copies in Caucasians and proposed that genetic variations in CCL3L1 might affect the susceptibility to and progression or severity of diseases such as HIV. More recently, Gonzalez and co-workers affirmed these interindividual differences and also found significant interpopulation differences among African, European, Middle and East Asian, and Oceanic populations in the gene encoding CCL3L1.[102] The possession of a *CCL3L1* copy number lower than the population average was associated with markedly enhanced susceptibility to AIDS. They believe the relationship between *CCL3L1* dose, HIV/AIDS pathogenesis, and susceptibility may constitute a genetic basis for variable responses to this disorder.

Structural chromosomal rearrangements often arise from nonallelic homologous recombination and unequal crossing over between genes, as in the case of GRA described above. If the recombination occurred within a gene, the structure, and likely the function of that gene would be disrupted. In the case of coagulation Factor VIII, a 9.5-kilobase DNA sequence in intron 22 is repeated twice in a region near the long arm terminus of the X chromosome.[103] The intrachromosomal recombination involving this repeated region disrupts the Factor VIII gene and accounts for at least half of hemophilia A cases.

Global Views of Cancer Genetics

The molecular classification of tumors is central to advances in the treatment of these cancers as a means of maximizing the efficacy and minimizing the toxicity of specific therapies targeted to distinct tumor types. Attempts to identify distinct tumor types by gene expression monitoring using DNA microarrays began in the 1990s. Joseph DeRisi and colleagues were among the first to demonstrate that such microarrays could provide a tool for cancer identification.[110] They used a high-density microarray composed of 1161 DNA elements to search for differences in gene expression associated with tumor suppression of a melanoma cell line and they identified a number of alterations in the expression of genes specific to the tumorigenic phenotype of those cells. Their results suggested that DNA microarrays could be used as a tool to define alterations in gene expression associated with a specific cancer, and that they might provide a deeper understanding of pathognomonic molecular derangements that contribute to its origin. Recognition of such alterations in gene expression thus might improve diagnoses and permit selection of most appropriate therapeutic strategies.

Microarrays, a Tool for Gaining Insight into Cancer Genomics

The potential of microarrays as a tool for assigning tumors to known classes of cancer (class prediction) and for identifying new classes of cancers (class discovery) quickly engaged the attention of investigators who used this technology to classify and subclassify leukemia, lymphoma, melanoma, and breast cancer.[111–118] Todd Golub and co-workers set out to develop a systematic analytical approach to class prediction using gene expression profiles to distinguish acute leukemia types whose histological appearance was highly similar.[111] Golub et al. prepared RNA from mononuclear cells isolated from bone marrow samples obtained from 27 acute lymphoblastic leukemia (ALL) and 11 acute myelogenous leukemia (AML) patients and produced microarrays containing probes for 6817 human genes. In this case, a microarray was designed to distinguish these two forms of leukemia. This distinction is critical to successful therapy because chemotherapy regimens for ALL generally contain corticosteroids, vincristine, methotrexate, and L-asparaginase, whereas most AML therapies rely on regimens that contain daunorubicin and cytarabine. The goal was to create an array consisting of 50 predictor genes based on all 38 samples. The 50 genes most highly correlated with the ALL–AML class distinction are shown in Figure 11.1 where the genes that distinguish ALL from AML (y-axis) are grouped separately for individuals tested (x-axis). This 50-gene predictor was then applied to an independent collection of 34 leukemia samples. Results demonstrated the feasibility of cancer classification based solely on gene expression monitoring, and suggested a general strategy for discovering and predicting cancer classes for other types of cancer, independent of previous biological knowledge.

Shortly after Golub's report appeared, Hedenfalk and co-workers reported the use of transcriptional profiling to obtain molecular signatures left by BRCA1 and BRCA2 genes in patients with breast cancer.[115] They used complementary DNA microarrays containing probes for 5361 genes to explore the patterns of gene expression in a sample of 22 primary breast tumors that had mutations in BRCA1, BRCA2, or neither gene. Their study demonstrated that significantly different groups of genes are expressed among BRCA1 mutation-positive tumors, BRCA2 mutation-positive tumors, and sporadic tumors. With respect to BRCA1 mutations, in one case an error was made. In that case, however, there was no BRCA1 mutation, but examination of this patient's germline DNA revealed that the transcriptional activity of her BRCA1 gene was silenced by abnormal methylation of the gene's promoter region. Thus the microarray analysis of her tumor was correct, because the function of BRCA1 was suppressed by an epigenetic mechanism that was not revealed by the sequence of the BRCA1 gene.

Predicting Outcome and Therapeutic Benefit from Molecular Profiles of Cancer

Cancer patients with the same stage of disease can have markedly different treatment responses and overall outcomes. In addition to better systems of cancer classification and clarification of pathways that are altered in neoplastic cells, the advent of microarray technology has also prompted investigators to explore gene expression as a means of predicting the prognosis and response to chemotherapeutic decisions.[116,117,119–122] Van't Veer and colleagues, for instance, have used microarray analysis to predict clinical outcomes of breast cancer. They identified a "poor prognosis" gene signature strongly predictive of distant metastases in

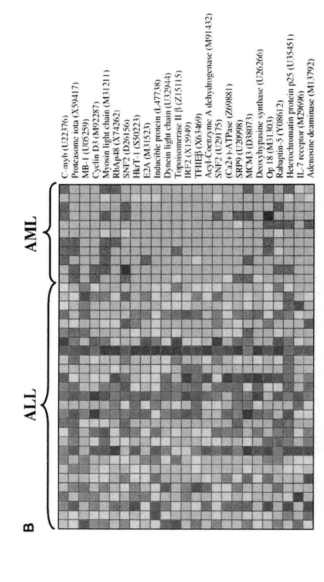

B

ALL   AML

C-myb (U22376)
Proteasome iota (X59417)
MB-1 (U05259)
Cyclin D3 (M92287)
Myosin light chain (M31211)
RbAp48 (X74262)
SNF2 (D26156)
HkrT-1 (S50223)
E2A (M31523)
Inducible protein (L47738)
Dynein light chain (U32944)
Topoisomerase II β (Z15115)
IRF2 (X15949)
TFIIEβ (X63469)
Acyl-Coenzyme A dehydrogenase (M91432)
SNF2 (U29175)
(Ca2+)-ATPase (Z69881)
SRP9 (U20998)
MCM3 (D38073)
Deoxyhypusine synthase (U26266)
Op 18 (M31303)
Rabaptin-5 (Y08612)
Heterochromatin protein p25 (U35451)
IL-7 receptor (M29696)
Adenosine deaminase (M13792)

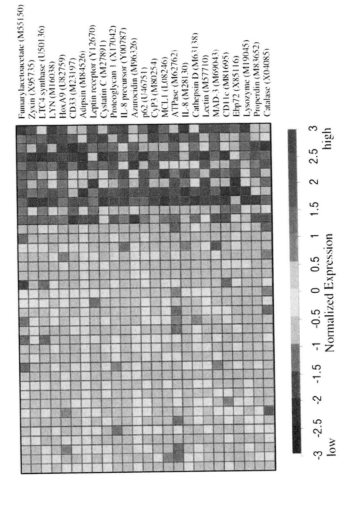

Figure 11.1 Gene expression patterns for acute lymphoblastic leukemia (ALL) and acute myelogenous leukemia (AML). With permission from the *New England Journal of Medicine*.

breast cancer patients without tumor cells in local lymph nodes (lymph node negative).[116] This finding provided a strategy to select patients who would benefit from adjuvant therapy. This prognostic profile could provide a tool to tailor adjuvant systemic treatment that could greatly decrease the risk of adverse side effects and health care expenditure. The study of van de Vijver and co-workers describes a gene expression signature as a predictor for breast cancer survival among a cohort of patients younger than 53 years of age (range <40–53 years) and with either stage I or II breast cancer.[117] The gene signature they identified is a powerful predictor of outcome in young patients. The data indicated that classification of patients into high-risk and low-risk subgroups according to their prognosis profile might be a useful guide to adjuvant therapy in patients with lymph node-positive breast cancer. Such an approach should also improve the selection of patients who would benefit from adjuvant systemic treatment, reducing the rate of both overtreatment and undertreatment.

Liu and colleagues examined the prognostic role of a gene signature from tumorigenic breast cancer cells.[122] Differentially expressed genes were used to generate a 186-gene "invasiveness gene signature" (IGS) for its association with overall survival and metastasis-free survival in patients with breast cancer and other types of cancer. They found a significant association between the IGS and both overall and metastasis-free survival ($p < 0.001$ for both) in patients with breast cancer, which was independent of established clinical and pathological variables. The IGS was also associated with the prognosis in medulloblastoma ($p = 0.004$), lung cancer ($p = 0.03$), and prostate cancer ($p = 0.01$). This genetic signature of tumorigenic breast cancer cells was more strongly associated with clinical outcomes when combined with wound response signature in breast cancer. The "wound response" signature is a 512-gene signature that correlates with overall survival and metastasis-free survival in breast cancer patients. The IGS and WR signatures are representations of different biological phenomena and are based on nonoverlapping lists of genes.

Molecular profiling to characterize tumors and predict outcomes is a major effort to improve the control of lung cancer, one of the deadliest cancers in human populations. Molecular studies of lung tumors began with single or relatively small groups of potential prognostic markers and have progressed to microarray analysis of thousands of genes in large numbers of tissue analyses. The recent study of small cell lung cancer, the most common form of lung cancer, in Chinese (Taiwanese) subjects, identified a five-gene signature that is closely associated with survival of this form of lung cancer.[123] Analysis of microarray data and risk scores of 185 frozen tissue specimens led to the identification of 16 genes that correlated with survival. Further analysis of five selected genes (DUSP6, MMD, STAT1, ERBB3, and LCK) that were submitted to decision-tree analysis showed them to be an independent predictor of relapse-free and overall survival. The model was validated with data from an independent cohort of 60 patients and with a set of published microarray data for 86 patients with small cell lung cancer.

Despite advances in the understanding of molecular pathways that are altered in cancerous cells, diagnosis and decisions regarding treatment still rely largely on classical histopathological and immunohistochemical techniques. Diagnosis and treatment would both benefit from a more quantitative approach. Molecular signatures of gene expression that correlate with the recurrence of breast cancer have been identified, but their clinical application has been limited by the requirement for fresh or snap frozen tissue and uncertainties about reproducibility, and few assays have been rigorously tested as prognostic or predictive in oncology. In 2004, Paik and colleagues resolved some of these issues by developing an assay to predict recurrence in patients with tamoxifen-treated, node-negative, breast cancer.[124] The levels of expression of 16 cancer-related genes and 5 reference genes were used in the prospectively defined algorithm to calculate the recurrence score and to determine a risk group (low, intermediate, high) for each patient. The recurrence score was validated in a large multicenter clinical trial as quantifying the likelihood of distant recurrence in tamoxifen-treated patients with node-negative, estrogen-positive breast cancer. The rates of distant recurrence at 10 years in the low-risk, intermediate-risk, and high-risk groups were 6.8%, 14.3%, and 30.5%. In addition, the rate in the low-risk group was significantly lower than that in the high-risk group ($p < 0.001$), and was independent of age and tumor size. In an extension of this work, Paik et al. subsequently examined the relationship of the recurrence score (RS) to benefit from chemotherapy.[125] The RS was measured in tumors from the tamoxifen-treated (227) and tamoxifen plus chemotherapy-treated patients (424) in the National Surgical Adjuvant Breast and Bowel Project (NSABP) B20 trial. Patients with high-RS tumors benefited greatly from chemotherapy whereas patients with low-RS tumors derived minimal, if any, benefit from chemotherapy. Patients with intermediate-RS tumors did not appear to derive a large benefit, but the uncertainty of the estimate could not exclude a clinically important benefit. The RS assay not only quantified the likelihood of breast cancer recurrence, but it also predicted the magnitude of the chemotherapy benefit. This methodology is now commercially available and is being used clinically.

From Molecular Signatures to Personalized Therapy

The research cited above reflects the maturation of cancer genomics. During the past two decades, they indicate that much progress has been made in the molecular taxonomy, experimental design, and analysis of patterns and pathways of cancer.[126–128] DNA microarrays have allowed investigators to develop expression-based classifications for many types of cancer including breast, brain, ovary, lung, colon, kidney, prostate, gastric, leukemia, and lymphoma.[126] A further advance has been the development of high-density microarrays for detecting regions of genomic amplification or deletion.[129,130] For example, Mullighan and co-workers discovered frequent deletions and loss-of-function mutations on chromosome 9 in the PAX5 gene in 30% of patients with childhood ALL. Deletions were also detected in TCF3 (also known as E2A), EBF1, LEF1, IKZF1 (IKAROS), and IKZF3 (AIOLOS). These findings suggested that direct disruption of pathways controlling B cell development and differentiation contributes to B progenitor ALL pathogenesis. Since cancer pathogenesis seems to follow a largely common path, regardless of the type of cell in which it originates, it is reasonable to expect that these findings may generalize to other forms of cancer.

However, many of the studies performed in support of molecular profiling of human diseases are retrospective, and it appears the field is now poised to begin its next phase—the conduct of prospective trials of adjuvant chemotherapy in patients with various early forms of cancer.[131] For breast cancer, the next phase has already begun with retrospective data indicating that adjuvant treatment is beneficial in patients with high-risk breast tumors.[125] Next, we might anticipate that cancer genomics will emphasize three areas: molecular profiles associated with response or resistance to targeted therapies, clinical trials based on molecular profiles that indicate beneficial effects from targeted therapies, and the evaluation of the significance of epigenetic phenomena (DNA methylation, histone modification) in cancer genomics. Several signaling pathways are associated with sensitivity or resistance to agents targeting these pathways. In lung cancer, one of the best examples concerns epidermal growth factor receptor (EGFR) mutations and amplification that identify patients with small cell lung cancer who respond to EGFR tyrosine kinase inhibitors. Given the recent approval of the EGFR inhibitor erlotinib and the angiogenesis inhibitor bevacizumab for lung cancer, it is important to create molecular tools to predict the response of these cancers to single agents or combination chemotherapies. The signature reported by Chen et al.[123] includes ERRB3, a gene associated with sensitivity to EGFR tyrosine kinase inhibitors. Additional examples of molecular markers of resistance include the expression of the excision repair cross-complementation group1 gene (ERCC1) (resistance to cisplatin-based adjuvant therapy) and ras mutations (resistance to cisplatin-based therapy and EGFR tyrosine kinase inhibitors).[131] It is expected that treatment of individual patients with early-stage cancers will be targeted on the basis of the molecular characteristics of the tumors.

Epigenetic changes often occur at tumor suppressor gene loci and are hypothesized to participate in cancer genomics. In an effort to identify new cancer-specific methylation markers, Shames et al.[132] employed high-throughput gene expression profiling of lung cancer cells and immortalized bronchial epithelial cells, and compared their expression phenotype before and after treatment with the methylation inducer 5-aza-2'-deoxycytidine. They identified multiple genes that are methylated with high penetrance in primary lung, breast, colon, and prostate cancers. Seven loci were frequently methylated in both breast and lung cancers, with four showing extensive methylation in all four epithelial tumors. The cross-tumor methylation pattern observed suggests that a partial promoter hypermethylation signature for these common malignancies may have been identified. The data suggest that while gene expression of tumors in different tissues vary substantially, there may be commonalities in their promoter methylation profiles that represent targets for early detection screening, diagnosis, or therapeutic intervention.

NEW DIMENSIONS IN DRUG DISCOVERY

The contribution of genetic engineering and gene-based approaches to innovative drug development was addressed in the previous chapter, but genomic studies currently in progress suggest additional leads to the discovery of new drugs.

RGS Proteins as Targets for Small Molecule Drugs

Regulators of G-protein signaling (RGS) are important components of signal transduction pathways initiated through G-protein-coupled receptors (GPCRs). Activation of GPCRs turns on signaling by inducing GTP exchange for GDP on Gα subunits, which then undergo an activating conformational change causing downstream events, such as channel opening, control of adenylcyclase, or hydrolysis of phosphoinositides. Upon hydrolysis of the bound GTP, the Gα subunit returns to its inactive, GDP-liganded form, terminating its signaling functions. The hydrolysis of GTP brought about by GTPase activity intrinsic to the Gα subunit (GAP activity) is very slow, but is accelerated by as much as 1000-fold by RGS proteins (Figure 10.3). As a result, the lifetime and the magnitude of signaling are reduced. In addition to these effects, RGS proteins can competitively inhibit effector coupling by Gα subunits.

Of the 20 well-known RGS proteins, 19 act on Gαi family signaling whereas at least 12 act on Gαq family signaling. Loss of RGS function *in vivo* also leads to markedly altered GPCR signaling.[133]

The structural and biochemical properties of the RGS proteins enable them to interact with a growing list of proteins with diverse cellular functions. Their ability to suppress or silence GPCR signaling pathways provides a compelling reason to investigate their role in human variation in the response to drugs and other exogenous chemicals. Information gained will not only make possible a broader understanding of the physiological roles of RGS proteins, but may also open new avenues to the discovery of more effective drugs and individualized drug therapy.[133,134] Because the targeting of GPCRs is the basis for many therapeutics, the RGS proteins have been proposed as drug targets. Reports suggest that RGS proteins may play a role in various disease states including schizophrenia, Parkinson's disease, hypertension, and addiction.[133,135] Inhibiting a specific RGS protein would potentiate the action of naturally occurring and exogenous agonists, and could enhance their tissue specificity by selectively increasing receptor activity in tissues that express particular RGS proteins.

Recently, David Roman, Richard Neubig, and colleagues screened a 3028-compound library to identify compounds capable of inhibiting RGS4/Gαo protein–protein interactions.[133] From this screen, five potential RGS4 inhibitors were identified, two of which had IC$_{50}$ values less that 10 μM. One compound (CCG-4986) inhibited RGS4 GAP activity and RGS4 activity on μ-opioid-mediated signaling. This is the first small molecule RGS inhibitor to be reported and it should prove to be a useful tool for studying the role of RGS in GPCR signaling.

Drug Target Discovery by Receptorome Screening

The receptorome encodes receptors that mediate responses to a large number of exogenous and endogenous substances, including the majority of medications used in the treatment of human disease.[136,137] It comprises at least 5% of the human genome. Screening the receptorome has been used as an efficient approach to drug target validation and discovery of new therapeutic drugs. Receptor screening has also been used to discover the molecular targets for serious drug side effects as the "fen-phen" story described below illustrates.

The "Fen-phen" Story: Serotonergic Mechanisms Determine Drug-Induced Valvular Heart Disease

Appetite suppressant medications have been used worldwide for decades for the treatment of obesity. One of the most widely prescribed anorectic agents was fenfluramine either alone or in combination with the noradrenergic drug phentermine ("fen-phen"). When used in combination, the drugs may be just as effective as either drug alone, with the added advantage of the need for lower doses of each agent and perhaps fewer side effects. Each drug received FDA approval individually in 1996, but the combination was not approved. In that year, the total number of prescriptions in the United States for fenfluramine and phentermine exceeded 18 million.

However, the situation changed abruptly in 1997 with a report by Heidi Connolly and co-workers of heart valve regurgitation in 24 women who had taken fenfluramine and phentermine for an average of 11 months (range 1–28 months).[138] Echocardiograms demonstrated unusual valvular morphology and regurgitation in all patients. Both right-sided and left-sided heart valves were involved, and the five patients who underwent cardiac surgery had valvular heart disease (VHD) with histological features resembling changes seen in carcinoid syndrome (a mitogenic, serotonin-secreting tumor), or ergotamine-induced valve disease. Eight of the patients also had newly documented pulmonary hypertension. In a population-based study of the appetite suppressants that was reported simultaneously, Hershel Jick and colleagues found there were 11 cases of valvular disorders after the use of fenfluramine including cases of aortic regurgitation, mitral regurgitation, and combined aortic and mitral regurgitation.[139] Notably, phentermine, which had long been used alone as an appetite suppressant, was not known to be associated with cardiopulmonary side effects, and in the study of Jick et al., none was found among those who took only phentermine. These cases aroused concern that fenfluramine–phentermine therapy might be associated with valvular heart disease and in 1997 the manufacturer voluntarily withdrew the combination of appetite suppressants from the market. However, the validity and magnitude of the association were left in doubt as this action was based on incomplete information.

In an attempt to understand the molecular basis of the side effects associated with these appetite suppressants, particularly with fenfluramine, researchers initially suspected that GPCRs, or ligand-gated ion channels, and/or monoamine transporters were likely to be involved. At that same time, "receptorome screening" of drugs and their metabolites held promise as a method to search for the mechanism responsible for drug-induced side effects, and to predict their occurrence. Then Rothman and colleagues performed a receptorome screen.

In light of the established role of serotonin (5-HT) as an mitogen, Rothman and colleagues performed a receptorome screen of fenfluramine and its *in vivo* metabolite norfenfluramine, along with the valvular heart disease- and pulmonary hypertension-associated ergoline methylsergide and its *in vivo* metabolite methylergonovine. The serotonin transporter inhibitor fluoxetine and its *in vivo* metabolite norfluoxetine were included as negative controls. Results of the receptorome screen and additional *in vitro* studies indicated that activation of the 5-HT_{2B} receptor was necessary to produce VHD, and that serotonergic medications that did not activate 5-HT_{2B} receptors were unlikely to produce VHD.[140] At about the same time Fitzgerald and co-workers independently reported that norfenfluramine was a potent 5-HT_{2B} agonist.[141] In contrast to its activity at 5-HT_{2B} receptors, norfenfluramine was devoid of appreciable activity at many other types of receptors that are plentiful in cardiac tissue, including known biogenic amine (α_1-, α_2-, and β-adrenergic) receptors and peptide receptors. Rothman et al. suggested that all clinically available medications with serotonergic activity and their active metabolites be screened for agonist activity at 5-HT_{2B} receptors and that clinicians consider suspending the use of medications with significant activity at 5-HT_{2B} receptors. In subsequent studies, several other valvulopathic drugs including ergotamine and methylergonovine were found to be 5-HT_{2B} agonists, further implicating the activation of 5-HT_{2B} receptors as a key step in drug-induced VHD. Later, Launay et al.[142] discovered that 5-HT_{2B} receptor activation is also responsible for fenfluramine-induced pulmonary hypertension.

Valvulopathic drugs have been shown to induce mitogenesis in cultured interstitial cells from human cardiac valves. Roth and co-workers have thus proposed that damage to heart valves induced by 5-HT_{2B} may involve inappropriate mitogenic stimulation of normally quiescent valve cells, resulting in overgrowth, although the signaling pathways whereby leaflet surfaces overgrow is not known.

Subsequently, Roth and co-workers found that two antiparkinsonian dopamine agonists, pergolide and cabergoline, were potent 5-HT_{2B} agonists. They were predicted to be valulopathic agents[143] and case reports of pergolide- and cabergoline-induced VHD soon appeared.[144] Recently, two large European studies have verified the association of VHD with these two drugs.[145,146]

The "fen-phen" story is an excellent example of how receptorome screening facilitated the discovery that the fenfluramine metabolite norfenfluramine is the agent causing VHD, and how the screen facilitated the discovery of the mechanism underlying fenfluramine-induced VHD.[143] A receptorome screen was also performed with MDMA (3,4-methylenedioxymethamphetamine, the recreational drug, also known as Ecstacy), which is a drug similar to fenfluramine. It was found that MDMA, and to a greater extent its N-demethylated metabolite 3,4-methylenedioxyamphetamine (MDA), are both 5-HT_{2B} agonists. Whether MDMA abuse is associated with VHD in humans is not known, but MDMA and MDA both elicit proliferative responses of heart valve cells *in vitro*, an activity similar to that which *in vivo* gives rise to fibrotic lesions that compromise valve function. Future studies revealing increased risk for VHD among chronic MDMA users would better validate the value of receptorome screening for the prediction of adverse drug responses.

Other Recent Receptorome-Based Discoveries

Receptorome screening of salvinorum A, a naturally occurring potent hallucinogen from the sage *Salvia divinorum*, revealed this compound has high affinity and is a potent agonist of the κ opioid receptor. This interaction is specific as salvinorum A does not have appreciable activity for either μ or δ opioid receptors, and unlike lysergic acid diethylamide (LSD), salvinorum A has no activity for the 5-HT$_{2A}$ receptor, which is associated with hallucinations and psychosis. Another recent receptorome screening study investigating the inhibition of human polyomavirus (JCV) infection by antipsychotics, highlighted the role of receptors in disease. The infection of oligodendrocytes by JCV results in neuronal demyelination, which is responsible for the fatal disease progressive multifocal leukencephalopathy (PML). Antipsychotic drugs such as clonazipine inhibit JCV infection suggesting that one of several receptors having affinity for such drugs might participate in this process. Receptorome screening plus additional experiments pointed to a subclass of serotonin receptors that helps internalize JCV as being in part responsible for the clonazipine-related inhibitory effect.[136]

Fresh Insights into Therapies for Trinucleotide Disorders

More than 30 human neurodegenerative diseases, including Huntington's disease, spinocerebellar ataxias, and fragile X syndrome, involve expanded polyglutamine [poly(Q)] repeats of trios of nucleotides, such as CAG and CGG. When they occur within coding regions of genes, the expanded poly(Q) domain may cause misfolding of the affected protein and its aggregation into visible abnormal nuclear inclusions. Repeat poly(Q) lengths are also unstable, undergoing shrinkage and expansion, in some cases involving tens of repeats, upon transmission from parent to child. Expansion of repeat lengths is associated with more severe disease, and in some cases their instability accounts for "genetic anticipation" in which disease symptoms in successive generations become progressively more severe.

Trinucleotide-repeat instability has been viewed largely as a matter of DNA metabolism, but recent data suggest that repeat instability may be influenced by poly(Q) protein toxicity. Jung and Bonini have shown that repeat instability can be replicated in the fruit fly, *Drosophila melanogaster,* and they exploited this organism to better understand the mechanism of instability. Their study provided fresh insights into the role of gene transcription, DNA repair, and the potential complicity of pathogenic poly(Q) proteins that underlie repeat instability.[147,148] By showing that changes in repeat length that require decades in humans could be monitored in weeks in the fly, the study opened the way for genetic analysis. Based on the idea that transcription of CAG repeats might be critical for generating instability, they reasoned that forcing a repeat-containing transgene to be active in germ cells might trigger changes in repeat length; they also expected that germline events would be transmitted from one generation to the next as occurs in "genetic anticipation." They suspected that previous fly models that were more suitable for studying the neurodegenerative phenomenon might have failed to uncover instability because they relied on the expression of repeats in either developing or fully differentiated tissues.

To test their idea, Jung and Bonini expressed a transgene bearing 51–78 CAG repeats in germ cells, and tracked transgenes over nine generations. They found that the overall rate of instability was 20% and that the majority of changes were small, involving expansion or shrinkage of one to three CAG units. However, 10% of changes involved larger (>10) repeat expansions or shrinkages, and expansions consistently outweighed shrinkages similar to what is observed in human poly(Q) diseases.

Jung and Bonini then asked how transcription might influence the size of trinucleotide repeats. They found that fly variants deficient in transcription-coupled DNA repair dampened rates of repeat instability, while decreased levels of adenosine 3,′ 5′-monophosphate (cAMP) response element-binding protein (CREB)-binding protein (CBP), a protein found in poly(Q) inclusions that regulates many transcription factors, increasing repeat instability. Because the inhibitory effect of pathogenic poly(Q) proteins on CBP was thought to be due to the loss of histone acetylase activity, the investigators expected that treating flies with histone deacetylase inhibitors to normalize acetylation levels might protect against poly(Q) protein pathogenesis. They found that flies treated with the histone deacetylase inhibitor trichostatin A countered the loss of CBP activity and protected against poly(Q) instability for maternal and paternal transmissions. Although trichostatin can affect multiple pathways, analysis of the pattern of repeat changes suggested that reduced instability was, at least in part, due to compensation for decreased CPB and/or histone acetylase activity because both *CBP* gene changes and trichostatin treatment preferentially modulated poly(Q) expansions relative to other events.

Jung and Bonini extended these findings by examining the effects of transcription and the contribution of CBP protein to models of Huntington's disease, and by examining instability in a model for CGG premutation expansions in fragile X syndrome, an unstable noncoding trinucleotide repeat. Repeat instability with germline transcription was enhanced in both models, from which they concluded that features of repeat instability, including transcriptional dependence, might be a fundamental property of trinucleotide instability seen in several disease models.

These studies recapitulate several features of human CAG repeat instability including the wide range of repeat changes and the strong bias toward repeat expansions. Finding that poly(Q) protein pathology, that is, a decrease of CBP activity via sequestration or inhibition, might enhance repeat instability was an important consequence of Jung and Bonini's work. They noted that CAG expansions occurred not only generationally, but also somatically in Huntington's disease, and pointed out that modifiers such as Msh2 modulate instability in both germline and somatic tissues. This suggested that findings with respect to germline instability might apply to somatic instability. Finally, Jung and colleagues suggested that repeat instability might be influenced by poly(Q) protein toxicity, and that treatments that restrict repeat instability might also provide an avenue to curb poly(Q) protein toxicity. Among these, histone deacetylase inhibitors are in clinical trials.[149]

Thwarting Nonsense-Mediated Decay

Nearly one-third of genetic defects are caused by nonsense mutations. When nonsense mutations are transcribed into messenger RNA, the ribosomal machinery interprets the "stop" codon as a signal to terminate production of the encoded protein prematurely. Nonsense mutations give rise to in-frame UAA, UAG, and UAA codons in the messenger RNA coding region; they also promote mRNA destabilization and lead to shortened versions of polypeptide products that may not function properly.[150] Inactivation of this, the NMD pathway, stabilizes nonsense-containing transcripts and promotes read-through of nonsense codons. Hence, nonsense-mediated transcripts might produce functional proteins if either their decay rate or the extent of premature termination is curtailed.[151–153]

It has long been known that aminoglycosides, such as gentamicin, can suppress stop codons by allowing an erroneous amino acid to be incorporated into the growing peptide. Suppression requires the aminoglycoside to bind to the decoding center of the ribosomal machinery during translation of nonsense transcripts, reducing both the accuracy of codon–anticodon pairing and the fidelity of translation. By increasing the frequency of erroneous insertions at the nonsense codon, translation continues to the end of the gene.[154]

Mutations in the cystic fibrosis transmembrane conductance regulator (CFTR) gene containing a premature termination signal cause a deficiency or absence of functional chloride channel activity. In 2003, Wilschanski and colleagues demonstrated that gentamicin treatment of patients with cystic fibrosis restored CFTR function in ∼90% of patients who had "stop" mutations in CFTR.[155] Treatment consisted of the application of two drops of gentamicin (3 mg/ml) applied into each nostril three times daily for two consecutive periods of 14 days. Translational "read-through" was achieved in patients who were homozygous and heterozygous for stop mutations, but not in patients who were homozygous for ΔF508, the most common mutation for cystic fibrosis.

In vitro quantitative histochemical studies of cells from cystic fibrosis patients treated with gentamicin have shown that 25–35% of the concentration of full-length CFTR was attained in cells transfected with wild-type CFTR complementary DNA, and that the concentration of CFTR increased as the dose of gentamicin administered was increased. Just how much CFTR activity is needed to prevent significant pulmonary morbidity is unclear, but Kerem has estimated that 10–35% might be necessary to avoid the principal manifestations of the disease.[156]

The success of aminoglycoside treatment of patients harboring nonsense mutations in CFTR that promote production of the CFTR protein has encouraged the use of aminoglycoside antibiotics as standard treatment for cystic fibrosis. However, lack of potency and the potential for renal and otic toxicities have limited the clinical usefulness of this approach, particularly in children. Ellen Welch and colleagues thus set out to identify an orally bioavailable, nontoxic, small molecule that promoted read-through of premature termination codons as a way to diminish the pathological features of nonsense-mediated diseases.[157] They performed high-throughput screens comprising ∼800,000 low-molecular-weight compounds to identify compounds that promoted UGA nonsense suppression. These analyses identified PTC124, an achiral, 1,2,4-oxadiazole analog of fluorobenzene and benzoic acid, as a candidate for development. The compound had no structural similarity to aminoglycosides, and despite low solubility, met requirements for oral bioavailability.

PTC124 proved to be a nonsense-suppressing agent more potent (by more than two orders of magnitude) than gentamicin in cell lines harboring nonsense coding alleles, and was capable of modulating the termination efficiency by 4- to 15-fold greater stimulation of read-through than controls. PTC124 promoted read-through of premature termination without affecting normal termination, even at drug exposures substantially greater than values achieving maximal activity. PTC124 was tolerated well in animals at plasma exposures substantially in excess of those required for nonsense suppression and human clinical trials of this agent have been initiated. This promising approach as a model for personalized medicine is among the first to focus on the treatment of a specific genetic defect in the treatment of disease.

WHEN GOOD DRUGS GO BAD, WHAT TO DO?

That adverse drug reactions (ADRs) account for a substantial proportion of acute hospitalizations is well accepted, although variation in the estimates is wide. In the Netherlands in 2001, for example, van der Hooft and colleagues found that 1.83% of 12,249 acute hospitalizations were ADR related.[158] From these admissions, intended forms of overdose, errors in administration, and therapeutic failures were excluded. The proportion of ADR-related admissions increased with age from 0.8% in the <18-year-old group to 3.2% in the >80-year-old group. Older age patients and female patients were both preferentially associated with ADR-related hospitalizations, and 6% overall had a fatal outcome. Considering that not all ADRs may be recognized or mentioned in discharge letters, the proportion of ADR-related hospitalizations was substantial. Van der Hooft et al. also estimated that only about 1% of ADR-related hospitalizations were reported to the national center for spontaneous ADR reporting. In other western countries including the United States, estimates of all hospital admissions attributed to ADRs were somewhat higher and varied widely between 2.4% and 6.4%.

It is also widely accepted that ADRs are underreported, and that reporting is selective and biased toward newer drugs for which intensive reporting is encouraged. Hazell and Shakir[159] investigated the extent of underreporting of ADRs to spontaneous reporting systems in the published literature, and whether there were differences between different types of ADRs. A literature search identified a total of 247 articles of which 210 were excluded because they made no numerical estimates of underreporting, were not available in English, or were irrelevant. The remaining 37 studies surveyed data from 12 western countries using various surveillance methods. The UK, France, Sweden, and the United States provided the highest number of studies. Across the 37 studies, the rate of underreporting ranged from 6% to 100% with a median underreporting rate of 94% (interquartile range 82–98%), but no difference in underreporting between general practice and hospital-based studies was found. For 19 studies investigating specific serious or severe ADR drug combinations, the median underreporting rate was lower but was still high at 85%.

Spontaneous reporting of adverse drug reactions (ADRs) by healthcare professionals is vital to pharmacovigilance. Without such an early warning system, the ability of the healthcare system to protect patients from unwanted or unexpected ADRs is severely limited. For example, when comparing the relative safety profiles of two drugs, underreporting limits the interpretation of the comparisons since it cannot be assumed that the underreporting rate is the same for both drugs. If underreporting is markedly different, any true difference in toxicity between the drugs may be masked or exaggerated.

Common reasons for underreporting include lack of time, different care priorities, uncertainty about the drug causing the ADR, difficulty in accessing reporting forms, lack of awareness of the requirements for reporting, and lack of understanding of the purpose of spontaneous reporting.[159] In some instances, physicians may not report ADRs because they believe that serious reactions will have been documented by the time the drug is marketed, or that one case will not contribute to medical knowledge.

Various strategies have been introduced to encourage and facilitate reporting such as greater accessibility to spontaneous databases through electronic and on-line reporting.[159] Prescribing medications is a very important responsibility for the practicing physician, pharmacist, or nurse, but reporting suspected ADRs and participation in ADR monitoring should also be promoted as a professional duty of similar importance. Education is the cornerstone for good reporting and should become a part of the continuing medical education and clinical governance. A recent survey of UK medical and pharmacy schools noted that 50% of the respondents provide undergraduate students with a guide to reporting ADRs, and that postgraduate educational resources in the form of learning modules are available but are not compulsory.

Others believe the promise of emerging genomic technologies offers an opportunity to alert and educate clinicians and the public about the problem of serious ADRs (SADRs). SADRs associated with beneficial drugs can lead to drug withdrawal, in some cases many years after the drug has received approval for marketing. As examples, Table 11.4 lists 19 drugs withdrawn from the U.S. market since 1998 because of unpredicted fatalities.

In their recent commentary on how best to reduce the risk of SADRs to marketed drugs, Giacomini and colleagues sense that a global pharmacogenomics network to study SADRs is needed.[160] They note that several multicenter networks such as the Canadian Genotypic Adjustment of Therapy in Childhood (GATC) project built upon Canada's national healthcare system and the EUDRAGENE project associated with and funded by the European Commission are in developmental stages. The latter project involves multicenter collaboration of 10 European countries and targets a potential population of 350 million patients. The United States has no national or regional programs for spontaneous reporting of ADRs to physicians. However, the PGRN (described above and in Table 11.1) has several established centers for studying genetic risk factors to SADRs, and is forming partnerships with healthcare systems in the United States and the U.S. FDA has initiated collaborations that focus on SADRs related to drug toxicities with major stakeholders including the National Institutes of Health, academic institutions, and the pharmaceutical industry. Giacomini et al. argue that because of the low frequency, the ethnic diversity, and the complexity of SADRs, often no single site or

Table 11.4 Drugs Withdrawn from the U.S. Market since 1998

Drug	Approved/ withdrawn	Indication	Risk
Pemoline	1975/2005	Attention deficit hyperactivity disorder	Liver failure
Astemizole	1985/1999	Antihistamine	Torsade de pointes Drug interactions
Etretinate	1986/1999	Psoriasis	Birth defects
Pergolide	1988/2007	Parkinson's disease	Valvulopathy
Cisapride	1993/2000	Heartburn	Torsade de pointes Drug interactions
Lovamethadyl	1993/2003	Opiate dependence	Fatal arrhythmia
Mibreftadil	1997/1998	High blood pressure, angina	Drug interactions
Bromfenac	1997/1998	NSAID	Acute liver failure
Terfenadine	1997/1998	Antihistamine	Torsade de pointes Drug interactions
Grepafloxacin	1997/1999	Antibiotic	Torsade de pointes
Troglitazone	1997/2000	Diabetes	Acute liver failure
Cerivastatin	1997/2001	Antilipidemic	Rhabdomyolysis Drug interactions
Rofecoxib	1999/2004	Pain relief	Heart attack, stroke
Rapacuronium	1999/2001	Anesthesia	Bronchospasm
Alosetron	2000/2000 (2002)	Irritable bowel (remarketed with restrictions)	Ischemic colitis Complications of constipation
Valdecoxib	2001/2005	Pain relief	Skin reactions (Stevens–Johnson syndrome)
Tegaserod	2002/2007	Irritable bowel syndrome with constipation	Angina, heart attack, stroke
Natalizumab	2004/2005 (2006)	Multiple sclerosis (remarketed with restrictions)	Brain infection
Technetium (^{99m}Tc) fanolesomab	2004/2005	Diagnostic aid	Cardiopulmonary arrest

Source: Modified from Giacomini et al.[160]

even a single country can generate enough cases for analysis. Hence, they propose establishing a global research network that would focus on the diagnosis, study design, and data analysis of specific, high-priority SADRs in genetically at-risk individuals and populations as a key first step to enhance the identification and reporting of SADRs, which may ultimately reduce the prevalence of these events.

SUMMARY

Pharmacogenetics is firmly focused on understanding how genetic variations in molecular processes in cells are linked to human drug responses. After biologists learned how cells read and express the information encoded in the genome, many new genes and gene-based drug targets were discovered, and new therapeutic agents were developed. Having reached a point at which many of the molecular complexities of human drug responses were understood, the field has been transformed in the last few years from a descriptive science to a predictive science. Pharmacogenetics, like most other biological fields, is primarily data driven, without which attempts at prediction would fail. Looking to the future, consideration is given in this chapter to a number of newer topics and recent observations that are likely to facilitate pharmacogenomic research, further the prospects and promise of personalized medicine, advance the understanding of human genetic variation, and expand the horizons of drug discovery.

REFERENCES

1. Altman RB, Flockhart DA, Sherry ST, Oliver DE, Rubin DL, Klein TE. Indexing pharmacogenetic knowledge on the World Wide Web. Pharmacogenetics 2003; 13(1):3–5.
2. Long RM. Planning for a national effort to enable and accelerate discoveries in pharmacogenetics: the NIH Pharmacogenetics Research Network. Clin Pharmacol Ther 2007; 81(3):450–454.
3. Giacomini KM, Brett CM, Altman RB, Benowitz NL, Dolan ME, Flockhart DA et al. The pharmacogenetics research network: from SNP discovery to clinical drug response. Clin Pharmacol Ther 2007; 81(3):328–345.
4. Hodge AE, Altman RB, Klein TE. The PharmGKB: integration, aggregation, and annotation of pharmacogenomic data and knowledge. Clin Pharmacol Ther 2007; 81(1):21–24.
5. Marshall A. Laying the foundations for personalized medicines. Nat Biotechnol 1997; 15(10):954–957.
6. Marshall A. Getting the right drug into the right patient. Nat Biotechnol 1997; 15(12):1249–1252.
7. Phillips KA, Veenstra DL, Oren E, Lee JK, Sadee W. Potential role of pharmacogenomics in reducing adverse drug reactions: a systematic review. JAMA 2001; 286(18):2270–2279.
8. Spear BB, Heath-Chiozzi M, Huff J. Clinical application of pharmacogenetics. Trends Mol Med 2001; 7(5):201–204.
9. Lazarou J, Pomeranz BH, Corey PN. Incidence of adverse drug reactions in hospitalized patients: a meta-analysis of prospective studies. JAMA 1998; 279(15):1200–1205.
10. Ernst FR, Grizzle AJ. Drug-related morbidity and mortality: updating the cost-of-illness model. J Am Pharm Assoc (Wash) 2001; 41(2):192–199.
11. Lichter JB, Kurth JH. The impact of pharmacogenetics on the future of healthcare. Curr Opin Biotechnol 1997; 8(6):692–695.
12. Veenstra DL, Higashi MK, Phillips KA. Assessing the cost-effectiveness of pharmacogenomics. AAPS PharmSci 2000; 2(3):E29.
13. Taube J, Halsall D, Baglin T. Influence of cytochrome P-450 CYP2C9 polymorphisms on warfarin sensitivity and risk of over-anticoagulation in patients on long-term treatment. Blood 2000; 96(5):1816–1819.
14. Thijssen HH, Verkooijen IW, Frank HL. The possession of the CYP2C9*3 allele is associated with low dose requirement of acenocoumarol. Pharmacogenetics 2000; 10(8):757–760.

15. Van Der WJ, Steijns LS, van Weelden MJ, de Haan K. The effect of genetic polymorphism of cytochrome P450 CYP2C9 on phenytoin dose requirement. Pharmacogenetics 2001; 11(4):287–291.

16. Brandolese R, Scordo MG, Spina E, Gusella M, Padrini R. Severe phenytoin intoxication in a subject homozygous for CYP2C9*3. Clin Pharmacol Ther 2001; 70(4):391–394.

17. Mamiya K, Kojima K, Yukawa E, Higuchi S, Ieiri I, Ninomiya H et al. Phenytoin intoxication induced by fluvoxamine. Ther Drug Monit 2001; 23(1):75–77.

18. Furuta T, Shirai N, Watanabe F, Honda S, Takeuchi K, Iida T et al. Effect of cytochrome P4502C19 genotypic differences on cure rates for gastroesophageal reflux disease by lansoprazole. Clin Pharmacol Ther 2002; 72(4):453–460.

19. Sallee FR, DeVane CL, Ferrell RE. Fluoxetine-related death in a child with cytochrome P-450 2D6 genetic deficiency. J Child Adolesc Psychopharmacol 2000; 10(1):27–34.

20. Dalen P, Frengell C, Dahl ML, Sjoqvist F. Quick onset of severe abdominal pain after codeine in an ultrarapid metabolizer of debrisoquine. Ther Drug Monit 1997; 19(5):543–544.

21. Gasche Y, Daali Y, Fathi M, Chiappe A, Cottini S, Dayer P et al. Codeine intoxication associated with ultrarapid CYP2D6 metabolism. N Engl J Med 2004; 351(27):2827–2831.

22. Rettie AE, Tai G. The pharmocogenomics of warfarin: closing in on personalized medicine. Mol Interv 2006; 6(4):223–227.

23. Van Kuilenburg AB, Muller EW, Haasjes J, Meinsma R, Zoetekouw L, Waterham HR et al. Lethal outcome of a patient with a complete dihydropyrimidine dehydrogenase (DPD) deficiency after administration of 5-fluorouracil: frequency of the common IVS14+1G>A mutation causing DPD deficiency. Clin Cancer Res 2001; 7(5):1149–1153.

24. Van Kuilenburg AB, Meinsma R, Zoetekouw L, van Gennip AH. High prevalence of the IVS14 + 1G>A mutation in the dihydropyrimidine dehydrogenase gene of patients with severe 5-fluorouracil-associated toxicity. Pharmacogenetics 2002; 12(7):555–558.

25. Iyer L, Das S, Janisch L, Wen M, Ramirez J, Karrison T et al. UGT1A1*28 polymorphism as a determinant of irinotecan disposition and toxicity. Pharmacogenomics J 2002; 2(1):43–47.

26. McLeod HL, Krynetski EY, Relling MV, Evans WE. Genetic polymorphism of thiopurine methyltransferase and its clinical relevance for childhood acute lymphoblastic leukemia. Leukemia 2000; 14(4):567–572.

27. Schutz E, Gummert J, Mohr F, Oellerich M. Azathioprine-induced myelosuppression in thiopurine methyltransferase deficient heart transplant recipient. Lancet 1993; 341(8842):436.

28. Daly AK, Cholerton S, Gregory W, Idle JR. Metabolic polymorphisms. Pharmacol Ther 1993; 57(2–3):129–160.

29. Wolf CR, Smith G, Smith RL. Science, medicine, and the future: Pharmacogenetics. BMJ 2000; 320(7240):987–990.

30. Kirchheiner J, Seeringer A. Clinical implications of pharmacogenetics of cytochrome P450 drug metabolizing enzymes. Biochim Biophys Acta 2007; 1770(3):489–494.

31. Sindrup SH, Brosen K. [Combination preparations of codeine and paracetamol]. Ugeskr Laeger 1998; 160(4):448–449.

32. Koren G, Cairns J, Chitayat D, Gaedigk A, Leeder SJ. Pharmacogenetics of morphine poisoning in a breastfed neonate of a codeine-prescribed mother. Lancet 2006; 368(9536):704.

33. Desta Z, Zhao X, Shin JG, Flockhart DA. Clinical significance of the cytochrome P450 2C19 genetic polymorphism. Clin Pharmacokinet 2002; 41(12):913–958.

34. Andersson T, Flockhart DA, Goldstein DB, Huang SM, Kroetz DL, Milos PM et al. Drug-metabolizing enzymes: evidence for clinical utility of pharmacogenomic tests. Clin Pharmacol Ther 2005; 78(6):559–581.

35. Goldstein JA. Clinical relevance of genetic polymorphisms in the human CYP2C subfamily. Br J Clin Pharmacol 2001; 52(4):349–355.

36. Miners JO, Birkett DJ. Cytochrome P4502C9: an enzyme of major importance in human drug metabolism. Br J clin Pharmacol 1998; 45(6):525–538.

37. Lee CR, Goldstein JA, Pieper JA. Cytochrome P450 2C9 polymorphisms: a comprehensive review of the in-vitro and human data. Pharmacogenetics 2002; 12(3): 251–263.

38. Loebstein R, Yonath H, Peleg D, Almog S, Rotenberg M, Lubetsky A et al. Interindividual variability in sensitivity to warfarin—Nature or nurture? Clin Pharmacol Ther 2001; 70(2):159–164.

39. Aithal GP, Day CP, Leathart JB, Daly AK. Relationship of polymorphism in CYP2C9 to genetic susceptibility to diclofenac-induced hepatitis. Pharmacogenetics 2000; 10(6):511–518.

40. Higashi MK, Veenstra DL, Kondo LM, Wittkowsky AK, Srinouanprachanh SL, Farin FM et al. Association between CYP2C9 genetic variants and anticoagulation-related outcomes during warfarin therapy. JAMA 2002; 287(13):1690–1698.

41. Caffee AE, Teichman PG. Improving anticoagulation management at the point of care. Fam Pract Manag 2002; 9(2):35–37.

42. Shetty HG, Routledge PA. Optimising the dose of oral anticoagulants. Ann Acad Med Singapore 1991; 20(1):161–164.

43. Fihn SD, McDonell M, Martin D, Henikoff J, Vermes D, Kent D et al. Risk factors for complications of chronic anticoagulation. A multicenter study. Warfarin Optimized Outpatient Follow-up Study Group. Ann Intern Med 1993; 118(7):511–520.

44. Daly AK, Day CP, Aithal GP. CYP2C9 polymorphism and warfarin dose requirements. Br J clin Pharmacol 2002; 53(4):408–409.

45. Higuchi S, MUramatsu T, Shigemori K, Saito M, Kono H, Dufour MC et al. The relationship between low Km aldehyde dehydrogenase phenotype and drinking behavior in Japanese. J Stud Alcohol 1992; 53(2):170–175.

46. Milano G, Etienne MC. Potential importance of dihydropyrimidine dehydrogenase (DPD) in cancer chemotherapy. Pharmacogenetics 1994; 4(6):301–306.

47. Weinshilboum R. Thiopurine pharmacogenetics: clinical and molecular studies of thiopurine methyltransferase. Drug Metab Dispos 2001; 29(4 Pt 2):601–605.

48. Lewis LD, Benin A, Szumlanski CL, Otterness DM, Lennard L, Weinshilboum RM et al. Olsalazine and 6-mercaptopurine-related bone marrow suppression: a possible drug-drug interaction. Clin Pharmacol Ther 1997; 62(4):464–475.

49. Lennard L, Lilleyman JS, Van Loon J, Weinshilboum RM. Genetic variation in response to 6-mercaptopurine for childhood acute lymphoblastic leukaemia. Lancet 1990; 336(8709):225–229.

50. Dubinsky MC, Lamothe S, Yang HY, Targan SR, Sinnett D, Theoret Y et al. Pharmacogenomics and metabolite measurement for 6-mercaptopurine therapy in inflammatory bowel disease. Gastroenterology 2000; 118(4):705–713.

51. Van Aken J, Schmedders M, Feuerstein G, Kollek R. Prospects and limits of pharmacogenetics: the thiopurine methyl transferase (TPMT) experience. Am J Pharmacogenomics 2003; 3(3):149–155.

52. Marshall E. Preventing toxicity with a gene test. Science 2003; 302(5645):588–590.

53. Stephens JC. Single-nucleotide polymorphisms, haplotype, and their relevance to pharmacogenetics. Mol Diagnosis 1999; 4(4):309–317.

54. Drysdale CM, McGraw DW, Stack CB, Stephens JC, Judson RS, Nandabalan K et al. Complex promoter and coding region beta 2-adrenergic receptor haplotypes alter receptor expression and predict in vivo responsiveness. Proc Natl Acad Sci U S A 2000; 97(19):10483–10488.

55. Tucker GT. Advances in understanding drug metabolism and its contribution to variability in patient response. Ther Drug Monit 2000; 22(1):110–113.

56. Kirchheiner J, et al., Brockmoller J. CYP2D6 and CYP2C19 genotype-based dose recommendations for antidepressants: a first step towards subpopulation-specific dosages. Acta Psychiatr Scand 2001; 104(Sep):173–192.

57. Kirchheiner J, Meinke I, Muller G, Roots I, Brockmoller J. Contributions of CYP2D6, CYP2C9, and CYP2C19 to the biotransformation of E- and Z-doxepin in healthy volunteers. Pharmacogenetics 2002; 12:571–580.

58. Kirchheiner J, Fuhr U, Brockmoller J. Pharmacogenetics-based therapeutic recommendations—ready for clinical practice? Nat Rev Drug Discov 2005; 4(8): 639–647.

59. Wilke RA, Musana A.K., Weber WW. Cytochrome P450 gene-based drug prescribing and factors impacting translation into routine clinical practice. Personalized Medicine 2005; 2(3):213–224.

60. Peltonen L, McKusick VA. Genomics and medicine. Dissecting human disease in the postgenomic era. Science 2001; 291(5507):1224–1229.

61. Frye RF, Matzke GR, Adedoyin A, Porter JA, Branch RA. Validation of the five-drug "Pittsburgh cocktail" approach for assessment of selective regulation of drug-metabolizing enzymes. Clin Pharmacol Ther 1997; 62(4):365–376.

62. Dierks EA, Stams KR, Lim HK, Cornelius G, Zhang H, Ball SE. A method for the simultaneous evaluation of the activities of seven major human drug-metabolizing cytochrome P450s using an in vitro cocktail of probe substrates and fast gradient liquid chromatography tandem mass spectrometry. Drug Metab Dispos 2001; 29(1):23–29.

63. Chainuvati S, Nafziger AN, Leeder JS, Gaedigk A, Kearns GL, Sellers E et al. Combined phenotypic assessment of cytochrome p450 1A2, 2C9, 2C19, 2D6, and 3A, N-acetyltransferase-2, and xanthine oxidase activities with the "Cooperstown 5+1 cocktail." Clin Pharmacol Ther 2003; 74(5):437–447.

64. Frye RF. Probing the world of cytochrome p450 enzymes. Mol Interv 2004; 4(3):157–162.

65. Morgan ET. Regulation of cytochromes P450 during inflammation and infection. Drug Metab Rev 1997; 29(4):1129–1188.

66. Morgan ET, Sewer MB, Iber H, Gonzalez FJ, Lee YH, Tukey RH et al. Physiological and pathophysiological regulation of cytochrome P450. Drug Metab Dispos 1998; 26(12):1232–1240.

67. Aitken AE, Richardson TA, Morgan ET. Regulation of drug-metabolizing enzymes and transporters in inflammation. Annu Rev Pharmacol Toxicol 2006; 46:123–149.

68. Furuta T, Ohashi K, Kobayashi K, Iida I, Yoshida H, Shirai N et al. Effects of clarithromycin on the metabolism of omeprazole in relation to CYP2C19 genotype status in humans. Clin Pharmacol Ther 1999; 66(3):265–274.

69. Schwab M, Schaeffeler E, Klotz U, Treiber G. CYP2C19 polymorphism is a major predictor of treatment failure in white patients by use of lansoprazole-based quad-

ruple therapy for eradication of Helicobacter pylori. Clin Pharmacol Ther 2004; 76(3):201–209.

70. Lehmann DF, Medicis JJ, Franklin PD. Polymorphisms and the pocketbook: the cost-effectiveness of cytochrome P450 2C19 genotyping in the eradication of Helicobacter pylori infection associated with duodenal ulcer. J Clin Pharmacol 2003; 43(12):1316–1323.

71. Wilke RA, Berg RL, Vidaillet HJ, Caldwell MD, Burmester JK, Hillman MA. Impact of age, CYP2C9 genotype and concomitant medication on the rate of rise for prothrombin time during the first 30 days of warfarin therapy. Clin Med Res 2005; 3(4):207–213.

72. You JH, Chan FW, Wong RS, Cheng G. The potential clinical and economic outcomes of pharmacogenetics-oriented management of warfarin therapy—a decision analysis. Thromb Haemost 2004; 92(3):590–597.

73. Wadelius M, Sorlin K, Wallerman O, Karlsson J, Yue QY, Magnusson PK et al. Warfarin sensitivity related to CYP2C9, CYP3A5, ABCB1 (MDR1) and other factors. Pharmacogenomics J 2004; 4(1):40–48.

74. Hillman MA, Wilke RA, Caldwell MD, Berg RL, Glurich I, Burmester JK. Relative impact of covariates in prescribing warfarin according to CYP2C9 genotype. Pharmacogenetics 2004; 14(8):539–547.

75. Gage BF, Eby C, Milligan PE, Banet GA, Duncan JR, McLeod HL. Use of pharmacogenetics and clinical factors to predict the maintenance dose of warfarin. Thromb Haemost 2004; 91(1):87–94.

76. McCarty CA, Nair A, Austin DM, Giampietro PF. Informed consent and subject motivation to participate in a large, population-based genomics study: the Marshfield Clinic Personalized Medicine Research Project. Community Genet 2007; 10(1):2–9.

77. Hillman MA, Wilke RA, Yale SH, Vidaillet HJ, Caldwell MD, Glurich I et al. A prospective, randomized pilot trial of model-based warfarin dose initiation using CYP2C9 genotype and clinical data. Clin Med Res 2005; 3(3):137–145.

78. Shikata E, Ieiri I, Ishiguro S, Aono H, Inoue K, Koide T et al. Association of pharmacokinetic (CYP2C9) and pharmacodynamic (factors II, VII, IX, and X; proteins S and C; and gamma-glutamyl carboxylase) gene variants with warfarin sensitivity. Blood 2004; 103(7):2630–2635.

79. Wilke RA, Reif DM, Moore JH. Combinatorial pharmacogenetics. Nat Rev Drug Discov 2005; 4(11):911–918.

80. Wilke RA, Moore JH, Burmester JK. Relative impact of CYP3A genotype and concomitant medication on the severity of atorvastatin-induced muscle damage. Pharmacogenet Genomics 2005; 15(6):415–421.

81. Collins FS, Green ED, Guttmacher AE, Guyer MS. A vision for the future of genomics research. Nature 2003; 422(6934):835–847.

82. Khoury MJ. The case for a global human genome epidemiology initiative. Nat Genet 2004; 36(10):1027–1028.

83. McCarty CA, Wilke RA, Giampietro PF, Wesbrook SD, Caldwell MD. Marshfield Clinic Personalized Medicine Research Project (PMRP): Design, methods and recruitment for alarge population-based biobank. Future Medicine 2005; 2(1):49–79.

84. Abrahams E, Ginsburg GS, Silver M. The personalized medicine coalition : goals and strategies. Am J Pharmacogenomics 2005; 5(6):345–355.

85. Duan J, Wainwright MS, Comeron JM, Saitou N, Sanders AR, Gelernter J et al. Synonymous mutations in the human dopamine receptor D2 (DRD2) affect mRNA stability and synthesis of the receptor. Hum Mol Genet 2003; 12(3):205–216.

86. Kimchi-Sarfaty C, Oh JM, Kim IW, Sauna ZE, Calcagno AM, Ambudkar SV et al. A "silent" polymorphism in the MDR1 gene changes substrate specificity. Science 2007; 315(5811):525–528.

87. Komar AA. Genetics. SNPs, silent but not invisible. Science 2007; 315(5811):466–467.

88. Nackley AG, Shabalina SA, Tchivileva IE, Satterfield K, Korchynskyi O, Makarov SS et al. Human catechol-O-methyltransferase haplotypes modulate protein expression by altering mRNA secondary structure. Science 2006; 314(5807):1930–1933.

89. Stankiewicz P, Lupski JR. Genome architecture, rearrangements and genomic disorders. Trends Genet 2002; 18(2):74–82.

90. Eichler EE, Nickerson DA, Altshuler D, Bowcock AM, Brooks LD, Carter NP et al. Completing the map of human genetic variation. Nature 2007; 447(7141):161–165.

91. Buckland PR. Polymorphically duplicated genes: their relevance to phenotypic variation in humans. Ann Med 2003; 35(5):308–315.

92. Ouahchi K, Lindeman N, Lee C. Copy number variants and pharmacogenomics. Pharmacogenomics 2006; 7(1):25–29.

93. Prody CA, Dreyfus P, Zamir R, Zakut H, Soreq H. De novo amplification within a "silent" human cholinesterase gene in a family subjected to prolonged exposure to organophosphorous insecticides. Proc Natl Acad Sci USA 1989; 86:690–694.

94. Allderdice PW, Gardner HA, Galutira D, Lockridge O, LaDu BN, McAlpine PJ. The cloned butyrylcholinesterase (BCHE) gene maps to a single chromosome site, 3q26. Genomics 1991; 11(2):452–454.

95. Johansson I, Lundqvist E, Bertilsson L, Dahl ML, Sjoqvist F, Ingelman-Sundberg M. Inherited amplification of an active gene in the cytochrome P450 CYP2D locus as a cause of ultrarapid metabolism of debrisoquine. Proc Natl Acad Sci U S A 1993; 90(24):11825–11829.

96. Dalen P, Dahl ML, Ruiz ML, Nordin J, Bertilsson L. 10-Hydroxylation of nortriptyline in white persons with 0, 1, 2, 3, and 13 functional CYP2D6 genes. Clin Pharmacol Ther 1998; 63(4):444–452.

97. Rabbani H, Pan Q, Kondo N, Smith CI, Hammarstrom L. Duplications and deletions of the human IGHC locus: evolutionary implications. Immunogenetics 1996; 45(2):136–141.

98. McLellan RA, Oscarson M, Alexandrie AK, Seidegard J, Evans DA, Rannug A et al. Characterization of a human glutathione S-transferase mu cluster containing a duplicated GSTM1 gene that causes ultrarapid enzyme activity. Mol Pharmacol 1997; 52(6):958–965.

99. Lifton RP, Dluhy RG, Powers M, Rich GM, Gutkin M, Fallo F et al. Hereditary hypertension caused by chimaeric gene duplications and ectopic expression of aldosterone synthase. Nat Genet 1992; 2(1):66–74.

100. Rich GM, Ulick S, Cook S, Wang JZ, Lifton RP, Dluhy RG. Glucocorticoid-remediable aldosteronism in a large kindred: clinical spectrum and diagnosis using a characteristic biochemical phenotype. Ann Intern Med 1992; 116(10):813–820.

101. Townson JR, Barcellos LF, Nibbs RJ. Gene copy number regulates the production of the human chemokine CCL3-L1. Eur J Immunol 2002; 32(10):3016–3026.

102. Gonzalez E, Kulkarni H, Bolivar H, Mangano A, Sanchez R, Catano G et al. The influence of CCL3L1 gene-containing segmental duplications on HIV-1/AIDS susceptibility. Science 2005; 307(5714):1434–1440.

103. Bowen DJ. Haemophilia A and haemophilia B: molecular insights. Mol Pathol 2002; 55(2):127–144.

104. Oscarson M, McLellan RA, Gullsten H, Agundez JA, Benitez J, Rautio A et al. Identification and characterisation of novel polymorphisms in the CYP2A locus: implications for nicotine metabolism. FEBS Lett 1999; 460(2):321–327.

105. Rao Y, Hoffmann E, Zia M, Bodin L, Zeman M, Sellers EM et al. Duplications and defects in the CYP2A6 gene: identification, genotyping, and in vivo effects on smoking. Mol Pharmacol 2000; 58(4):747–755.

106. Pink JJ, Wu SQ, Wolf DM, Bilimoria MM, Jordan VC. A novel 80 kDa human estrogen receptor containing a duplication of exons 6 and 7. Nucleic Acids Res 1996; 24(5):962–969.

107. Pink JJ, Fritsch M, Bilimoria MM, Assikis VJ, Jordan VC. Cloning and characterization of a 77-kDa oestrogen receptor isolated from a human breast cancer cell line. Br J Cancer 1997; 75(1):17–27.

108. Franchina M, Kay PH. Allele-specific variation in the gene copy number of human cytosine 5-methyltransferase. Hum Hered 2000; 50(2):112–117.

109. Ledesma MC, Agundez JA. Identification of subtypes of CYP2D gene rearrangements among carriers of CYP2D6 gene deletion and duplication. Clin Chem 2005; 51(6):939–943.

110. DeRisi J, Penland L, Brown PO, Bittner ML, Melzer PS, Ray M et al. Use of a cDNA microarray to analyse gene expression patterns in human cancer. Nature Genetics 1996; 14:457–460.

111. Golub TReal. Molecular classification of cancer: Class discovery and class prediction by gene expression monitoring. Science 1999; 286(15 oct):531-xxx.

112. Alizadeh AA, Eisen MB, Davis RE, Ma C, Lossos IS, Rosenwald A et al. Distinct types of diffuse large B-cell lymphoma identified by gene expression profiling. Nature 2000; 403(6769):503–511.

113. Bittner M, Meltzer P, Chen Y, Jiang Y, Seftor E, Hendrix M et al. Molecular classification of cutaneous malignant melanoma by gene expression profiling. Nature 2000; 406(6795):536–540.

114. Perou CM, et al. BD. Molecular portraits of human breast tumours. Nature 2000; 406(17 Aug):747–752.

115. Hedenfalk I, Duggan D, Chen Y, Radmacher M, Bittner M, Simon R et al. Gene-expression profiles in hereditary breast cancer. N Engl J Med 2001; 344(8):539–548.

116. Van't Veer LJ, Dai H, van de Vijver MJ, He YD, Hart AA, Mao M et al. Gene expression profiling predicts clinical outcome of breast cancer. Nature 2002; 415(6871):530–536.

117. Van de Vijver MJ, He YD, van't Veer LJ, Dai H, Hart AA, Voskuil DW et al. A gene-expression signature as a predictor of survival in breast cancer. N Engl J Med 2002; 347(25):1999–2009.

118. Robetoyre RS, Bohling SD, MOrgan JW, Fillmore GC, Lim MS, Elenitoba-Johnson KSJ. Microarray analysis of B-cell lymphoma cell lines with the t(14;18). J Mol Diagn 2002; 4(3):123–136.

119. Bild AH, Yao G, Chang JT, Wang Q, Potti A, Chasse D et al. Oncogenic pathway signatures in human cancers as a guide to targeted therapies. Nature 2006; 439(7074):353–357.

120. Bild AH, Potti A, Nevins JR. Linking oncogenic pathways with therapeutic opportunities. Nat Rev Cancer 2006; 6(9):735–741.

121. Fan C, Oh DS, Wessels L, Weigelt B, Nuyten DS, Nobel AB et al. Concordance among gene-expression-based predictors for breast cancer. N Engl J Med 2006; 355(6):560–569.

122. Liu R, Wang X, Chen GY, Dalerba P, Gurney A, Hoey T et al. The prognostic role of a gene signature from tumorigenic breast-cancer cells. N Engl J Med 2007; 356(3):217–226.

123. Chen HY, Yu SL, Chen CH, Chang GC, Chen CY, Yuan A et al. A five-gene signature and clinical outcome in non-small-cell lung cancer. N Engl J Med 2007; 356(1):11–20.

124. Paik S, Shak S, Tang G, Kim C, Baker J, Cronin M et al. A multigene assay to predict recurrence of tamoxifen-treated, node-negative breast cancer. N Engl J Med 2004; 351(27):2817–2826.

125. Paik S, Tang G, Shak S, Kim C, Baker J, Kim W et al. Gene expression and benefit of chemotherapy in women with node-negative, estrogen receptor-positive breast cancer. J Clin Oncol 2006; 24(23):3726–3734.

126. Chung CH, Bernard PS, Perou CM. Molecular portraits and the family tree of cancer. Nat Genet 2002; 32 Suppl:533–540.

127. Churchill GA. Fundamentals of experimental design for cDNA microarrays. Nat Genet 2002; 32 Suppl:490–495.

128. Slonim DK. From patterns to pathways: gene expression data analysis comes of age. Nat Genet 2002; 32 Suppl:502–508.

129. Golub TR. Genomics: global views of leukaemia. Nature 2007; 446(7137):739–740.

130. Mullighan CG, Goorha S, Radtke I, Miller CB, Coustan-Smith E, Dalton JD et al. Genome-wide analysis of genetic alterations in acute lymphoblastic leukaemia. Nature 2007; 446(7137):758–764.

131. Herbst RS, Lippman SM. Molecular signatures of lung cancer—toward personalized therapy. N Engl J Med 2007; 356(1):76–78.

132. Shames DS, Girard L, Gao B, Sato M, Lewis CM, Shivapurkar N et al. A genome-wide screen for promoter methylation in lung cancer identifies novel methylation markers for multiple malignancies. PLoS Med 2006; 3(12):e486.

133. Roman DL, Talbot JN, Roof RA, Sunahara RK, Traynor JR, Neubig RR. Identification of small-molecule inhibitors of RGS4 using a high-throughput flow cytometry protein interaction assay. Mol Pharmacol 2007; 71(1):169–175.

134. Roof RA, Jin Y, Roman DL, Sunahara RK, Ishii M, Mosberg HI et al. Mechanism of action and structural requirements of constrained peptide inhibitors of RGS proteins. Chem Biol Drug Des 2006; 67(4):266–274.

135. Traynor JR, Neubig RR. Regulators of G protein signaling & drugs of abuse. Mol Interv 2005; 5(1):30–41.

136. Armbruster BN, Roth BL. Mining the receptorome. J Biol Chem 2005; 280(7):5129–5132.

137. Strachan RT, Ferrara G, Roth BL. Screening the receptorome: an efficient approach for drug discovery and target validation. Drug Discov Today 2006; 11(15–16):708–716.

138. Connolly HM, Crary JL, McGoon MD, Hensrud DD, Edwards BS, Edwards WD et al. Valvular heart disease associated with fenfluramine-phentermine. N Engl J Med 1997; 337(9):581–588.

139. Jick H, Vasilakis C, Weinrauch LA, Meier CR, Jick SS, Derby LE. A population-based study of appetite-suppressant drugs and the risk of cardiac-valve regurgitation. N Engl J Med 1998; 339(11):719–724.

140. Rothman RB, Baumann MH, Savage JE, Rauser L, McBride A, Hufeisen SJ et al. Evidence for possible involvement of 5-HT(2B) receptors in the cardiac valvulopathy associated with fenfluramine and other serotonergic medications. Circulation 2000; 102(23):2836–2841.

141. Fitzgerald LW, Burn TC, Brown BS, Patterson JP, Corjay MH, Valentine PA et al. Possible role of valvular serotonin 5-HT(2B) receptors in the cardiopathy associated with fenfluramine. Mol Pharmacol 2000; 57(1):75–81.

142. Launay JM, Herve P, Peoc'h K, Tournois C, Callebert J, Nebigil CG et al. Function of the serotonin 5-hydroxytryptamine 2B receptor in pulmonary hypertension. Nat Med 2002; 8(10):1129–1135.

143. Setola V, Roth BL. Screening the receptorome reveals molecular targets responsible for drug-induced side effects: focus on 'fen-phen.' Expert Opin Drug Metab Toxicol 2005; 1(3):377–387.

144. Roth BL. Drugs and valvular heart disease. N Engl J Med 2007; 356(1):6–9.

145. Schade R, Andersohn F, Suissa S, Haverkamp W, Garbe E. Dopamine agonists and the risk of cardiac-valve regurgitation. N Engl J Med 2007; 356(1):29–38.

146. Zanettini R, Antonini A, Gatto G, Gentile R, Tesei S, Pezzoli G. Valvular heart disease and the use of dopamine agonists for Parkinson's disease. N Engl J Med 2007; 356(1):39–46.

147. Jung J, Bonini N. CREB-binding protein modulates repeat instability in a Drosophila model for polyQ disease. Science 2007; 315(5820):1857–1859.

148. Fortini ME. Medicine. Anticipating trouble from gene transcription. Science 2007; 315(5820):1800–1801.

149. Marx J. Neurodegeneration. Huntington's research points to possible new therapies. Science 2005; 310(5745):43–45.

150. Mendell JT, Sharifi NA, Meyers JL, Martinez-Murillo F, Dietz HC. Nonsense surveillance regulates expression of diverse classes of mammalian transcripts and mutes genomic noise. Nat Genet 2004; 36(10):1073–1078.

151. Holbrook JA, Neu-Yilik G, Hentze MW, Kulozik AE. Nonsense-mediated decay approaches the clinic. Nat Genet 2004; 36(8):801–808.

152. Ainsworth C. Nonsense mutations: running the red light. Nature 2005; 438(7069):726–728.

153. Howard M, Frizzell RA, Bedwell DM. Aminoglycoside antibiotics restore CFTR function by overcoming premature stop mutations. Nat Med 1996; 2(4):467–469.

154. Schmitz A, Famulok M. Chemical Biology: ignore the nonsense. Nature 2007; 447(7140):42–43.

155. Wilschanski M, Yahav Y, Yaacov Y, Blau H, Bentur L, Rivlin J et al. Gentamicin-induced correction of CFTR function in patients with cystic fibrosis and CFTR stop mutations. N Engl J Med 2003; 349(15):1433–1441.

156. Kerem E. Pharmacologic therapy for stop mutations: how much CFTR activity is enough? Curr Opin Pulm Med 2004; 10(6):547–552.

157. Welch EM, Barton ER, Zhuo J, Tomizawa Y, Friesen WJ, Trifillis P et al. PTC124 targets genetic disorders caused by nonsense mutations. Nature 2007; 447(7140):87–91.

158. Van der Hooft CS, Sturkenboom MC, van Grootheest K, Kingma HJ, Stricker BH. Adverse drug reaction-related hospitalisations: a nationwide study in The Netherlands. Drug Saf 2006; 29(2):161–168.

159. Hazell L, Shakir SA. Under-reporting of adverse drug reactions : a systematic review. Drug Saf 2006; 29(5):385–396.

160. Giacomini KM, Krauss RM, Roden DM, Eichelbaum M, Hayden MR, Nakamura Y. When good drugs go bad. Nature 2007; 446(7139):975–977.

Synthesis

Pharmacogenetics provides a rich legacy of research that has intensified concerns about the safety and efficacy of drugs used in the treatment of human disease. Although these are complex issues, it has long been apparent that the combined influence of the environment and genetics is the primary source of these problems. The only way to eliminate such risks is to identify their causes and use this information to prevent their occurrence.

This book uses the principles of pharmacology and genetics as points of departure for analyzing and explaining the unexpected consequences of human responses to therapeutic drugs and other environmental toxicants. Historically, pharmacogenetics has roots that date back more than 150 years, but it is best to begin with the 1950s when a small number of pharmacologists created the field by incorporating genetics into their studies of adverse responses to therapeutic drugs. Responses to these agents, like many other physical and mental traits, trace to our genes, and pharmacogenetics bridges the gap between pharmacology and genetics by providing the experimental framework for dissecting the causes of genetic variations of these responses. The growth of pharmacogenetics has resulted in the accumulation of a vast store of knowledge, firmly establishing the importance of heredity to human drug responses and greatly enriching the discipline of pharmacology.

By the mid-1980s, the question of interest was no longer whether human drug responses were genetically determined but to what extent. Since then, many of the most significant advances in biology have occurred in the field of genomics. The invention of tools for analyzing genetic variation and the completion of the human genome initiative have provided a wealth of primary genetic information and functional genomic data to further fuel our understanding of genetic variation. In just 5 years we moved from mapping the first complete nucleotide sequence of a free-living organism, *Haemophilus influenzae,* to a working draft of the human genome. Initially, and for many years afterward, pharmacogenetics was limited to an investigation of the effects of a single gene on patterns of drug response in small groups of individuals, their families and ethnic populations mainly in a research setting. But now, such investigations engage a broad spectrum of basic and clinical biomedical scientists in testing multiple genetic loci that span a large fraction of the human genome in many patients and healthy persons.

Until recently, changes in genomic DNA sequences were regarded as the sole mechanism of heritable variation, but the emergence of epigenetics revealed that heritable changes in gene expression are transmitted by direct modification of DNA and chromatin. New knowledge of the chemical nature of these modifications demonstrated that methylation of cytosines and numerous modifications of chromatin are intimately connected to gene expression. It follows that "epigenetic inheritance," which implies modification of gene expression without modifying DNA sequence and is proposed as a mechanism complementing genetic inheritance, properly belongs within the scope of pharmacogenetic inquiry.

The scope of pharmacogenetics is expanding rapidly and is undergoing redefinition. Today, pharmacogenetics is often referred to as pharmacogenomics, although the distinction between the two terms is not always evident. Currently, pharmacogenetics encompasses a worldwide network of well-integrated academic and industrial scientists seeking to identify genetic/genomic variations and to learn whether and how they connect to drug response. But its legacy extends well beyond the present as we contemplate ways to use genomic information proactively to design new, more effective therapeutics and predict the likely occurrence of unwanted side effects of these agents in susceptible human subjects of all ages.

Ideally, drugs approved for medical treatment are intended to achieve predictable therapeutic responses, but physicians as well as their recipients know that for a drug to be safe and effective for everyone is rare. Because responses to standard doses of a drug can vary so much from one person to another, drug therapy is still regarded as a medical art. Adverse drug reactions of a serious nature are likely to occur more frequently than is generally recognized, costing far more than U.S. $100 billion annually and ranking among the leading causes of hospitalization and death. A recent epidemiological study that measured the effectiveness of major drugs commonly used for a variety of diseases found, for instance, that for COX2 inhibitors used to treat pain, the highest percentage of patients who responded was 80%, while responses to drugs used to treat cancer ranked lowest at 25%. Successful drugs employed in the treatment of major diseases, such as diabetes, cardiovascular disease, incontinence, migraine, and osteoporosis, work in only 40–75% of patients, but for those the drug usually retains its effectiveness throughout their life.

The physician who encounters an unusual or an unexpected response in practice would be well advised to question whether the responses might have a genetic basis, whether the patient might carry a known pharmacogenetic variant that could explain the response, and whether responses of such patients to other drugs might be affected. Such observations should be examined carefully to document their authenticity and to test whether heredity compared to other potential effects might influence their expression. It is time for physicians in clinical practice to apply the fundamentals of pharmacogenetic analysis to better understand individual variability in drug responses to be able to select the drug and the dose that will provide the optimal benefit and safety appropriate for individual patients.

Appendix A

SUPPLEMENTARY INFORMATION ON THE RANGE OF PHARMACOGENETICS

Table A.1 The Range of Pharmacogenetics: The Gene Targeted and Trait Summary

Polymorphic Trait	Gene Targeted	Trait Summary	Key References[a]	
			Variant discovery	Recent reference
		Drug-Metabolizing Enzyme and Transporter Proteins		
CYP2C19 mephenytoin polymorphism	*CYP2C19*	CYP2C19 polymorphism was originally described for the metabolism of mephenytoin (anticonvulsant). Approximately 15% of prescribed drugs are subject to this trait. Mephenytoin is a racemic mixture of *R* and *S* enantiomers. In most persons *S* mephenytoin is eliminated by hydroxylation more efficiently than *R* mephenytoin. The urinary *R/S* ratio of 4-hydroxy (4-OH) mephenytoin is a determinant of CYP2C19 phenotypes, called EMs and PMs. CYP2C19 PMs may suffer acute side effects and chronic toxicity on usual drug doses. For mephenytoin these include drowsiness (acute) and skin rash, fever, and blood dyscrasias (chronic). Other drugs that are subject to CYP2C19 polymorphism are proguanil (antimalarial), omeprazole and lansoprazole (antacids), and some barbiturates (hypnotics). In persons with gastric ulcers, *Helicobacter pylori* eradication and response to therapy are reduced in EMs compared to PMs.	1–3	4–6

(continued)

Table A.1 (continued)

Polymorphic Trait	Gene Targeted	Trait Summary	Key References[a]	
			Variant discovery	Recent reference
CYP2C9 polymorphism	CYP2C9	Warfarin therapy is complicated by wide variations in anticoagulant response. The CYP2C9 polymorphism affects some 15% of prescribed drugs, including warfarin. Between 5% and 40% of persons carry at least one copy of either of two major variants with reduced enzymatic activity for S-warfarin and many other drug substrates. Inappropriate dosing with warfarin leads to excessive and occasionally life-threatening bleeding, especially during the initiation of therapy. CYP2C9 explains that approximately 6–10% of the variation in dose and genotyping prior to warfarin treatment could benefit patients by reducing the risk of bleeding, especially during the high-risk period of therapy initiation. Other drugs that are subject to this polymorphism include phenytoin, tolbutamide, nonsteroidal antiinflammatory drugs (NSAIDs), and angiotensin-converting enzyme (ACE) inhibitors.	7	5, 6, 8
Vitamin K epoxide reductase complex 1	VKORC1	VKORC1 is the target of coumarin anticoagulant drugs such as warfarin and is emerging as an important genetic factor influencing dose and response to these drugs. The VKORC1 gene contains three exons coding for an 18-kDa integral membrane protein. It is located on the short arm of chromosome 16 at 16p11.2. Common polymorphisms in regulatory regions correlate strongly with warfarin response. At least 10 noncoding haplotypes and 5 major haplotypes have been identified. Patients with varying degrees of warfarin resistance carry mutations in one copy of VKORC1, and can be stratified into low-, intermediate-, and high-dose warfarin groups based on their VKORC1 haplotypes. The low-dose and intermediate-dose haplotype explain approximately 25% of the variance in dose. A single allelic site, 1173T/C, in intron 1 assigns European-American subjects to either the low or intermediate groups, and the well-recognized reduction in average maintenance warfarin dose for Asians is largely a consequence of the paucity of the high-dose-associated 1173T allele in this ethnic population.	9–13	14

(continued)

Aldehyde dehydrogenase 2 polymorphism	ALDH2	Mitochondrial ALDH2 polymorphism was initially described in Asians and is present in 8–45% of Asian and South American Indian populations of Mongoloid origin. This dominantly inherited trait results from an inactive form of ALDH2 due to substitution of lysine for glutamate at codon 487 and it predisposes individuals to impaired metabolism of ethanol. The deficiency is absent from or occurs at very low levels among Caucasian and Negroid populations. Family studies show that phenotypically ALDH2-deficient persons possess one or two mutant alleles—i.e., are either heterozygous or homozygous—indicating the autosomal dominant inheritance of this trait. Japanese men and women who have the "Asian" type of ALDH2 drink less and suffer less from the aversive effects of alcohol than those with the active "Caucasian" ALDH2. Vasomotor dilation as revealed by "facial flushing" is an acute reaction to ethanol that occurs in individuals homozygous and heterozygous for the "Asian" type of ALDH2 variant while those homozygous for the usual ALDH2 are nonflushers.	15–17	18
Succinylcholine sensitivity	SeChE	Discovery of low serum pseudocholinesterase in two Cypriot brothers that resulted in prolonged apnea (paralysis of breathing) after succinylcholine ("succinylcholine sensitivity") first suggested that the enzyme deficiency was familial and possibly hereditary. It is known to be hydrolyzed by serum cholinesterase. It is a low potency drug with very fast clearance. It produces skeletal muscle paralysis and apnea. Succinylcholine sensitivity is inherited as a relatively rare (1/2500 Caucasians) autosomal codominant trait. Persons homozygous for the mutant (atypical) form of serum cholinesterase gene have low serum cholinesterase activity and are susceptible to this disorder. At least six other low-activity hereditary variants have also been identified in association with succinylcholine sensitivity.	19	20
Acetylation polymorphism	NAT2	N-Acetyltransferase (NAT2) polymorphism was originally described for the metabolism of isoniazid (antituberculotic). Other drug substrates for NAT2 polymorphism affect the metabolism of aromatic amine and hydrazine drugs including hydralazine, antimicrobial sulfonamides, sulfasalazine, and procainamide as well as aromatic amine carcinogens (β-naphthylamine, 4-aminobiphenyl, and benzidine) and dietary mutagens. Individuals can be	21, 22	23–26

Table A.1 (continued)

Polymorphic Trait	Gene Targeted	Trait Summary	Key References[a]	
			Variant discovery	Recent reference
		divided into two phenotypes: rapid and slow acetylators. Slow acetylators are more susceptible to semiacute and chronic toxicity of the nervous system and chemical hepatitis from these drugs and xenobiotics.		
Thiopurine methyltransferase (TPMT) deficiency	TPMT	TPMT deficiency is ascribed to two major single-nucleotide polymorphisms (SNPs) (at least eight have been identified) that result in low TPMT activity. TPMT deficiency is associated with life-threatening acute and delayed intolerance to immunosuppressive and antileukemic drugs (6-mercaptopurine, 6-thioguanine, azathioprine) and bleeding from cephalosporin antibiotics (moxalactam and cephamandole). In contrast, high levels of TPMT may result in failure to respond to antimetabolite therapy and leukemic relapse.	27	28–32
Dihydropyrimidine dehydrogenase (DPD) polymorphism	DPD	DPD deficiency occurs in 1–3% of cancer patients with solid tumors of the head, neck, stomach, intestine, and breast. A homozygous DPD-deficient person given 5-fluorouracil (5-FU) exhibits altered 5-FU metabolism resulting in severe 5-FU toxicity. A splice site G > A mutation yields a completely nonfunctional form of DPD in sufficiently high frequency (1.8% of heterozygotes) to warrant genetic screening for the presence of this DPD variant in cancer patients before 5-FU administration.	33–38	39–43
Glucuronyltransferase polymorphism	UGT1A1	Polymorphism of the promoter of UGT1A1, designated UGT1A1*28, is responsible for impaired glucuronidation activity. UGT1A1*28 is associated with Gilbert's syndrome, a mild nonpathogenic hyperbilirubinemic, often undiagnosed disorder that occurs in up to 19% of individuals. Additionally, persons with UGT1A1*28 given irinotecan suffer severe diarrhea and leukopenia (low white blood cell counts). Irinotecan is an anticancer prodrug that is initially converted to SN-38, a highly toxic intermediate metabolite that requires glucuronidation for efficient excretion. SN-38 glucuronidation is	44	45, 46

			48
			47, 48
Fish malodor syndrome	FMO3		
			49
			53, 54
Multidrug resistance-related protein (MRP2)	ABCC2		

impaired by UGT1A1*28. The polymorphism is due to an additional TA repeat in the TATA sequence of the UGT1A1 promoter [(TA)₇TAA, instead of (TA)₆TAA]. The frequency of UGT1A1*28 is 20%. UGT1A1*28 serves as a marker predictive of patients predisposed to irinotecan-induced gastrointestinal and bone marrow toxicity.

The fish malodor syndrome is an example of a person-to-person variation in response to foods that yield trimethylamine as a breakdown product. Limited studies suggest autosomal recessive (or codominant) transmission of this trait. Its expression causes affected persons to exude the odor of rotting fish in sweat, breath, and urine. This trait is attributed to a variant form of flavin monooxygenase (FMO3). Two polymorphisms, P153L and E305X, that inactivate FMO3 appear to account for the majority of cases. Other mutations have been identified in FMO3 that determine modified and less severe forms of the condition. Affected persons can suffer devastating educational, economic, and social consequences. Management remains empirical. The usual recourse is to reduce the intake of eggs, liver, marine fish, and other trimethylamine precursors.

MRP2 is one of at least nine isoforms of the multidrug resistance-related protein family of transporters.[49] MPR2 functions as an ATP-dependent export pump for conjugates of lipophilic compounds with anionic residues such as glutathione and glucuronate. The genomic structure of the human MRP2 gene was determined in 1996,[50] and mapped to chromosome 10q24.[51,52] MPR2 is present both in basolateral and canalicular plasma membranes from normal human liver. The normal hepatic localization of MPR isoforms is altered in Dubin–Johnson syndrome, a recessive hereditary defect in hepatobiliary transport described in humans of several races and in several animal models that results in predominantly conjugated hyperbilirubinemia following its conjugation with glutathione in hepatocytes and transport to blood. The selective absence of this transport protein from the hepatocyte canalicular membrane is associated with the presence of a MRP2 isoform in the lateral plasma membrane. Several genetic variations are known to result in loss of MRP2 transporter function and aberrant RNA splicing with the majority

(continued)

397

Table A.1 (*continued*)

Polymorphic Trait	Gene Targeted	Trait Summary	Key References[a]	
			Variant discovery	Recent reference
		resulting in the absence of immunochemically detectable MRP2. The discovery that canalicular MRP2 is lacking in Dubin–Johnson syndrome liver is consistent with deficient unidirectional export of amphiphilic organic substrates into bile. The occurrence of the Dubin–Johnson syndrome in all races and ethnic backgrounds raises the question of whether this trait may be associated with a biological advantage under certain conditions.[53]		
Organic anion transporting polypep-tide (OATP-C) (OATP1B1)	*SLCO1B1*	One large family of uptake transporters with members expressed in hepatocytes is the OATP family of organic anion transporters. At least 11 human OATPs have been identified as described by the HUGO Gene Nomenclature Committee at www.kpt.unizh.ch/oatp/. OATP-C (also designated as LST-1 and OATP2) is a major solute carrier specific to liver located at the basolateral membrane of human hepatocytes. Like other members of the organic anion transporter family, OATP-C has broad substrate selectivity, transporting various anionic compounds including bile acids, sulfate and glucuronide conjugates, estrogens, thyroid hormones, and peptides. OATP-C also has selectivity for drugs such as pravastatin, methotrexate, rifampin, and the endothelin A receptor antagonist. The genomic structure of SLCO1B1 has been determined by several groups of investigators.[49] Several genetic changes in the SLCO1B1 gene have been described, three of which, N130D (338A → G), V174A (521T → C), and G488A (1463G → A), may have altered function. However, reduced activity of OATP1B1 V174A protein has been observed consistently for several substrates.[55,56] Genotypic analyses of subjects of European-American and African-American descent indicate that variants of OATP-C are common and racially dependent[57]. A novel allele of the OATP-C gene, called OATP-C*15, contains both N130D and V174A single nucleotide polymorphisms, and has a frequency in Japanese subjects	60	49, 61

		of 3%.[55] Individuals carrying the OATP-C*15 allele [a haplotype consisting of OATP-C*1B (Asp-130)] had increased pravastatin plasma levels as compared to individuals carrying only the OATP-C*1B allele (Asp-130-Val-174).[58] Much of the functional loss associated with the OATP-C*15 haplotype is related to the V174A polymorphism. Various carriers of functionally deficient OATP-C variants exhibit reduced hepatocellular uptake of rifampin suggesting that such persons may demonstrate reduced capacity for rifampin-mediated induction of hepatic drug-metabolizing enzymes and transporters.[59]	

Drug Receptor Targets

Malignant hyperthermia	RYR1	Malignant hyperthermia is a rare, clinically heterogeneous disorder associated with a high frequency of anesthetic deaths. This trait is inherited as an autosomal dominant disorder. It is elicited by inhalation anesthetics such as halothane when given in combination with the muscle relaxant, succinylcholine. Malignant hyperthermia is characterized by an acute onset of elevated temperatures, hypermetabolism, and muscle rigidity. Some cases appear to be due to a point mutation in the ryanodine (calcium release channel) receptor that renders the muscle susceptible to disturbances in calcium regulation. If therapy is not administered immediately, the patient may die within minutes from ventricular fibrillation, or a few hours later from pulmonary edema and renal failure. The introduction of *dantrolene* a muscle relaxant, as a prophylactic or therapeutic agent dramatically improves the outcome. The genetics of malignant hyperthermia are complex, because this disease shows substantial locus and allelic heterogeneity. Every pregnant woman with a self or family history should be offered the option of molecular genetic investigations of umbilical cord blood.	62 63, 64
CCR5 polymorphism	CCR5	The CCR5 gene encodes a seven transmembrane, G-protein-coupled T-lymphocyte surface receptor that is required for attachment and infectivity of viruses such as HIV-1. A 32-bp deletion mutant of CCR5 (CCR5Δ32) occurs disproportionately among persons who are frequently exposed to HIV-1. The defective gene is severely truncated and not expressed at the cell surface. Persons homozygous for the CCR5Δ32 allele are highly protected from	65–67 68

(*continued*)

Table A.1 (*continued*)

Polymorphic Trait	Gene Targeted	Trait Summary	Key References[a]	
			Variant discovery	Recent reference
		contracting HIV infection, and progression of AIDS is slower in individuals who are heterozygous for the deletion or carry a partial deletion of the gene. The CCR5Δ32 allele occurs at a frequency of 0.1–0.2 in Caucasian and Western European populations but is absent among native African, American Indian, and East Indian ethnic groups.		
Toll receptor 4 polymorphism	TLR4	TLR4 represents an ancient self-defense mechanism that has emerged as a conduit for endotoxic shock in humans and other mammals. The endotoxic principle is a bacterial lipopolysaccharide (LPS), which is an abundant component of Gram-negative bacteria, comprising a toxic lipid moiety (lipid A) and several other nontoxic moieties of highly variable structure. LPS is of pharmacogenetic interest because Gram-negative infection claims thousands of lives in the United States, and genetic studies suggest that variations in the recognition of this toxin are important for containment and eradication of Gram-negative infection. Identification of LPS-resistant mice and cloning of the responsible gene from resistant mice provided the clues that Tlr4 was the gene product of the LPS locus, and when defective, resulted in hyporesponsiveness (LPS resistance). While the studies of mice were in progress, five human toll-like receptors including the human homolog (TLR4) of mouse Tlr4 were cloned. Currently, at least 10 members of the Toll superfamily of receptors are known.[69] Except for a single anecdotal case,[70] no human models of hyporesponsiveness have been described. However, human exposure to endotoxin in the environment is associated with various airway disorders including asthma.[71,72] Arbour and co-workers provided the first direct evidence that one (Asp-299-Gly) of two sequence polymorphisms in exon 4 of TLR4 was associated with an endotoxin hyporesponsive phenotype in humans.[73] Because not all subjects who were	69–72	73

hyporesponsive to LPS had mutations in TLR4, this mutation is thought to act in concert with other genetic or acquired factors to influence the response to LPS.

Other Drug Target Proteins

Glucose-6-phosphate dehydrogenase (G6PD) deficiency	*G6PD*	G6PD is one of the enzymatic components of the pentose phosphate pathway that is required to maintain glutathione in a reduced state for the maintenance of RBC integrity. A deficiency of G6PD can cause the red blood cell disorder, hemolytic anemia. Numerous drugs, dietary substances, and some oxidative chemicals induce hemolytic anemia in G6PD-deficient persons. Drugs that cause hemolytic anemia in susceptible persons include antimalarial 8-aminoquinolines (pamaquine, pentaquine, isopentaquine, primaquine), sulfones, sulfonamides, quinidine, nitrofurans, chloramphenicol, and vitamin K analogs. Consumption of fava beans and certain other vegetables can cause G6PD-induced hemolysis. G6PD deficiency is a sex-linked trait. The gene that encodes G6PD is on chromosome Xq28 and lies between the genes for clotting factor VIII and color vision. More than 400 million people worldwide have G6PD deficiency.	74 75, 76
α_1-Antitrypsin deficiency	α_1-*Antitrypsin*	Persons with α_1-antitrypsin deficiency are predisposed to abnormally rapid degradation of the lung, joints, kidneys, and vasculature. Susceptibility to lung disease of homozygotes is due to low plasma levels of the SNP Z variant of α_1-antitrypsin, permitting destruction of lung elastin by neutrophile elastase. Smoking is particularly detrimental to the lungs of affected persons, predisposing them at an early age to lung disease and emphysema. The survival rates for α_1-antitrypsin-deficient smokers was 22% compared to 83% for nonsmokers. The high frequency of PiMZ heterozygotes in many populations (2–5%) is also of interest because PiMZ smokers show some loss of elastic lung recoil. The loss for heterozygote smokers is about equal to that of homozygous nonsmokers.	77 78
Glucocorticoid remediable aldosteronism (GRA)	*CYP11B1/CYP11B2*	GRA is a form of mineralocorticoid hypertension characterized by hypokalemia, a moderate overproduction of aldosterone, and suppressed plasma renin activity. Normally aldosterone production is controlled by angiotensin II, but in GRA it is controlled by ACTH. Affected persons are	79, 80 81

(continued)

401

Table A.1 (*continued*)

Polymorphic Trait	Gene Targeted	Trait Summary	Key References[a] Variant discovery	Recent reference
	A chimeric gene fusing the 5' hormone response element of 11β-hydroxylase to the coding sequence of aldosterone synthase on chromosome 8q	usually diagnosed with hypertension at a young age, and 50% of family members may die of cardiovascular accidents before 45 years of age. The biochemical phenotype is characterized by overproduction of aldosterone and the aberrant adrenal steroids 18-oxocortisol and 18-hydroxycortisol. They have 18-oxocortisol and 18-hydroxycortisol:aldosterone ratios that may be more than 10 standard deviations above the means of unaffected family members. Blood pressure control of GRA using standard antihypertensive agents is poor, but is remediated effectively with glucocorticoids. A recent genetic study shows that some patients may have dexamethasone-suppressible aldosteronism without the chimeric CYP11B1/CYP11B2 gene, and that the diagnosis must be confirmed with a definitive genetic test for the chimeric gene before proceeding to therapy.		
Lactose intolerance (lactase nonpersistence syndrome)	Lactase-phlorizin hydrolase (lactase)	Milk drinking in early life is one of the defining characteristics of mammals and most humans are born with this trait. Intolerance to milk is caused by an inability to digest lactose by the enzyme lactase and results in flatulence and watery diarrhea due to fermentation of unabsorbed, dietary carbohydrates by intestinal flora.[82] Lactase nonpersistence is an autosomal recessive trait in Europeans determined by a polymorphic gene (*LCT*). This polymorphism determines whether some humans express lactase and are lactose tolerant while others lose lactase expression and are lactose intolerant. Lactase activity declines rapidly after weaning in most humans, but persists into adulthood in many others, particularly those individuals descended from agrarian populations of the Middle East and North Africa that developed cattle domestication 7500–9000 years ago. In certain Caucasian populations lactase activity remains at or slightly below gestational levels throughout adulthood. The age of onset of lactose intolerance ranges from 1 to 2 years	83, 84, 86, 87	88, 89

Hereditary fructose intolerance	Aldolase B	among the Thai to 10 to 20 years among Finns.[83] The ethnic distribution of adult lactase phenotypes in human populations varies widely: Asians, 7%; whites, 22%; blacks, 65%; American Indians, 95%; Vietnamese, 100%.[84] There is a north-to-south gradient (cline) in the distribution of Caucasian haplotypes from north to south Europe.[85] Fructose intolerance is characterized by severe abdominal pain, vomiting, and other effects including hypoglycemia that may be fatal on ingesting fructose. This underdiagnosed trait (1/20,000) is inherited as an autosomal codominant character. Aldolase B, which is expressed in liver, kidney, and small intestine, is the primary aldolase isozyme used during the incorporation of diet-derived fructose into the glycolytic and gluconeogenic pathways. Two mutant alleles affecting protein stability (A149P and A174D) and one mutation affecting the carboxy-terminal tail (N334K) are responsible for 84% of the aldolase B variants in Europeans. The trait is widely distributed in European populations. The absence of consanguinity in most parents of affected persons suggests that mutant alleles for aldolase B may be relatively common in populations at large. Recognition of this disorder is important because exclusion of fructose and related sugars from the diet usually leads to dramatic recovery. Continued ingestion of fructose or its congeners is required to establish the disease, but the widespread distribution of these sugars in human foods places genetically susceptible persons at constant risk to an avoidable disorder.	90, 91
			92
Long QT syndrome.	*KCNQ1* and others	The long QT syndrome is a rare familial congenital disorder that is characterized by QT prolongation on the electrocardiogram—a sign of abnormal cardiac repolarization—syncope, seizures, and sudden death from ventricular arrhythmias. The long QT syndrome is a genetically complex disorder whose molecular basis has not been fully elucidated. Molecular studies reveal point mutations (SNPs) on at least four different chromosomes associated with defective potassium and sodium channels affecting cardiac function. Persons with hereditary long QT syndrome may die suddenly during excitement or stress. Sudden death occurred at an average of 16 years in nine persons of one affected family over a 30-year period. Affected persons are	93–96
			97

(continued)

Table A.1 (*continued*)

Polymorphic Trait	Gene Targeted	Trait Summary	Key References[a] Variant discovery	Recent reference
		also highly susceptible to ventricular arrhythmias induced by certain drugs (quinidine, chlorpromazine, tricyclic antidepressants, and HI antihistaminics). The antihistamines terfenadine and astemizole, especially in the presence of P450 inhibition, now both withdrawn, have produced such a response in susceptible persons.		
Retinoic acid resistance and acute promyelocytic leukemia (APL)	*PML-RARα*	APL is a distinct clinical, morphological, and cytogenetic subtype of acute myelogenous leukemia that is characterized by a balanced translocation between chromosomes 15 and 17 in APL cells. This specific translocation (q15;17) (q22;q11.2–12) has not been observed in any other subtype of acute myelogenous leukemia or in any other malignant disease. The translocation results in a head-to-tail fusion to form a chimeric PML-RARα gene under the transcriptional control of the PML promoter. The hybrid PML-RARα protein appears to block terminal differentiation in APL cells. Upon treatment with all-*trans*-retinoic acid (ATRA), APL cells are induced to differentiate. The therapeutic effect of ATRA may be due to its capacity to restore the normal nuclear organization. APL is the first example of a human cancer successfully treated with differentiation therapy. Use of ATRA results in a 85–90% remission rate among APL patients.	98, 99	100
Aminoglycoside antibiotic-induced deafness (AAID)	Mitochondrial *12srRNA*	AAID is a form of nonsyndromic hearing loss that is a major cause of deafness in persons receiving antibiotics such as streptomycin and gentamicin. A point mutation (SNP) in the mitochondrial genome is associated with this defect in Chinese and Arab-Israeli pedigrees. Because the mutation is transmitted maternally, the most immediate clinical significance is to avoid aminoglycosides for any maternal relative with maternally inherited AAID.	101	102, 103

| | | | 104 | 105, 106 |

Thrombophilia (deep vein thrombosis) — Factor V

Thrombophilia, also known as "activated protein C (APC) resistance," is an autosomal dominant trait that is associated with a point mutation (SNP) in coagulation factor V. The variant clotting factor is detectable by the activated partial prothrombin times (APPT) test but is not associated with a change in plasma levels of factor V. The trait causes a 7-fold increase in susceptibility to deep vein thrombosis, especially at younger ages. Persons who harbor the variant protein may never suffer thrombosis. Nevertheless, they may be lifelong candidates for anticoagulant therapy and its attendant risks (see CYP2C9 polymorphism), a fact that must be weighed against the benefits of preventing infrequent but potentially devastating thrombotic risks.

| | | | 107 | 108 |

Major histocompatability (MHC) polymorphism — Ancestral haplotype *HLA-B*5701*, *HLA-DR7*, and *HLA-DQ3*

Abacavir is a potent HIV-1 nucleoside reverse transcriptase inhibitor used in the treatment of AIDS. A life-threatening hypersensitivity is the drug's main toxic effect. Recently, its use in 200 AIDS patients was associated with 18 cases (9%) of potentially life-threatening hypersensitivity. Mapping of candidate MHC susceptibility loci within this cohort revealed an ancestral haplotype (HLA-B*5701, HLA-DR7, and HLA-DQ3) that was present in 13 (72%) of hypersensitive patients and only 5 (3%) of tolerant patients. Within the entire patient sample, the presence of these three loci had a positive predictive value for hypersensitivity of 100% and a negative predictive value of 97%. The findings are consistent with a direct role for MHC-specific alleles in the pathogenesis of abacavir hypersensitivity and provide a plausible basis for testing the safe use of the drug.

REFERENCES

1. Wrighton SA, Stevens JC, Becker GW, VandenBranden M. Isolation and characterization of human liver cytochrome P450 2C19: Correlation between 2C19 and S-mephenytoin 4'-hydroxylation. Arch Biochem Biophys 1993; 306(1):240–245.

2. de Morais SM, Wilkinson GR, Blaisdell J, Nakamura K, Meyer UA, Goldstein JA. The major genetic defect responsible for the polymorphism of S-mephenytoin metabolism in humans. J Biol Chem 1994; 269(22):15419–15422.

3. de Morais SM, Wilkinson GR, Blaisdell J, Meyer UA, Nakamura K, Goldstein JA. Identification of a new genetic defect responsible for the polymorphism of (S)-mephenytoin metabolism in Japanese. Mol Pharmacol 1994; 46(4):594–598.

4. Sim SC, Risinger C, Dahl ML, Aklillu E, Christensen M, Bertilsson L, et al. A common novel CYP2C19 gene variant causes ultrarapid drug metabolism relevant for the drug response to proton pump inhibitors and antidepressants. Clin Pharmacol Ther 2006; 79(1):103–113.

5. http://www.imm.ki.se/. 2006.

(continued)

Table A.1 (*continued*)

6. http://medicine.iupui.edu/flockhart. 2006.

7. Rettie AE, Wienkers LC, Gonzalez FJ, Trager WF, Korzekwa KR. Impaired (S)-warfarin metabolism catalysed by the R144C allelic variant of CYP2C9. Pharmacogenetics 1994; 4(1):39–42.

8. Aquilante CL, Langaee TY, Lopez LM, Yarandi HN, Tromberg JS, Mohuczy D, et al. Influence of coagulation factor, vitamin K epoxide reductase complex subunit 1, and cytochrome P450 2C9 gene polymorphisms on warfarin dose requirements. Clin Pharmacol Ther 2006; 79(4):291–302.

9. Li T, Chang CY, Jin DY, Lin PJ, Khvorova A, Stafford DW. Identification of the gene for vitamin K epoxide reductase. Nature 2004; 427(6974):541–544.

10. Veenstra DL, You JH, Rieder MJ, Farin FM, Wilkerson HW, Blough DK, et al. Association of vitamin K epoxide reductase complex 1 (VKORC1) variants with warfarin dose in a Hong Kong Chinese patient population. Pharmacogenet Genomics 2005; 15(10):687–691.

11. Rieder MJ, Reiner AP, Gage BF, Nickerson DA, Eby CS, McLeod HL, et al. Effect of VKORC1 haplotypes on transcriptional regulation and warfarin dose. N Engl J Med 2005; 352(22):2285–2293.

12. Harrington DJ, Underwood S, Morse C, Shearer MJ, Tuddenham EG, Mumford AD. Pharmacodynamic resistance to warfarin associated with a Val66Met substitution in vitamin K epoxide reductase complex subunit 1. Thromb Haemost 2005; 93(1):23–26.

13. Bodin L, Horellou MH, Flaujac C, Loriot MA, Samama MM. A vitamin K epoxide reductase complex subunit-1 (VKORC1) mutation in a patient with vitamin K antagonist resistance. J Thromb Haemost 2005; 3(7):1533–1535.

14. Rettie AE, Tai G. The pharmacogenomics of warfarin: Closing in on personalized medicine. Mol Interv 2006; 6(4):223–227.

15. Yoshida A, Huang IY, Ikawa M. Molecular abnormality of an inactive aldehyde dehydrogenase variant commonly found in Orientals. Proc Natl Acad Sci USA 1984; 81(1):258–261.

16. Hsu LC, Tani K, Fujiyoshi T, Kurachi K, Yoshida A. Cloning of cDNAs for human aldehyde dehydrogenases 1 and 2. Proc Natl Acad Sci USA 1985; 82(11):3771–3775.

17. Crabb DW, Edenberg HJ, Bosron WF, Li TK. Genotypes for aldehyde dehydrogenase deficiency and alcohol sensitivity. The inactive ALDH2(2) allele is dominant. J Clin Invest 1989; 83(1):314–316.

18. Matsuo K, Wakai K, Hirose K, Ito H, Saito T, Tajima K. Alcohol dehydrogenase 2 His47Arg polymorphism influences drinking habit independently of aldehyde dehydrogenase 2 Glu487Lys polymorphism: Analysis of 2,299 Japanese subjects. Cancer Epidemiol Biomarkers Prev 2006; 15(5):1009–1013.

19. McGuire MC, Nogueira CP, Bartels CF, Lightstone H, Hajra A, Van der Spek AF, et al. Identification of the structural mutation responsible for the dibucaine-resistant (atypical) variant form of human serum cholinesterase. Proc Natl Acad Sci USA 1989; 86(3):953–957.

20. Roy JJ, Donati F, Boismenu D, Varin F. Concentration-effect relation of succinylcholine chloride during propofol anesthesia. Anesthesiology 2002; 97(5):1082–1092.

21. Blum M, Demierre A, Grant DM, Heim M, Meyer UA. Molecular mechanism of slow acetylation of drugs and carcinogens in humans. Proc Natl Acad Sci USA 1991; 88(12):5237–5241.

22. Vatsis KP, Martell KJ, Weber WW. Diverse point mutations in the human gene for polymorphic N-acetyltransferase. Proc Natl Acad Sci USA 1991; 88(14):6333–6337.

23. Upton AM, Mushtaq A, Victor TC, Sampson SL, Sandy J. Smith DM, et al. Arylamine N-acetyltransferase of Mycobacterium tuberculosis is a polymorphic enzyme and a site of isoniazid metabolism. Mol Microbiol 2001; 42(2):309–317.

24. Gu J, Liang D, Wang Y, Lu C, Wu X. Effects of N-acetyl transferase 1 and 2 polymorphisms on bladder cancer risk in Caucasians. Mutat Res 2005; 581(1–2):97–104.

25. Boukouvala S, Sim E. Structural analysis of the genes for human arylamine N-acetyltransferases and characterisation of alternative transcripts. Basic Clin Pharmacol Toxicol 2005; 96(5):343–351.

26. http://www.louisville.edu/medschool/pharmacology/NAT. 2006.

27. Krynetski EY, Schuetz JD, Galpin AJ, Pui CH, Relling MV, Evans WE. A single point mutation leading to loss of catalytic activity in human thiopurine S-methyltransferase. Proc Natl Acad Sci USA 1995; 92(4):949–953.

28. Weinshilboum RW. Inheritance and drug response. N Engl J Med 2003; 348(Feb 6):529–552.

29. Wang L, Sullivan W, Toft D, Weinshilboum R. Thiopurine S-methyltransferase pharmacogenetics: Chaperone protein association and allozyme degradation. Pharmacogenetics 2003; 13:555–564.

30. Weinshilboum R, Wang L. Pharmacogenetics: Inherited variation in amino acid sequence and altered protein quantity. Clin Pharmacol Ther 2004; 75(4):253–258.

31. Corominas H. Is thiopurine methyltransferase genetic polymorphism a major factor for withdrawal of azathioprine in rheumatoid arthritis patients? Rheumatology 2003; 42:40–45.

32. van Aken J, Schmedders M, Feuerstein G, Kollek R. Prospects and limits of pharmacogenetics. The thiopurine methyl transferase (TPMT) experience. Am J Pharmacogenom 2003; 3(3):149–155.

33. Wei X, McLeod HL, McMurrough J, Gonzalez FJ, Fernandez-Salguero P. Molecular basis of the human dihydropyrimidine dehydrogenase deficiency and 5-fluorouracil toxicity. J Clin Invest 1996; 98(3):610–615.

34. Vreken P, Van Kuilenburg AB, Meinsma R, van Gennip AH. Dihydropyrimidine dehydrogenase (DPD) deficiency: Identification and expression of missense mutations C29R, R886H and R235W. Hum Genet 1997; 1013):333–338.

35. van Gennip AH, De Abreu RA, Van Lenthe H, Bakkeren J, Rotteveel J, Vreken P, et al. Dihydropyrimidinase deficiency: Confirmation of the enzyme defect in dihydropyrimidinuria. J Inherit Metab Dis 1997; 20(3):339–342.

36. Vreken P, Van Kuilenburg AB, Meinsma R, van Gennip AH. Identification of novel point mutations in the dihydropyrimidine dehydrogenase gene. J Inherit Metab Dis 1997; 20(3):335–338.

37. Van Kuilenburg AB, Vreken P, Beex LV, Meinsma R, Van Lenthe H, De Abreu RA, et al. Heterozygosity for a point mutation in an invariant splice donor site of dihydropyrimidine dehydrogenase and severe 5-fluorouracil related toxicity. Eur J Cancer 1997; 33(13):2258–2264.

38. Johnson MR, Hageboutros A, Wang K, High L, Smith JB, Diasio RB. Life-threatening toxicity in a dihydropyrimidine dehydrogenase-deficient patient after treatment with topical 5-fluorouracil. Clin Cancer Res 1999; 5(8):2006–2011.

39. Johnson MR, Wang K, Diasio RB. Profound dihydropyrimidine dehydrogenase deficiency resulting from a novel compound heterozygote genotype. Clin Cancer Res 2002; 8(Mar):768–774.

(continued)

Table A.1 (*continued*)

40. Van Kuilenburg AB, Meinsma R, Zoetekouw L, van Gennip AH. High prevalence of the IVS14 + 1G<A mutation in the dihydropyrimidine dehydrogenase gene of patients with severe 5-fluorouracil-associated toxicity. Pharmacogenetics 2002; 12(7):555–558.

41. Eliason JF, Megyeri A. Potential for predicting toxicity and response of fluoropyrimidines in patients. Curr Drug Targets 2004; 5(4):383–388.

42. Ezzeldin H, Johnson MR, Okamoto Y, Diasio R. Denaturing high performance liquid chromatography analysis of the DPYD gene in patients with lethal 5-fluorouracil toxicity. Clin Cancer Res 2003; 9(8):3021–3028.

43. http://www.dpdenzyme.com/. 2006.

44. Monaghan G, Ryan M, Seddon R, Hume R, Burchell B. Genetic variation in bilirubin UPD-glucuronosyltransferase gene promoter and Gilbert's syndrome. Lancet 1996; 347(9001):578–581.

45. Innocenti F, Iyer L, Ratain MJ. Pharmacogenetics of anticancer agents: Lessons from amonafide and irinotecan. Drug Metab Dispos 2001; 29(4 Pt 2):596–600.

46. Hsieh TY, Shiu TY, Huang SM, Lin HH, Lee TC, Chen PJ, et al. Molecular pathogenesis of Gilbert's syndrome: Decreased TATA-binding protein binding affinity of UGT1A1 gene promoter. Pharmacogenet Genomics 2007; 17(4):229–236.

47. Dolphin CT, Janmohamed A, Smith RL, Shephard EA, Phillips IR. Missense mutation in flavin-containing mono-oxygenase 3 gene, FMO3, underlies fish-odour syndrome. Nat Genet 1997; 17(4):491–494.

48. Treacy EP, Akerman BR, Chow LM, Youil R, Bibeau C, Lin J, et al. Mutations of the flavin-containing monooxygenase gene (FMO3) cause trimethylaminuria, a defect in detoxication. Hum Mol Genet 1998; 7(5):839–845.

49. Marzolini C, Tirona RG, Kim RB. Pharmacogenetics of drug transporters. In: Kalow W, Meyer UA, Tyndale RF, editors. Pharmacogenomics. Boca Raton: Taylor & Francis, 2005: 109–155.

50. Toh S, Wada M, Uchiumi T, Inokuchi A, Makino Y, Horie Y, et al. Genomic structure of the canalicular multispecific organic anion-transporter gene (MRP2/cMOAT) and mutations in the ATP-binding-cassette region in Dubin-Johnson syndrome. Am J Hum Genet 1999; 64(3):739–746.

51. Taniguchi K, Wada M, Kohno K, Nakamura T, Kawabe T, Kawakami M, et al. A human canalicular multispecific organic anion transporter (cMOAT) gene is overexpressed in cisplatin-resistant human cancer cell lines with decreased drug accumulation. Cancer Res 1996; 56(18):4124–4129.

52. van Kuijck MA, Kool M, Merkx GF, Geurts vK, Bindels RJ, Deen PM, et al. Assignment of the canalicular multispecific organic anion transporter gene (CMOAT) to human chromosome 10q24 and mouse chromosome 19D2 by fluorescent in situ hybridization. Cytogenet Cell Genet 1997; 77(3–4):285–287.

53. Kartenbeck J, Leuschner U, Mayer R, Keppler D. Absence of the canalicular isoform of the MRP gene-encoded conjugate export pump from the hepatocytes in Dubin-Johnson syndrome. Hepatology 1996; 23(5):1061–1066.

54. Cole SP, Bhardwaj G, Gerlach JH, Mackie JE, Grant CE, Almquist KC, et al. Overexpression of a transporter gene in a multidrug-resistant human lung cancer cell line. Science 1992; 258(5088):1650–1654.

55. Nozawa T, Nakajima M, Tamai I, Noda K, Nezu J, Sai Y, et al. Genetic polymorphisms of human organic anion transporters OATP-C (SLC21A6) and OATP-B (SLC21A9): Allele frequencies in the Japanese population and functional analysis. J Pharmacol Exp Ther 2002; 302(2):804–813.

56. Michalski C, Cui Y, Nies AT, Nuessler AK, Neuhaus P, Zanger UM, et al. A naturally occurring mutation in the SLC21A6 gene causing impaired membrane localization of the hepatocyte uptake transporter. J Biol Chem 2002; 277(45):43058–43063.

57. Tirona RG, Leake BF, Merino G, Kim RB. Polymorphisms in OATP-C: Identification of multiple allelic variants associated with altered transport activity among European- and African-Americans. J Biol Chem 2001; 276(38):35669–35675.

58. Nishizato Y, Ieiri I, Suzuki H, Kimura M, Kawabata K, Hirota T, et al. Polymorphisms of OATP-C (SLC21A6) and OAT3 (SLC22A8) genes: Consequences for pravastatin pharmacokinetics. Clin Pharmacol Ther 2003; 73(6):554–565.

59. Tirona RG, Leake BF, Wolkoff AW, Kim RB. Human organic anion transporting polypeptide-C (SLC21A6) is a major determinant of rifampin-mediated pregnane X receptor activation. J Pharmacol Exp Ther 2003; 304(1):223–228.

60. Tamai I, Nezu J, Uchino H, Sai Y, Oku A, Shimane M, et al. Molecular identification and characterization of novel members of the human organic anion transporter (OATP) family. Biochem Biophys Res Commun 2000; 273(1):251–260.

61. Katz DA, Carr R, Grimm DR, Xiong H, Holley-Shanks R, Mueller T, et al. Organic anion transporting polypeptide 1B1 activity classified by SLCO1B1 genotype influences atrasentan pharmacokinetics. Clin Pharmacol Ther 2006; 79(3):186–196.

62. Gillard EF, Otsu K, Fujii J, Duff C, De Leon S, Khanna VK, et al. Polymorphisms and deduced amino acid substitutions in the coding sequence of the ryanodine receptor (RYR1) gene in individuals with malignant hyperthermia. Genomics 1992; 13(4):1247–1254.

63. Robinson R, Hopkins P, Carsana A, Gilly H, Halsall J, Heytens L, et al. Several interacting genes influence the malignant hyperthermia phenotype. Hum Genet 2003; 112(2):217–218.

64. Girard T, Johr M, Schaefer C, Urwyler A. Perinatal diagnosis of malignant hyperthermia susceptibility. Anesthesiology 2006; 104(6):1353–1354.

65. Liu R, Paxton WA, Choe S, Ceradini D, Martin SR, Horuk R, et al. Homozygous defect in HIV-1 coreceptor accounts for resistance of some multiply-exposed individuals to HIV-1 infection. Cell 1996; 86(3):367–377.

66. Samson M, Libert F, Doranz BJ, Rucker J, Liesnard C, Farber CM, et al. Resistance to HIV-1 infection in Caucasian individuals bearing mutant alleles of the CCR-5 chemokine receptor gene. Nature 1996; 382(6593):722–725.

67. Dean M, Carrington M, Winkler C, Huttley GA, Smith MW, Allikmets R, et al. Genetic restriction of HIV-1 infection and progression to AIDS by a deletion allele of the CKR5 structural gene. Hemophilia Growth and Development Study, Multicenter AIDS Cohort Study, Multicenter Hemophilia Cohort Study, San Francisco City Cohort, ALIVE Study. Science 1996; 273(5283):1856–1862.

68. Hedrick PW, Verrelli BC. 'Ground truth' for selection on CCR5-Delta32. Trends Genet 2006; 22(6):293–296.

69. Beutler B, Poltorak A. The sole gateway to endotoxin response: How LPS was identified as Tlr4, and its role in innate immunity. Drug Metab Dispos 2001; 29(4 Pt 2):474–478.

70. Kuhns DB, Long Priel DA, Gallin JI. Endotoxin and IL-1 hyporesponsiveness in a patient with recurrent bacterial infections. J Immunol 1997; 158(8):3959–3964.

71. Michel O, Kips J, Duchateau J, Vertongen F, Robert L, Collet H, et al. Severity of asthma is related to endotoxin in house dust. Am J Respir Crit Care Med 1996; 154(6 Pt 1):1641–1646.

72. Schwartz DA, Thorne PS, Yagla SJ, Burmeister LF, Olenchock SA, Watt JL, et al. The role of endotoxin in grain dust-induced lung disease. Am J Respir Crit Care Med 1995; 152(2):603–608.

73. Arbour NC, Lorenz E, Schutte BC, Zabner J, Kline JN, Jones M, et al. TLR4 mutations are associated with endotoxin hyporesponsiveness in humans. Nat Genet 2000; 25(2):187–191.

(*continued*)

Table A.1 (*continued*)

74. Vulliamy TJ, D'Urso M, Battistuzzi G, Estrada M, Foulkes NS, Martini G, et al. Diverse point mutations in the human glucose-6-phosphate dehydrogenase gene cause enzyme deficiency and mild or severe hemolytic anemia. Proc Natl Acad Sci USA 1988; 85(14):5171–5175.

75. Kaplan M, Renbaum P, Levy-lahad E, Hammerman C, Laghad A, Beutler E. Gilbert syndrome and glucose-6-phosphate dehydrogenase deficiency: A dose-dependent genetic interaction crucial to neonatal hyperbilirubinemia. Proc Natl Acad Sci USA 1997; 94(Oct):12128–12132.

76. Tagarelli A, Piro A, Bastone L, Condino F, Tagarelli G. Reliability of quantitative and qualitative tests to identify heterozygotes carrying severe or mild G6PD deficiency. Clin Biochem 2006; 39(2):183–186.

77. Jeppsson JO. Amino acid substitution Glu leads to Lys alpha1-antitrypsin PiZ. FEBS Lett 1976; 65(2):195–197.

78. Wu Y, Foreman RC. The molecular genetics of alpha 1 antitrypsin deficiency. BioEssays 1991; 13(4):163–169.

79. Lifton RP, Dluhy RG, Powers M, Rich GM, Gutkin M, Fallo F, et al. Hereditary hypertension caused by chimaeric gene duplications and ectopic expression of aldosterone synthase. Nat Genet 1992; 2(1):66–74.

80. Rich GM, Ulick S, Cook S, Wang JZ, Lifton RP, Dluhy RG. Glucocorticoid-remediable aldosteronism in a large kindred: Clinical spectrum and diagnosis using a characteristic biochemical phenotype. Ann Intern Med 1992; 116(10):813–820.

81. Fardella CE, Pinto M, Mosso L, Gomez-Sanchez C, Jalil J, Montero J. Genetic study of patients with dexamethasone-suppressible aldosteronism without the chimeric CYP11B1/CYP11B2 gene. J Clin Endocrinol Metab 2001; 86(10):4805–4807.

82. Weijers HA, van de Kamer JH. Aetiology and diagnosis of fermentative diarrhoeas. Acta Paediatr 1963; 52:329–337.

83. Enattah NS, Sahi T, Savilahti E, Terwilliger JD, Peltonen L, Jarvela I. Identification of a variant associated with adult-type hypolactasia. Nat Genet 2002; 30(2):233–237.

84. Flatz G. The genetic polymorphism of intestinal lactase activity in adult humans. In: Scriver CR, Beaudet AL, Sly WS, Valle D, editors. The Metabolic and Molecular Bases of Inherited Disease. New York: McGraw-Hill, 1995: 4441–4450.

85. Harvey CB, Hollox EJ, Poulter M, Wang Y, Rossi M, Auricchio S, et al. Lactase haplotype frequencies in Caucasians: Association with the lactase persistence/non-persistence polymorphism. Ann Hum Genet 1998; 62 (Pt 3):215–223.

86. Montgomery RKB. Lactose intolerance and the genetic regulation of intestinal lactase-phlorizin hydrolase. FASEB 1991; 5:2824–2832.

87. Swallow DM, Poulter M, Hollox EJ. Intolerance to lactose and other dietary sugars. Drug Metab Dispos 2001; 29(4 Pt 2):513–516.

88. Tishkoff SA, Reed FA, Ranciaro A, Voight BF, Babbitt CC, Silverman JS, et al. Convergent adaptation of human lactase persistence in Africa and Europe. Nat Genet 2007; 39(1):31–40.

89. Wooding SP. Following the herd. Nat Genet 2007; 39(1):7–8.

90. Cross NC, Tolan DR, Cox TM. Catalytic deficiency of human aldolase B in hereditary fructose intolerance caused by a common missense mutation. Cell 1988; 53(6):881–885.

91. Tolan DR. Molecular basis of hereditary fructose intolerance: Mutations and polymorphisms in the human aldolase B gene. Hum Mutat 1995; 6(3):210–218.

92. Wong D. Hereditary fructose intolerance. Mol Genet Metab 2005; 85(3):165–167.

93. Keating M, Atkinson D, Dunn C, Timothy K, Vincent GM, Leppert M. Linkage of a cardiac arrhythmia, the long QT syndrome, and the Harvey ras-1 gene. Science 1991; 252(5006):704–706.

94. Keating M, Dunn C, Atkinson D, Timothy K, Vincent GM, Leppert M. Consistent linkage of the long-QT syndrome to the Harvey ras-1 locus on chromosome 11. Am J Hum Genet 1991; 49(6):1335–1339.

95. Wang Q, Curran ME, Splawski I, Burn TC, Mulholland JM, et al. Positional cloning of a novel potassium channel gene: KVLQT1 mutations cause cardiac arrhythmias. Nat Genet 1996; 12:17–23.

96. Wang Q, Shen J, Splawski I, Atkinson D, Li Z, Robinson JL, et al. SCN5A mutations associated with an inherited cardiac arrhythmia, long QT syndrome. Cell 1995; 80(5):805–811.

97. Towbin JA, Wang Z, Li H. Genotype and severity of long QT syndrome. Drug Metab Dispos 2001; 29(4 Pt 2):574–579.

98. de The H, Lavau C, Marchio A, Chomienne C, Degos L, Dejean A. The PML-RAR alpha fusion mRNA generated by the t(15;17) translocation in acute promyelocytic leukemia encodes a functionally altered RAR. Cell 1991; 66(4):675–684.

99. Kakizuka A, Miller WH Jr, Umesono K, Warrell RP Jr, Frankel SR, Murty VV, et al. Chromosomal translocation t(15;17) in human acute promyelocytic leukemia fuses RAR alpha with a novel putative transcription factor, PML. Cell 1991; 66(4):663–674.

100. Takeshita A, Shinjo K, Naito K, Matsui H, Sahara N, Shigeno K, et al. Two patients with all-trans retinoic acid-resistant acute promyelocytic leukemia treated successfully with gemtuzumab ozogamicin as a single agent. Int J Hematol 2005; 82(5):445–448.

101. Fischel-Ghodsian N, Prezant TR, Bu X, Oztas S. Mitochondrial ribosomal RNA gene mutation in a patient with sporadic aminoglycoside ototoxicity. Am J Otolaryngol 1993; 14(6):399–403.

102. Fischel-Ghodsian N. Genetic factors in aminoglycoside toxicity. Pharmacogenomics 2005; 6(1):27–36.

103. Li X, Zhang LS, Fischel-Ghodsian N, Guan MX. Biochemical characterization of the deafness-associated mitochondrial tRNASer(UCN) A7445G mutation in osteosarcoma cell cybrids. Biochem Biophys Res Commun 2005; 328(2):491–498.

104. Bertina RM, Koeleman BP, Koster T, Rosendaal FR, Dirven RJ, de Ronde H, et al. Mutation in blood coagulation factor V associated with resistance to activated protein C. Nature 1994; 369(6475):64–67.

105. Gehring NH, et al. Increased efficiency of mRNA 3′ end formation: A new genetic mechanism contributing to hereditary thrombophilia. Nat Genet 2001; 28(Aug):389–392.

106. Nurk E, Tell GS, Refsum H, Ueland PM, Vollset SE. Factor V Leiden, pregnancy complications and adverse outcomes: The Hordaland Homocysteine Study. QJM 2006; 99(5):289–298.

107. Mallal S, Nolan D, Witt C, Masel G, Martin AM, Moore C, et al. Association between presence of HLA-B*5701, HLA-DR7, and HLA-DQ3 and hypersensitivity to HIV-1 reverse-transcriptase inhibitor abacavir. Lancet 2002; 359(9308):727–732.

108. Martin A, Nolan D, Almeida CA, Rauch A, Mallal S. Predicting and diagnosing abacavir and nevirapine drug hypersensitivity: From bedside to bench and back again. Pharmacogenomics 2006; 7(1):15–23.

Probe Substrates for Drug-Metabolizing Enzyme Traits

Table B.1 Drugs and Other Substances Useful as Selective Probe Substrates for Phenotyping Drug-Metabolizing Enzyme Traits[a]

Phase 1 Enzymes
Oxidation

Aldehyde dehydrogenase (acetaldehyde)
Alcohol dehydrogenase (ethanol)
Catalase (hydrogen peroxide)
Cytochrome P450
CYP1A1 (benzo[a]pyrene)
CYP2A6 (coumarin, nicotine)
CYP2B6 (buproprion, bufurolol, cyclophosphamide)
CYP2C8 (phenytoin)
CYP2C9 (warfarin, diclofenac, tolbutamide)
CYP2C19 (mephenytoin, omeprazole)
CYP2D6 (Dextromethorphan, debrisoquine, sparteine)
CYP2E1 (chloroxazone, caffeine)
CYP3A4 (erythromycin, midazolam, testosterone)
Dihydropyrimidine dehydrogenase (5-fluorouracil)
Dopamine β-hydroxylase (dopamine)
Monoamine oxidase B (serotonin, dopamine)

Reduction

NAD(P)H:quinone oxidoreductase/DT diaphorase (ubiquinones)

Hydrolysis

Butyrylcholine esterase (benzoylcholine, butrylcholine)
Paraoxonase/arylesterase (paraoxon)

Table B.1 (*continued*)

Phase 2 Enzymes
Conjugation

N-Acetyltransferases: NAT1 (*p*-aminosalicylic acid)
NAT2 (isoniazid, sulfamethazine, caffeine)
Catechol-*O*-methyltransferase (adrenaline, L-DOPA, methyldopa)
Glutathione-*S*-transferase: GSTM1 (*trans*-stilbene oxide)
GSTT1 (methylbromide)
Histamine methyltransferase (histamine)
Phenol sulfotransferase (*p*-nitrophenol, phenol)
Thiomethyltransferase (6-mercaptopurine, 6-thioguanine, 8-azathioprine)
UDP-Glucuronosyltransferases: UGT1A (bilirubin)
UGT2B7 (Oxazepam, ketoprofen, estradiol)
UGT2B15 (dihydrotestosterone. naringenin)

---

[a]Probe substrates can be used alone and in various combinations ("cocktails") to assess the contribution of different metabolic pathways simultaneously. Several such cocktails are reported in the literature (2). Recently, the "Cooperstown 5 + 1" cocktail was developed to assess the activity of P450 1A2, 2C9, 2C19, 2D6, and 3A, NAT2, and xanthine oxidase (1).

REFERENCES

1. Frye RF. Probing the world of cytochrome p450 enzymes. Mol Interv 2004; 4(3): 157–162.
2. Chainuvati S, Nafziger AN, Leeder JS, Gaedigk A, Kearns GL, Sellers E, et al. Combined phenotypic assessment of cytochrome p450 1A2, 2C9, 2C19, 2D6, and 3A, N-acetyltransferase-2, and xanthine oxidase activities with the "Cooperstown 5+1 cocktail." Clin Pharmacol Ther 2003; 74(5):437–447.

Appendix C

REFERENCES FOR TABLE 9.1 ON PAGES 280–286

1. Waymire KG, Mahuren JD, Jaje JM, Guilarte TR, Coburn SP, MacGregor GR. Mice lacking tissue non-specific alkaline phosphatase die from seizures due to defective metabolism of vitamin B-6. Nat Genet 1995; 11(1):45–51.
2. Reaume AG, de Sousa PA, Kulkarni S, Langille BL, Zhu D, Davies TC et al. Cardiac malformation in neonatal mice lacking connexin43. Science 1995; 267(5205):1831–1834.
3. Bi L, Lawler AM, Antonarakis SE, High KA, Gearhart JD, Kazazian HH, Jr. Targeted disruption of the mouse factor VIII gene produces a model of haemophilia A. Nat Genet 1995; 10(1):119–121.
4. Harvey M, Vogel H, Morris D, Bradley A, Bernstein A, Donehower LA. A mutant p53 transgene accelerates tumour development in heterozygous but not nullizygous p53-deficient mice. Nat Genet 1995; 9(3):305–311.
5. Huang PL, Huang Z, Mashimo H, Bloch KD, Moskowitz MA, Bevan JA et al. Hypertension in mice lacking the gene for endothelial nitric oxide synthase. Nature 1995; 377(6546):239–242.
6. Lindberg RL, Porcher C, Grandchamp B, Ledermann B, Burki K, Brandner S et al. Porphobilinogen deaminase deficiency in mice causes a neuropathy resembling that of human hepatic porphyria. Nat Genet 1996; 12(2):195–199.
7. Cormier RT, Hong KH, Halberg RB, Hawkins TL, Richardson P, Mulherkar R et al. Secretory phospholipase Pla2g2a confers resistance to intestinal tumorigenesis. Nat Genet 1997; 17(1):88–91.
8. Gabriel SE, Brigman KN, Koller BH, Boucher RC, Stutts MJ. Cystic fibrosis heterozygote resistance to cholera toxin in the cystic fibrosis mouse model. Science 1994; 266(5182):107–109.
9. Shih DM, Gu L, Xia YR, Navab M, Li WF, Hama S et al. Mice lacking serum paraoxonase are susceptible to organophosphate toxicity and atherosclerosis. Nature 1998; 394(6690):284–287.
10. Ioffe E, Moon B, Connolly E, Friedman JM. Abnormal regulation of the leptin gene in the pathogenesis of obesity. Proc Natl Acad Sci U S A 1998; 95(20):11852–11857.
11. Nebigil CG, Choi DS, Dierich A, Hickel P, Le Meur M, Messaddeq N et al. Serotonin 2B receptor is required for heart development. Proc Natl Acad Sci U S A 2000; 97(17):9508–9513.

12. Launay JM, Herve P, Peoc'h K, Tournois C, Callebert J, Nebigil CG et al. Function of the serotonin 5-hydroxytryptamine 2B receptor in pulmonary hypertension. Nat Med 2002; 8(10):1129–1135.
13. Nuyens D, Stengl M, Dugarmaa S, Rossenbacker T, Compernolle V, Rudy Y et al. Abrupt rate accelerations or premature beats cause life-threatening arrhythmias in mice with long-QT3 syndrome. Nat Med 2001; 7(9):1021–1027.
14. Rego EM, Wang ZG, Peruzzi D, He LZ, Cordon-Cardo C, Pandolfi PP. Role of promyelocytic leukemia (PML) protein in tumor suppression. J Exp Med 2001; 193(4):521–529.
15. Hogema BM, Gupta M, Senephansiri H, Burlingame TG, Taylor M, Jakobs C et al. Pharmacologic rescue of lethal seizures in mice deficient in succinate semialdehyde dehydrogenase. Nat Genet 2001; 29(2):212–216.
16. Jonker JW, Wagenaar E, Mol CA, Buitelaar M, Koepsell H, Smit JW et al. Reduced hepatic uptake and intestinal excretion of organic cations in mice with a targeted disruption of the organic cation transporter 1 (Oct1 [Slc22a1]) gene. Mol Cell Biol 2001; 21(16):5471–5477.
17. Wang DS, Jonker JW, Kato Y, Kusuhara H, Schinkel AH, Sugiyama Y. Involvement of organic cation transporter 1 in hepatic and intestinal distribution of metformin. J Pharmacol Exp Ther 2002; 302(2):510–515.
18. Xie W, Stribley JA, Chatonnet A, Wilder PJ, Rizzino A, Mccomb RD et al. Postnatal developmental delay and supersensitivity to organophosphate in gene-targeted mice lacking acetylcholinesterase. J Pharmacol Exp Ther 2000; 293(3):896–902.
19. Xie W, Barwick JL, Downes M, Blumberg B, Simon CM, Nelson MC et al. Humanized xenobiotic response in mice expressing nuclear receptor SXR. Nature 2000; 406(6794):435–439.

Index